PRAISE FOR

THE DEPRESSION CURE

"Those who have suffered recurring, meaningless bouts of depression might want to reach for *The Depression Cure* rather than *Unstuck*, especially those sick of hearing how they should search their mental illness for wisdom."

—Bookslut Founder Jessa Crispin in *The Smart Set*

"Intriguing. Author Stephen S. Ilardi seems to be onto something when he points out that our ancestors didn't sit at a desk all day and fight traffic to go home stressed-out . . . Pick up a copy of *The Depression Cure*. With your doctor's blessing, a fair amount of effort, and this book, 'snapping out of it' might be a snap."

—"The Bookworm Sez" (nationally syndicated column)

"[Ilardi's] program helps patients reclaim six ancient lifestyle elements that can improve or eradicate depression. These include a diet rich in omega-3 fatty acids, the critical building blocks for brain structure and function; enjoyable activities that keep us from dwelling on negative thoughts; exercise that stimulates important brain chemicals; sufficient sunlight exposure to keep the body's clock in sync; social support to avoid isolation; and healthy sleep habits that allow the brain and body to recover. It works for me and it will work for you!"

—Bookviews.com

"A very good self help book. Ilardi writes clearly, avoiding jargon, and speaking eloquently about many topics. His depiction of negative lifestyle influences on people's emotions and actions are on target . . . this is a splendid book because the recommendations made should lead to a healthier lifestyle for most people . . . Overcoming depression is not a simple challenge but one, I suspect, has a chance of success by reading this book."

—Metapsychology Online Reviews

"Ilardi's theory draws on discoveries in cognitive neuroscience and evolutionary psychology, which add heft to his common-sense advice . . . *The Depression Cure* arrays data that may inspire action."

—*Kansas Alumni*

"Has a number of physical tips for staving off the mental wear and tear."

—*Day Spa Magazine*

"A realistic, fine guide, this is a recommendation for any general lending or health library." —Midwest Book Review

STEPHEN S. ILARDI, PhD

THE DEPRESSION CURE

The 6-Step Program to Beat Depression without Drugs

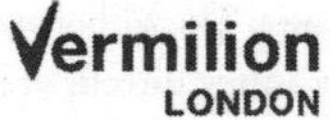

1 3 5 7 9 10 8 6 4 2

Published in 2010 by Vermilion, an imprint of Ebury Publishing
First published in the USA by Da Capo Press, a member of the Perseus Books Group, in 2009

Ebury Publishing is a Random House Group company

The Random House Group Limited Reg. No. 954009

Addresses for companies within the Random House Group can be found at:
www.rbooks.co.uk

A CIP catalogue record for this book is available from the British Library

The Random House Group Limited supports The Forest Stewardship Council (FSC), the leading international forest certification organisation. All our titles that are printed on Greenpeace approved FSC certified paper carry the FSC logo. Our paper procurement policy can be found at:
www.rbooks.co.uk/environment

Printed and bound in the UK by CPI Mackays, Chatham, ME5 8TD

ISBN 9780091929817

Copies are available at special rates for bulk orders. Contact the sales development team on 020 7840 8487 for more information.

To buy books by your favourite authors and register for offers, visit www.rbooks.co.uk

The informati[illegible] relation to the specific su[illegible] r medical, healthcare, [illegible] ances and in specific locati[illegible] g any medical treatment. S[illegible] to date as at May 2010. Pr[illegible] ain up to date professiona[illegible] as far as the [illegible]

Contents

PART THREE
MAKING THE CHANGE

Introduction

Depression is a devastating illness. It robs people of their energy, their sleep, their memory, their concentration, their vitality, their joy, their ability to love and work and play, and—sometimes—even their will to live. As a clinical psychologist, I've worked with hundreds of patients to help heal depression's debilitating effects, so I will never underestimate this treacherous foe. From the day I first walked onto a psychiatric unit at Duke Medical Center two decades ago, I've devoted my career to fighting the disorder: I know it far too well to make any blanket promises of a one-size-fits-all cure.

Yet here's what I *can* say with complete confidence: Depression is beatable. And the six-step program outlined in *The Depression Cure* is the most promising treatment for depression I've ever witnessed in my years of clinical research and practice. Admittedly, this is a bold claim—one I never would have imagined making when I began developing the program a few years ago.* But it's based on three important observations:

- The program—*Therapeutic Lifestyle Change* (TLC)—has proven remarkably effective in a large treatment study at my university. Patients were randomly assigned to receive either TLC or treatment-as-usual in the community (mostly medication), and

* With the help of several talented graduate students.

fewer than 25% of those in community-based treatment got better.* But the response rate among TLC patients was over three times higher. In fact, *every single patient who put the full program into practice got better*, even though most had already failed to get well on antidepressant medications.

- All six components of the TLC program—omega-3 fatty acids, engaging activity, physical exercise, sunlight exposure, social connection, and enhanced sleep—have antidepressant properties. We know this from mountains of published research. But TLC is the only approach that combines these separate elements into an integrated package—a comprehensive, step-by-step program that's more potent than any single component used on its own.
- Most important, TLC addresses the modern depression epidemic at its source: the fact that *human beings were never designed for the poorly nourished, sedentary, indoor, sleep-deprived, socially isolated, frenzied pace of twenty-first-century life*. The program provides a long-overdue, common sense remedy for a contemporary American lifestyle that's drifted dangerously off course.

In recent years, I've been invited to speak with thousands of people—patients, therapists, psychiatrists, students, and many others—about this lifestyle-based approach to healing depression. The question I'm most frequently asked is: Who might benefit from the program?

My reply: Everyone. This usually draws some laughter, as most people think I'm joking—a bit of ironic, self-mocking exaggeration. But I'm actually quite serious. At least four groups of people can benefit from the TLC program, and together they include just about everyone.

---

* "Getting better" was defined in the study as: experiencing at least a 50% reduction in depressive symptoms and no longer meeting diagnostic criteria for major depressive disorder by the end of treatment.

- The program was initially designed to help those suffering from clinical depression—whether or not they're already receiving some other form of treatment. TLC is highly effective when used on its own, but the program can also be combined with antidepressant medication or traditional psychotherapy.
- Then again, you don't have to be diagnosed with full-blown depression to benefit from TLC. The protocol can also help those who are simply feeling blue or fighting milder symptoms of the disorder.
- Likewise, the program offers protection to anyone who wants to minimize the risk of depression in the future.
- And a few years ago, psychologist Harriet Lerner—the bestselling author of influential books like *The Dance of Anger*—observed something else about the TLC program that I had never considered: Each step involves something that's good for us, no matter how well we may be doing already. As Harriet put it, "Your program isn't just about depression. It's something *everyone* can use to their benefit."

She's right, of course. There's a wealth of research on the physical and psychological benefits of the program's core elements: weight loss, increased energy, lower blood pressure, improved cardiac health, better immune function, reduced inflammation, greater mental clarity, and an enhanced sense of well-being. These are treatment "side effects" worth signing up for, and they represent another important reason for embracing the TLC program.

Despite the treatment's beneficial effects, it's still advisable to get a physical exam before you start putting the protocol into practice. In my own clinical research at the University of Kansas, I don't let anyone begin the full program until they've first seen a doctor. This policy may surprise you, but it's based on sound reasoning. For one thing, it's always a good idea to check with a physician before embarking on a new exercise program. The same goes for taking high-dose nutritional supplements or increasing sun exposure. Since these are all core elements of the TLC program, it's important to get your doctor's okay before you begin.

In addition, people occasionally write me to ask if they can stop taking their antidepressant medications once they begin putting the TLC program into practice. My advice is always short and simple: They *must* make any such medication-related decisions only in close consultation with their own prescribing physician. In fact, it can be dangerous to discontinue an antidepressant without close medical supervision, because in some cases difficult withdrawal symptoms—including a worsening of depression—can occur if the medication is stopped too abruptly.

Finally, depression can be triggered by many common medical conditions—diabetes, sleep apnea, thyroid disorder, heart disease, chronic infection, and hormonal imbalance, to name a few—and the disorder can be very difficult to treat effectively until such underlying medical problems are addressed. Several drugs also carry the potential to cause depression (ironically, even some common psychiatric drugs), and your doctor can help you consider this possibility, as well.

In the chapters that follow, I'll describe the Therapeutic Lifestyle Change program in clear, step-by-step detail. And I'll share countless stories of those who've used the program to overcome depression and find their way to lasting recovery. My hope is that by putting TLC into practice in your own life—one step at a time—you, too, will begin living the depression cure.

PART ONE

UNDERSTANDING DEPRESSION

1

The Epidemic and the Cure

"I don't know what's wrong with me. All I want to do is close my eyes and never have to wake up again. It's like my whole life is slipping away, and there's nothing I can do about it. Everybody keeps telling me I just need to 'snap out of it.' Don't they know how cruel that is? I mean, do they think I want to be like this? Sometimes I just start crying and I don't even know what I'm crying about. People stare at me like I'm crazy, like: 'Look at that poor guy. That poor, pathetic . . .'" Phil's voice trailed off as he slumped forward in his chair and cradled his head in his hands.* He fixed his gaze on the office floor and whispered, "I'm sorry." He repeated the phrase over and over, like a mantra.

Even though I was all too familiar with the devastating effect of depression, I still found it difficult to picture what Phil had been like just a few months earlier, before his illness struck. Phil's wife, who phoned to set up his first appointment, described him as "a confident, fun-loving guy." He was someone who ran a successful business, enjoyed a strong marriage, and adored his two kids. His wife said, "You would have looked at Phil and thought, 'Here's a guy who has it all.'"

* All names and other potentially indentifying information for each patient have been altered to preserve confidentiality.

And yet there he was in my office, struck down by depression in the prime of his life. Over the span of a few short months, he had lost his energy, his memory, his sex drive, his confidence, his ability to sleep through the night, and his concentration. He could no longer function effectively at work. He had completely withdrawn from his friends and his family. Lately, he had even lost his will to live.

Like many of the patients I treat, Phil had been taking antidepressant medications for a few months before he came to see me. Unfortunately, the drugs hadn't helped very much—an outcome that's more common than most people realize. Although medications are certainly valuable in some cases, they work for fewer than half the depressed patients who try them. (And many quit taking their meds anyway due to difficult side effects like sexual dysfunction or weight gain.)

Even though antidepressant use has skyrocketed in recent years, the rate of depression in the United States hasn't declined: It's *increased.* According to the latest research, about one in four Americans—over seventy million people—will meet the criteria for major depression at some point in their lives. Ominously, the rate of depression has been on the rise for decades. It's roughly ten times higher today than it was just two generations ago. How can people possibly be so much more vulnerable to depression now? What has changed?

It's clearly not a matter of genetics, since the collective gene pool simply can't change that quickly. It has to be something else. That something else, I believe, is lifestyle. Consider the following:

- Only one known group of Americans hasn't been hit by the modern depression epidemic: the Amish. Still clinging tenaciously to their eighteenth-century way of life, Amish communities have a rate of depression dramatically lower than that of the general population.

- In developing (third-world) countries, the lifetime rate of depression is often a fraction of that observed in the West. However, the prevalence of depression has begun to go up in those countries where people are shifting from more traditional to more Americanized lifestyles.
- The risk of depression has increased relentlessly in recent years across the entire industrialized world (such as Britain, Germany, Australia, New Zealand, and South Korea). It's not just an American phenomenon.
- Modern-day hunter-gatherer bands—such as the Kaluli people* of the New Guinea highlands—have been assessed by Western researchers for the presence of mental illness. Remarkably, *clinical depression is almost completely nonexistent among such groups*, whose way of life is similar to that of our remote ancestors. Despite living very hard lives—with none of the material comforts or medical advances we take for granted—they're largely immune to the plague of depressive illness that we see ruining lives all around us. (In perhaps the most telling example, anthropologist Edward Schieffelin lived among the Kaluli for nearly a decade and carefully interviewed over two thousand men, women, and children regarding their experience of grief and depression; he found only one person who came close to meeting our full diagnostic criteria for depressive illness.)

* The Kaluli subsist on a combination of hunting, foraging, and gardening, so they are also sometimes referred to as horticulturalists.

Such cross-cultural studies make one thing quite clear: the more "modern" a society's way of life, the higher its rate of depression. It may seem baffling, but the explanation is simple: *The human body was never designed for the modern post-industrial environment.* Until about twelve thousand years ago—when people invented farming and began domesticating livestock—everyone on the planet made their living by hunting and foraging for food. People lived as hunter-gatherers for the vast majority of human history.

And our genes still reflect this history: They've changed very little since the days of our hunter-gatherer forebears. Our genes are still beautifully calibrated to that ancient environment and are still building—in effect—Stone Age bodies. Unfortunately, when Stone Age body meets modern environment, the health consequences can be disastrous.

Consider the runaway epidemic of obesity. A staggering 65% of American adults are now clinically overweight. Why? Because our appetites are still fine-tuned to the Stone Age. Our hunter-gatherer ancestors faced a fluctuating, seasonal food supply—with the prospect of hunger and starvation ever just around the corner. So it made sense for them to crave sweets, starches, and fatty foods—the richest calorie sources available—and to binge whenever those rare, nutrient-rich foods happened to be on hand.

Our brains are still programmed with this sensibility. We, too, find it virtually impossible to resist the urge to feast on calorie-rich foods. When we savor, say, a slice of cheesecake (a sweet, starchy, fatty trifecta), our Stone Age brains gleefully register the satisfaction of storing away many, many calories for a rainy day—no matter how much energy we might already have tucked away in our fat reserves.

But over the past several decades, for the first time in human history, high-calorie foods have become available 24/7. Because the brain was never designed to regulate appetite in the face of such perpetual abundance, daily calorie consumption has gone through the roof. We see the food, and our brains can't "just say no." To make matters worse, this nutritional bonanza has coincided with a sharp drop in the number of calories people burn each day, as conveniences like the automobile, electrical appliances, and television have gradually turned us into a nation of couch potatoes. The result? A modern epidemic completely explained by recent changes in lifestyle.

Let's turn our attention back to the Amish, duly famous for their resistance to lifestyle changes over the past two centuries. Their rate of obesity? A recent study puts it at a mere 4%. As for modern-day hunter-gatherers, their obesity level is approximately 0.

But can the modern epidemic of depression, like that of obesity, really be explained by changes in the way people live? A wealth of scientific evidence says it can, and it goes far beyond cross-cultural studies. As we'll see in the next section, this evidence has important implications that may forever change the way we understand and treat depression.

THE ANTIDEPRESSANT LIFESTYLE

In many respects, modern Americans should be among the happiest people in the history of the world. Whether we look at rates of infant mortality, hunger, medical care, life expectancy, or material comforts, Americans are better off (on average) than the vast majority of people who have ever lived. Doesn't it follow, then, that we should also be among the least likely to get depressed? Shouldn't we, at the very least, have lower rates of depression than contemporary hunter-gatherers, whose lives are so much harder than our own? After all, they're much more likely than we are to experience tragic events like the death of a child, crippling illness, or violent assault—events that can serve as powerful triggers of depression.

Yet even as they suffer these disastrous events, hunter-gatherers rarely become clinically depressed. For some reason, they're much more resilient than we are. (It's a good thing, too, because if they *weren't*, the human species probably would have become extinct back in the days of our remote ancestors.)

But how are hunter-gatherers able to weather life's storms so effectively? That's the question I kept coming back to when I began wrestling with this mystery a few years ago. What emerged from my quest, after poring over hundreds of published studies in search of clues, was a finding so clear—and so obvious in hindsight—I was amazed no one had ever noticed it:* *The hunter-gatherer lifestyle is profoundly antidepressant.* As they go about their daily lives, hunter-gatherers naturally wind up doing many things that keep them from getting depressed. They do things that change the brain more powerfully than any medication.

For most of human history, everyone benefited from the antidepressant effect of these ancient lifestyle elements. As a result, people were able to cope with circumstances vastly more difficult than most of us ever face today. But over the past few hundred years, technological evolution has proceeded at a relentless pace, and many protective features of that ancient way of life have gradually disappeared. Accordingly, the rate of depression has begun to spiral out of control. Our Stone Age brains just weren't designed to handle the sedentary,

* At least, after reviewing the relevant scientific literature, I couldn't determine that anyone had noticed it. Science journalist Robert Wright does hint at the possibility, however, in his 1995 *Time* magazine article, "The Evolution of Despair."

isolated, indoor, sleep-deprived, fast-food-laden, stressed-out pace of twenty-first-century life.

In the chapters that follow, we'll look at the potent antidepressant effects of six major protective lifestyle elements that we all need to reclaim from our ancestors:

- Dietary omega-3 fatty acids
- Engaging activity
- Physical exercise
- Sunlight exposure
- Social support
- Sleep

These six elements form the core of a breakthrough treatment for depression, Therapeutic Lifestyle Change (TLC), developed by my clinical research team at the University of Kansas. TLC is a natural approach to healing depression, with no side effects and no insurance forms to file. And in our preliminary clinical trials, TLC has yielded exceptional results—far superior to those typically observed with medication. Among our study patients, the rate of favorable response to TLC has been *over three times higher* than that of antidepressant "treatment as usual" in the community. And we've yet to see someone put the entire TLC protocol into practice without experiencing significant improvement.

Omega-3 Fatty Acids

Did you know your brain is mostly made up of fat? It sounds like a straight line from a stand-up comedy routine, but it's true—the human brain is about 60% fat by dry weight. Fat molecules (sometimes called *fatty acids*) play a crucial role in the construction of brain cells and the insulation of nerve fibers. Fortunately, the body is able to make many of the fat molecules the brain needs. But there are some forms that the body can't manufacture on its own; these fats can be obtained only from our diet. And among the most important dietary fats is a group called *omega-3* fatty acids—critical building blocks for brain structure and function.

Omega-3 fatty acids are found mainly in fish, wild game, nuts, seeds, and leafy vegetables, all things found in abundance in the hunter-gatherer diet. *Our distant ancestors ate five to ten times more omega-3 fat than we do.* In fact, omega-3s have gradually disappeared from the American diet over the past century.

In the days of our great-grandparents, for example, beef cattle fed on the free range, where they ate grasses and wild plant sources of omega-3. Remarkably, beef used to be good for us. Today's cattle, in contrast, are mostly grain-fed, and they have little beneficial omega-3 content. The same is true with our grain-fed, farm-raised fish (most of the fish now consumed in America).

Because the brain needs a steady supply of omega-3s to function properly, people who don't eat enough of these fats are at increased risk for many forms of mental illness, including depression. Across the globe, countries with the highest levels of omega-3 consumption typically have the lowest rates of depression.

Clinical researchers have even started using omega-3 supplements to treat depression, and the results so far have been highly encouraging. For example, British researchers recently studied a group of depressed patients who had failed to recover after taking antidepressant medication for eight weeks. All study patients stayed on their meds as prescribed, but some also took an omega-3 supplement. About 70% of those who received the supplement* went on to recover, compared with only 25% of patients who kept taking only the medication. This study—along with a handful of others like it—suggests that omega-3s may be among the most effective antidepressant substances ever discovered.

Engaging Activity

Depression is closely linked to a toxic thought process called *rumination*—the habit of dwelling on negative thoughts, turning them over and over in your mind. We've probably all ruminated at some point. It's a perfectly natural response to upsetting events. And when rumination lasts for only a short while, it can even be useful, helping us figure out what went wrong and how we might work to correct things in the future.

The problem comes when people start ruminating for long stretches of time, going over the same thoughts again and again and again. Such chronic rumination actually cranks up the intensity of our negative mood, making it unbearably painful. Unfortunately, many depressed individuals spend literally hours ruminating every day.

The first time I introduced the concept of rumination to patients in a TLC group, it was as if a light went on for many people in the room. "I do that all the time!" one patient exclaimed. "And it definitely makes me feel worse." Someone else chimed in, "You mean there are people who *don't* ruminate all the time? I thought it was just something everyone did." Another smiled knowingly and said,

* Study patients were randomly assigned to various omega-3 dosage levels. I've presented here the results for those who received the supplement at the dose recommended in the TLC protocol: 1,000 mg per day of the active omega-3 molecule.

"It's so cool that there's actually a *name* for it. But how do you *stop* ruminating?"

How, indeed? For one thing, people only ruminate when they have free time on their hands, when their minds aren't occupied with some reasonably engaging activity. Sitting stuck in traffic, watching a boring TV show, eating a meal alone, staring off into space . . . those are the times when rumination typically takes over. The biggest risk factor for rumination is simply spending time alone, something Americans now do all the time.

When you're interacting with another person, your mind just doesn't have a chance to dwell on repetitive negative thoughts. But, really, any sort of engaging activity can work to interrupt rumination. It can even be something simple.

Dana, a forty-something accountant in one of our recent TLC groups, told us the following story: "You guys had just covered rumination, and literally as I was driving out of the parking lot after group, I noticed I was doing it! The negative thoughts were right there, going around and around in my head. I mean, I had no idea I was doing it that often. Anyway, I pulled the car over and just sat there in the parking lot and thought about how I could stop it. All I could think of was to turn on the radio and find a good song to focus on instead, so that's what I did. And it worked. I didn't ruminate for the entire drive home. Before I learned about this, I would have just stewed in those negative thoughts and pulled into my garage feeling like crap, but now I think I know how to turn it around. It feels like I finally have some control."

In Chapter 5, we'll go over the link between rumination and depression in much greater detail. We'll also cover several key strategies for helping you break the rumination habit.

Physical Exercise

Hunter-gatherers are in remarkably good shape. They get hours of exercise every day, with a fitness routine rivaling that of elite athletes. They commonly walk five to ten miles each day just to find food and water, which they then have to haul back to the rest of the group. They erect their own dwellings and routinely handle logs weighing hundreds of pounds. They perform ritual dances that last for hours.

In effect, the hunter-gatherer life is an intense cross-training regimen—one that involves lots of lifting, carrying, sprinting, climbing, walking, and stretching on a daily basis. Modern life, on the other hand, is notoriously sedentary, and most Americans are woefully out of shape. Many can run no farther than the distance from the sofa to the refrigerator. This is unfortunate, because exercise is a remarkably potent antidepressant.

Researchers have compared aerobic exercise and Lustral (a commonly prescribed antidepressant medication) head-to-head in the treatment of depression. Even at a low "dose" of exercise—thirty minutes of brisk walking three times a week—patients who worked out did just as well as those who took the medication. Strikingly, though, the patients on Lustral were about three times more likely than exercisers to become depressed again over a ten-month follow-up period.

There are now over a hundred published studies documenting the antidepressant effects of exercise. Activities as varied as walking, biking, jogging, and weight lifting have all been found to be effective. It's also becoming clear just *how* they work. *Exercise changes the brain.* It increases the activity level of important brain chemicals such as dopamine and serotonin (the same neurochemical targeted by popular drugs like Lustral and Prozac). Exercise also increases the brain's production of a key growth hormone called BDNF. Because levels of this hormone plummet in depression, some parts of the brain start to shrink over time, and learning and memory are impaired. But exercise reverses this trend, protecting the brain in a way nothing else can.

Chloe, a twenty-one-year-old college student with a shy smile, was a patient in one of our TLC treatment groups two years ago. Introducing herself at the first session, she told us, "I've struggled with depression—on and off—for pretty much my whole life." Abandoned by her mother and raised by an alcoholic father who often left her to fend for herself, Chloe confessed that feelings of loneliness and sadness were constant fixtures of her childhood and adolescence. Things got even worse when she went off to college, where she fell into a debilitating episode of clinical depression. By the time she started treatment, she had stopped attending her classes and instead spent much of her time holed up alone in her apartment.

I spoke with Chloe early on in her treatment about the therapeutic value of exercise, but she said she'd never enjoyed working out. She also expressed a strong distaste for "the whole gym scene." I reassured her that our goal was to help her find some kind of physical activity she could enjoy. "I guess I used to like riding my bike as a kid," she recalled, "but I haven't done anything like that in years." With a little encouragement, she agreed to make a trip home to pick up her old bike and bring it back to campus. The following week, Chloe started going out for short rides, mostly just exploring the streets around her neighborhood. But before long she was pedaling all over town, often riding for over an hour each day.

Within a few weeks, Chloe began noticing a bit of improvement in her mood, her energy, and her sleep. Even though she was still depressed, this modest turn for the better seemed to spark a glimmer of hope. So, despite her continued symptoms, she kept on riding. And things slowly kept getting better. The following week, buoyed by her increased energy (a typical side effect of regular exercise), she worked up the courage to venture out shopping with some girls who lived next door in her apartment complex. Chloe found—much to her surprise—that she actually enjoyed herself. Soon, it was like a vicious cycle in reverse: exercise led to increased energy, which led to a better mood, which led to greater social activity, which led to more exercise (since she rode her bike to most social engagements), which led to increased energy, and so on.

The more we learn about the beneficial effects of physical activity, the more the following truth comes clearly into focus: *Exercise is medicine.* Literally. Just like a pill, it reliably changes brain function by altering the activity of key brain chemicals and hormones. This is a crucial point, but one that's often missed. For when people hear that depression is linked to a chemical imbalance, they usually conclude, "Well, if *that's* true, people with depression obviously need to take a drug—another chemical—to straighten out the imbalance." It's an understandable assumption, but it's dead wrong. Medication isn't the only way to correct brain abnormalities in depression. Physical exercise also brings about profound changes in the brain—changes that rival those seen with the most potent antidepressant medications.

In Chapter 6, I'll explain how you can start and maintain an exercise program to bring about these important benefits. You'll find a way to work out that doesn't feel like *work*—an exercise routine you can actually enjoy. After all, isn't that the best way to make sure you'll stick with it? And I can reassure you at the outset: Antidepressant exercise is much more doable than most people imagine, and it doesn't require an expensive gym membership. It can be as easy as going for a walk with a friend or taking a bike ride in the park. Physical activity is something we were designed to find enjoyable.

Sunlight Exposure

Millions of Americans and Europeans get depressed every year, almost like clockwork, during the dark, dreary months of winter. They suffer from a disorder aptly named SAD (for *seasonal affective disorder*)—a condition triggered by reduced light exposure during the short, cold, cloudy days that run from November through February or March (depending on where you live). Predictably, SAD hits people particularly hard in northern latitudes, where winter daylight is scarce (residents of New England, for example, are afflicted much more often than those living in Florida).

Although simply going outside on a sunny day can brighten your mood, an even deeper link exists between light exposure and depression—one involving the body's internal clock. As it turns out, the brain gauges the amount of light you get each day, and it uses that information to reset your body clock. Without enough light exposure, the body clock eventually gets out of sync, and when that happens, it throws off important *circadian rhythms* that regulate energy, sleep, appetite, and hormone levels. The disruption of these important biological rhythms can, in turn, trigger clinical depression.

Because natural sunlight is so much brighter than indoor lighting—over a hundred times brighter, on average—a half hour of sunlight is enough to reset your body clock. Even the natural light of a gray, cloudy day is several times brighter than the inside of most people's houses, and a few hours of exposure provide just enough light to keep circadian rhythms well regulated. But people who are inside from dawn to dusk often find their body clocks starting to malfunction.

Of course, thousands of years ago our ancestors were outside all day every day, so they always had enough light exposure to boost mood and prevent SAD. Likewise with modern-day hunter-gatherers. Even Americans of a few generations ago typically spent at least a few hours outside each day. For us, though, the situation is different. Increasingly, we just aren't bothering to go outside at all. And even if we wanted to, most of us don't have the luxury of spending hours at a time outside on a regular basis.

Fortunately, when getting enough sunlight isn't a realistic option (during the shorter days of winter, for example), you can use an elegant, high-tech solution that's effective in elevating mood and resetting the body's internal clock. In Chapter 7, we'll cover a range of options—both natural and high-tech—for getting adequate light exposure year-round and keeping mood and circadian rhythms in sync.

Social Support

Anthropologists who visit modern foraging tribes invariably notice something peculiar about their hosts' social lives: *Hunter-gatherers almost never spend time alone.* Even though the typical village consists of only fifty to two hundred people, it seems that just about every activity is a social occasion. Hunting, cooking, eating, playing, foraging, sleeping, grooming—they're all carried out in the company of close friends and loved ones. Loneliness and social isolation are virtually unknown.

The contrast with our way of life is profound. We often struggle to carve out the smallest blocks of face time with the very people we hold most dear. Not only do we spend much less time than previous generations interacting with our friends, neighbors, and extended family, but we're even less likely to connect with others in church or synagogue, or in civic groups like the Rotary Club or Girl Scouts.

Sadly, many Americans now spend the bulk of their leisure time walled up in their homes, parked in front of a TV or computer screen—alone. They spend hours each week sitting in traffic—alone. They often eat alone. And now they can even go online and do their shopping alone.

In many cases, technology promotes our increasing social isolation. For example, until a few months ago, I used to enjoy bumping into my friends and neighbors at the local video rental store. But that doesn't happen anymore, now that I can log in to an online service that delivers DVDs right to my mailbox. And even on the university campus where I teach—a place where people are still forced to get out and walk in public—many are now oblivious to the social world around them as they march along to the beat of an iPod. Sadly, our coolest new gadgets always seem to wind up cutting us off from each other.

As if we weren't becoming isolated enough, one of the great tragedies of depression is that it causes people to withdraw even further from the people around them.

Jane, a middle-aged divorcee with downcast eyes, was one of the more socially withdrawn patients we've ever treated in a TLC group. She used to shuffle unobtrusively in to each session, staring at her feet and speaking (only when spoken to) in a barely audible voice. Since depression had taken hold of her life the year before, she'd become increasingly reclusive, pulling away from her friends and loved ones, and even avoiding her adult children who lived in the area. But as my co-therapist and I learned more about Jane over the first few TLC sessions, it became clear that before her depression struck she'd been a vibrant, socially confident woman. A few weeks into treatment, we gently challenged her to think about friends or loved ones she might try to reconnect with, and she promised to "think about it." As fate would have it, her daughter contacted her shortly afterward to see if Jane might be willing to watch her two-year-old grandson every night after work that week. Reluctantly, she agreed.

After just a few days of this "grandson therapy," Jane noticed her mood starting to lift slightly and a little bit of her energy returning. The shift was subtle, but she said it felt like "somehow life wasn't quite so awful." So she took the fateful step of volunteering to watch her grandson the following week as well, and the improvement in her mood and energy slowly continued.

Jane was surprised by this clear connection between social contact and mood, but she couldn't deny her own experience. Gradually, with our encouragement, she started reaching out to reconnect with other people as well—an old friend, a neighbor, a coworker, a daughter. She said it felt like she was learning to reconnect with her old self in the process, to rediscover the person she used to be before depression robbed her of her social world. Inspired by her progress on this front, Jane grew determined to put other TLC elements into practice: She began getting regular exercise, taking an omega-3 supplement, and seeking out daily sunlight exposure. Over time, this process catalyzed further improvement—her sleep, her concentration, her appetite, and her confidence all slowly began to return. Fourteen weeks after she began treatment, Jane's depression was in full remission.

The research on this issue is clear: When it comes to depression, relationships matter. People who lack a supportive social network face an increased risk of becoming depressed, and of remaining depressed once an episode strikes. Fortunately, we can do a great deal to improve the quality and depth of our connections with others, and this can have a huge payoff in terms of fighting depression and reducing the risk of recurrence. In Chapter 8, I'll help you assess the strength of your social support networks, and provide a set of strategies for enhancing the quality of your connections with others.

Sleep

As you've likely discovered from your own experience, sleep and mood are intimately connected. After just a few nights of poor sleep, most people are noticeably less upbeat. Many of us start to get downright cranky. And when sleep deprivation continues for days or weeks at a time, it can interfere with our ability to think clearly. It can even bring about serious health consequences. Disrupted sleep is one of the most potent triggers of depression, and there's evidence that most episodes of mood disorder are preceded by at least several weeks of subpar slumber.

Not only can poor sleep cause depression, but depression can cause poor sleep. (Talk about a vicious cycle.) Fully 80% of depressed patients experience some form of sleep disturbance. While some have trouble drifting off at night, most have even greater difficulty *staying* asleep. Often, they'll find themselves wide awake in the middle of the night, tossing and turning until daybreak. Even worse, depression also affects sleep *quality,* depriving people of the deepest, most rejuvenating sleep phase (known as *slow-wave sleep*).

Despite its obvious importance, a good night's sleep is something most of us rarely get. It's a distinctly modern problem. Hunter-gatherers—whose sleep cycles are closely bound to the natural ebb and flow of darkness and daylight—have been observed to sleep about 10 hours a night. Even American adults of the nineteenth century averaged a good 9 hours. And now? We clock in at a paltry 6.7 hours per night. Not surprisingly, most of us walk around in a state of perpetual drowsiness, masked only by our collective caffeine habit (about 90% of Americans now consume it on a daily basis) and the widespread use of other stimulants.

Fortunately, as we'll cover in Chapter 9, you can take numerous steps to improve both the quality and quantity of your sleep. Not only can these strategies help improve mood and many other symptoms of depression, but they can also prevent the chronically disturbed sleep that so often ushers in an episode of full-blown depressive illness.

THERAPEUTIC LIFESTYLE CHANGE: AN IDEA WHOSE TIME HAS COME

The way we live can powerfully affect the way we feel. It's a simple observation, but one with profound implications when it comes to fighting depression. For as we've seen, six distinct lifestyle elements—ranging from exercise to nutrition (omega-3 fats) to social support to light exposure—can fight depression as effectively as any medication. They can even bring about important changes in the brain. Modern-day hunter-gatherers benefit from each of these lifestyle factors in abundance, and this explains why they rarely get depressed, despite leading very difficult lives. And although the world has changed a great deal since the days of our ancestors, these protective lifestyle elements were still present in American life—to a somewhat lesser extent—right up until the past century. In recent decades, though, they have steadily disappeared, and the rate of depression has skyrocketed in lockstep with their departure—not just in this country but around the globe.

When I first began to put all this together a few years ago, I started encouraging my depressed patients—folks I was treating at the time with a more traditional form of psychotherapy—to incorporate these antidepressant lifestyle elements into their daily routines. Not only did I find that most patients were surprisingly eager to make such lifestyle changes, but the clinical results were stunning. Even patients who had not responded to drugs or traditional therapy began recovering—*quickly*.

Such dramatic clinical results took me by surprise. Sure, I thought a lifestyle-based strategy might be helpful in some cases of depression, but I had no idea just how powerful it would prove to be. I caught an early glimpse of its effectiveness, however, in the experience of the first patient I ever worked with on these principles of therapeutic lifestyle change.

A tall, soft-spoken man in his mid-forties, Bill had been severely depressed for over four years. Other than a few brief periods of remission, he had been continuously depressed since his early teens. When we started working together, he had already been on depression medication for well over a year with little meaningful improvement.

In one of our first sessions together, Bill casually mentioned that although he didn't exercise regularly, he'd noticed in the past that working out sometimes made him feel a little better, at least for a short while. Since I'd recently been immersed in the research literature on exercise and depression, I was intrigued by his comment and decided to push him a bit on the point. "Bill, would you be willing to try working out on a regular basis? Dozens of published studies show it can help with symptoms of depression." Although his energy level was pretty low, he agreed to try jogging three times a week, either outside or on the small treadmill stored in his basement. (Like most pieces of home exercise equipment, it had been gathering dust for years.)

At our next session, Bill reported a small but noticeable improvement in his ability to sleep through the night, and he attributed this to the exercise. The following week brought a noticeable upswing in his energy level. Encouraged by this development, I decided to see if he was willing to crank things up a notch on the lifestyle front. So we spent the next few sessions talking about the clinical benefits of omega-3 supplementation, the toxic effects of time spent alone ruminating, and the importance of getting adequate sunlight exposure, social support, and sleep. To his immense credit, Bill gradually began putting into practice every major therapeutic lifestyle element we discussed. And within two months, his depressive symptoms were gone. Completely gone. It was nothing short of remarkable.

It's now been over five years since we began working together, and Bill is still fully recovered—the first stretch of continuous recovery in his adult life. In fact, we still touch base by phone every so often for a quick checkup, and during our most recent conversation Bill told me, "Steve, these past four years have been by far the best of my life."

Over the past few years, many others like Bill—people who had given up hope of ever beating their depression—have overcome the dreaded illness as well. The great majority of patients in our clinical trials have escaped depression's grip, and the response rate to Therapeutic Lifestyle Change has been considerably higher than researchers typically see with antidepressant medication.

I realize this is a surprising claim. After all, depression is a serious illness—one that robs people of their vitality, their hope, their sleep, their play, their friends, their work, and sometimes even their very lives. Can this debilitating disorder really be fought more effectively with a set of basic lifestyle changes than with powerful antidepressant drugs?

It *is* hard to believe. But I've seen firsthand the dramatic improvements that typically follow in the wake of these simple changes, even among those who haven't responded to medication.

Despite the best efforts of mental health professionals, depression continues to destroy millions of lives each year. This simply cannot continue. As we begin to reclaim the natural antidepressant benefits of the life we were all designed for, I believe we can put an end to the modern depression epidemic once and for all.

2

Making Sense of Depression

Mysteriously and in ways that are totally remote from normal experience, the gray drizzle of horror induced by depression takes on the quality of physical pain. But it is not an immediately identifiable pain, like that of a broken limb. It may be more accurate to say that despair, owing to some evil trick played upon the sick brain by the inhabiting psyche, comes to resemble the diabolical discomfort of being imprisoned in a fiercely overheated room. And because no breeze stirs this caldron, because there is no escape from the smothering confinement, it is entirely natural that the victim begins to think ceaselessly of oblivion.

—**William Styron**, ***Darkness Visible***

Wendy, a thirty-four-year-old middle school teacher from Kansas City, enrolled in one of our Therapeutic Lifestyle Change groups a few years ago after struggling with depression for the better part of a year. Like many of the patients we've worked with, she said her friends and family didn't really understand the disorder that had her in its grip. During the group's first session, as we reviewed the hallmark symptoms of depression and the devastation the illness leaves in its wake, Wendy turned to me and said, "You guys—you psychiatrists or psychologists or whatever—really need to come up with a better name for this thing. *Depression* just doesn't cut it. I mean, everyone knows the word, so they think they get what it's all about. But most of them have no idea."

She has a point. Depression *is* a problematic word, the source of so much needless confusion and misunderstanding. Here's the problem: Depression has two very different meanings—depending on the context—and people mix them up all the time.

In casual, everyday conversation, depression serves as a good synonym for *sadness.* In this sense, it's simply a mood state we all experience from time to time, typically after we've brushed up against one of life's inevitable setbacks or disappointments. For example, I've heard people say they were depressed after watching their favorite team lose a big game, or even after ripping a hole in a good pair of blue jeans. Such "depression" doesn't last for long, and it rarely affects our ability to function.

In a clinical context, however, the word has a radically different meaning. It refers to a profoundly debilitating form of mental illness. (The precise diagnostic label is *major depressive disorder*, but most clinicians simply call it *depression* for short.) It's a syndrome that deprives people of their energy, sleep, concentration, joy, confidence, memory, sex drive—their ability to love and work and play. It can even rob them of their will to live. Over time, depression damages the brain and wreaks havoc on the body. It's a treacherous illness—a shudder-inducing foe that no one in their right mind would ever take lightly, certainly not if they understood the disorder's capacity to destroy life.

Unfortunately, despite an encouraging increase in public awareness in recent years, confusion about depression abounds. In short, people still confuse the two vastly different meanings of the word. That's why so many believe the disorder is no big deal, that those cut down by the illness are just making mountains out of molehills. As one of my unenlightened students put it in class a few years ago, "I've always assumed these people are just a bunch of slackers—whiners who simply need to suck it up and snap out of it."

Over the years, I've found that such harsh, critical judgments usually stem from ignorance. Fortunately, once people grasp the true nature of depression, they usually develop a strong sense of compassion for those who fall under the disorder's tragic sway. The same basic principle also applies to one's *own* experience of depression: Knowledge can serve as a powerful defense against the destructive impulse of self-blame.

So, although this is a book about strategies for treating depression, I think it's useful to pause first to reflect on what the disorder is all about, and to address the most important questions people commonly raise. How is depression diagnosed? What are its telltale symptoms? What causes people to get depressed? Doesn't stress play a big role? What about genetics? And is depression really just a matter of chemical imbalance? It is to these questions that we now turn.

THE SYMPTOMS AND THE DIAGNOSIS

In the often-mysterious world of mental health practice, diagnoses are made according to the criteria laid out in a byzantine reference book called the *Diagnostic and Statistical Manual of Mental Disorders, Fourth Edition.* Most of us in the field simply call it the *DSM-IV,* for short. The book serves like a sort of diagnostic Bible, with a set of elaborate rules for deciding exactly who does and doesn't qualify to be diagnosed with any given disorder. When it comes to the diagnosis of depression (*major depressive episode* in technical diagnostic language), fortunately, the criteria are pretty straightforward.

First, the *DSM-IV* lays out a set of nine core diagnostic symptoms:

1. Depressed mood
2. Loss of interest or pleasure in all (or nearly all) activities
3. A large increase or decrease in appetite/weight
4. Insomnia or hypersomnia (greatly increased sleep)
5. Slowing of physical movements, or severe agitation
6. Intense fatigue
7. Excessive feelings of guilt or worthlessness
8. Difficulty concentrating or making decisions
9. Frequent thoughts of death, or suicidality

A diagnosis requires at least *five** of these hallmark symptoms to be present most of the day, nearly every day, for two weeks or more. These core symptoms also have to cause functional impairment or severe distress. In addition, the *DSM* includes some common sense guidelines to help clinicians distinguish between authentic cases of depression and other syndromes that can mimic the disorder—such as poor thyroid function, chronic fatigue syndrome, or some forms of substance abuse.† Likewise, the *DSM* urges clinicians to delay making a diagnosis for up to two months when someone has suffered the death of a family member or close friend, as it's normal to experience at least some depressive symptoms—including sad mood,

* And at least one of these symptoms has to be either depressed mood or loss of interest/pleasure.
† In essence, if the depressive symptoms can be explained by a medical illness or the effects of substance use (or withdrawal), the diagnosis needs to reflect that.

thoughts of death, and sleep disturbance—when we've just lost a loved one.*

Although the *DSM-IV* does a pretty good job of laying out the most common symptoms of depression, it leaves much to be desired when it comes to conveying what the disorder actually *feels like.* For example, in talking with hundreds of patients over the years, I've been struck by how often they use the word *pain* to describe the experience. (The word is nowhere to be found in the diagnostic criteria.) Several have told me the emotional anguish of depression far outstrips anything they've endured in the way of physical pain. They say it's worse, by orders of magnitude, than the prolonged agony of natural childbirth, spinal injury, or passing a kidney stone.

Back when I was a rookie psychology intern at Duke Medical Center, one of my patients helped me gain a much-needed sense of perspective on the intense suffering depression entails. He said right before he was hospitalized, he spent an entire day curled up in a fetal position on the floor of his apartment, sobbing, with no energy to move and powerless to get up. But then he finally noticed a little improvement in the evening. So he forced himself to get up and make a long-neglected trip to the grocery store. As he ambled up and down the aisles, he noticed a haggard man perched in a wheelchair near the checkout line. The man had visibly shriveled legs, and one of his arms had been amputated just below the shoulder. After passing him, many customers would glance back in pity. Taking in the scene, my patient began

* However, if the bereaved individual is suicidal or suffers from major functional impairment, a depression diagnosis may be given after only two weeks.

brooding: "I've been in agony for months, but no one else can see it. As far as they know, there's nothing to be concerned about and nothing to pity. But if they could actually see what I'm going through, they'd know that I'd give my right arm to be free from this depression, and I'd do it in a heartbeat. *I would give literally anything—even my limbs—just to escape this pain.*"

DEPRESSION ON THE BRAIN

As it turns out, some of the brain pathways that register physical pain serve double-duty by signaling emotional pain as well. These important neural hubs—with obscure Latin names such as *subgenual cingulate, thalamus*, *amygdala,* and *orbitofrontal cortex*—light up every time they detect something harmful happening to the body, and they don't always distinguish between physical and emotional sources of injury. As far as the brain is concerned, the experience of depression is very much like an excruciating physical sensation that never goes away. The illness brings relentless suffering, week after torturous week.

To make matters worse, depression also locks the brain into a gloomy, biased mode of thinking, shifting our perceptions in an extremely negative direction. Because it causes us to view things in the darkest possible terms, most depressed patients come to believe things will never get better. They genuinely believe their pain will never end, despite all the evidence to the contrary. That's why many eventually look to death in a desperate bid to escape their (seemingly endless) suffering. Each year, depression accounts for one million lives lost to suicide worldwide—a tragedy of unimaginable proportions.

The Stress Response

The toxic effects of depression on the brain are pervasive, going far beyond the function of pain circuits and biased thinking. It's impossible to truly understand the disorder—and equally impossible to treat it effectively—without factoring into the equation the myriad crucial events taking place in our gray matter. Although the neurological underpinnings of depression are astonishingly complex, involving dozens of neurotransmitters (brain chemicals), hundreds of specific brain regions, and billions of individual neurons, one of the most important discoveries on this front is remarkably intuitive: *a key trigger for depression is the brain's runaway stress response.*

Like death and taxes, stress is an unavoidable part of life. Most of us endure at least a few stressors every day: getting stuck in heavy traffic, quarreling with a family member, facing a tight deadline at work, opening an unexpectedly large bill—the list goes on and on. And when we face such strains, the brain springs into action with a clever set of adaptations that prepare us to rise to the occasion. But here's the thing: The brain's stress response system is ancient (in evolutionary terms). It's designed to help us deal with the sort of intense, short-term challenges faced by our remote ancestors. It's poorly suited to the stressors we face today.

When our hunter-gatherer forebears experienced stress, it often involved an immediate *fight-or-flight* response—evading a predator, fending off an attack from a hostile neighboring tribe, or scurrying for shelter in the face of an oncoming storm. In that ancient environment, *stress signaled the immediate need for vigorous physical activity.* And the brain's stress response is still calibrated to those ancestral conditions, mobilizing a cascade of physical reactions that quickly prepare the body for an intense burst of action.

For starters, when we're stressed, our bodies release potent hormones such as adrenaline and cortisol, which set in motion a host of other reactions. The liver dumps its stores of sugar into the bloodstream, providing booster fuel for the muscles. The lungs ramp up their intake of oxygen (another muscle fuel). The heart beats faster and stronger, sending more nutrient-rich blood throughout the body. And the immune system shifts into tissue repair mode to get ready for any injuries that might happen during a fight-or-flight encounter.

Bizarrely, when the stress response lasts into the night, it even prompts the brain to change the structure of our sleep. It shifts us out of the deep, restorative slumber the body needs and pushes us instead into a much shallower, restless, dream-filled sleep—not nearly as healthy for the body, but easier to wake up from in the case of encroaching danger.

Such changes are beautifully calibrated to an ancient world in which each stressor called for a robust physical response to a short-term threat. And even though the stress response can wreak havoc on the body if it ever lasts longer than a few days, ancestral life included several built-in safeguards to make sure that didn't happen. For example, intense physical exercise—once part of nearly every fight-or-flight encounter—provides direct feedback to the brain, prompting it to slam the brakes on its stress circuitry. (The basic message to the brain is: "A big burst of activity just took place, so there's no need to keep gearing up for more.") Likewise, the protective presence of loved ones—which our forebears experienced for the better part of each day—gives the brain a strong, primal signal that we're probably no longer in any immediate danger, so it ratchets down the stress response accordingly.

With such protective mechanisms in place, our hunter-gatherer ancestors were well-equipped to face the stressful events that came their way. They could instantly mobilize for activity in a crisis and just as quickly find their way back to a state of calm when the challenge had passed. How can we know? We can study modern-day hunter-gatherers, whose way of life is similar to that of our remote ancestors. And in one telling investigation, contemporary hunter-gatherers were found to have low levels of circulating stress hormones—considerably lower, on average, than those of the typical American.

Then again, modern life seems almost perversely designed to keep the brain's stress response in high gear, with a relentless procession of day-to-day pressures and hassles. However, while these routine, everyday strains certainly *can* usher in an episode of depression, they usually don't. Instead, the illness is most often triggered by the added stress of more painful, high-impact events—divorce, separation, job loss, sickness, failure, rejection, physical assault, or geographic relocation. For people who are vulnerable to depression (we'll take a careful look at who they are in the next section), such traumatic events can kick the brain's stress circuitry into such a high state of overdrive that it simply can't be turned off.

How, exactly, does the runaway stress response cause the full-blown syndrome of depression—with symptoms like social withdrawal and lethargy and loss of concentration and sleep disturbance? The short answer: It's complicated. Thousands of talented researchers from all over the world have been working for decades to fully unravel the causes of depressive illness. Every year, the picture comes a bit more clearly into focus. Two areas of the brain that play particularly important roles are the *frontal cortex,* which regulates mood and behavior, and the specialized neural circuits that coordinate sleep. We'll consider each in turn.

Frontal Assault

The frontal cortex is the outer part of the brain that sits right behind the eye sockets and forehead. It's the hub of conscious mental life, where the sense of self is made flesh. And, like many other regions of the brain, the frontal cortex is split down the middle. It's divided into separate-but-equal hemispheres (left and right) that play distinct, complementary roles in shaping our mood and behavior.

The frontal cortex is also richly interconnected with a little almond-shaped area deep in the brain called the *amygdala*—it's the brain's generator of strong emotions. The two hemispheres of the frontal cortex work with the amygdala to steer and direct our deepest feelings. When the left frontal hemisphere grows more active than the right, for example, our mood shifts in a positive direction and we experience a strong impulse to pursue our goals.* On the other hand, when the left hemisphere shuts down, mood takes a sharply negative turn, goal pursuit stops, and we become focused instead on avoiding harm. People who have suffered major damage to the left frontal cortex typically experience depressed mood, along with a profound decline in goal-directed activities. Frequently, they meet the full diagnostic criteria for depression.

As you may have guessed, the brain's runaway stress response—that important neurological trigger for depression—also causes a dramatic decrease in left frontal cortex activity. This, in turn, sends mood and activity levels plummeting.

Stress hormones like cortisol also have an important effect on another key function of the frontal cortex: memory. In the short-term, these stress hormones can enhance our ability to store new memo-

* This is the case, at least, for those who are right-handed. Among lefties, the brain's hemispheres can be wired the other way around.

ries, increasing the odds that we'll learn from our stressful experiences and, with luck, put such knowledge to good use in the future. But when the stress response goes on for weeks at a time—as it typically does before an episode of depression—cortisol begins to exact a toxic toll on the memory circuits of the frontal cortex. These areas of the brain actually start *shrinking*, and mental function grows less efficient: concentration, memory, attention, and abstract reasoning are all affected. Not surprisingly, depressed patients often complain that their minds don't seem to work as well as they did before the onset of the illness.

The Sleeping Brain

As we saw previously, when the brain's stress circuits are fully engaged, they can profoundly alter the structure of sleep. Specifically, there is a steady disappearance of the deep, restful form of slumber known as *slow-wave sleep*—the phase of sleep the brain needs to keep brain chemicals and hormones in balance, and to coordinate things such as tissue repair.

When laboratory rats are experimentally deprived of slow-wave sleep for several days at a time, their brains start to malfunction and they become seriously ill. Humans react in much the same way. After just a few nights of slow-wave sleep deprivation, most people report intense, aching fatigue. After a few more days, they begin to feel physically ill. They also start moving and speaking more slowly. Many people even complain of a sensation of physical pain (even though they can't quite tell where it's coming from). In this sleep-altered state, mood turns despondent, social interest disappears, thoughts turn negative, appetite becomes erratic, and concentration wanes. In other words, with the disappearance of slow-wave sleep, the core symptoms of depression quickly emerge.

RISK FACTORS

We've briefly touched on the fact that some people are much more vulnerable to depression than others. But what actually puts a person at risk? And what makes others resilient, allowing them to remain unaffected by the illness even in the face of unimaginably stressful circumstances? Let's briefly review some of the major known risk factors, as well as the things known to confer protection.

Genes. Much has been written in the popular press about the role of genes in depression. This prominent coverage has led some people to conclude—mistakenly—that the disorder is somehow "all genetic." Genes are far from the whole story. However, they certainly play an important role in determining who is at risk. We know this from several converging lines of evidence. For example, identical twins—with exactly the same genes—are much more similar in their susceptibility to depression than fraternal twins, who share only half their genes in common. Likewise, the biological (genetic) children of depressed parents are at greatly increased risk, but their adopted children generally are not. Based on such studies, geneticists have even been able to estimate how much of the risk for depression is directly linked to our genes. And the best studies have come back with a result of about 40%. In other words, faulty genes account for a little less than half the story of who gets depressed and who does not.

The most interesting link on this front comes from a stretch of DNA known as the *serotonin transporter gene*. As its name suggests, this gene affects the function of serotonin, a chemical messenger that plays a major role in shutting off the brain's stress response circuits and reducing anxiety. (As we'll see in Chapter 3, popular drugs like Lustral, Efexor, and Prozac directly target serotonin function in the brain. Likewise, serotonin abnormality is what most people seem to have in mind when they refer to depression as a matter of "chemical imbalance.")

The serotonin transporter gene comes in two versions,* dubbed *long* and *short,* and people with short versions of the gene have less effective serotonin function. As a result, they're more prone to feeling anxious, and to suffering a runaway stress response. From early childhood, such individuals are frequently anxiety-prone, and they are also highly vulnerable to depression. In a recent large-scale study of New Zealanders, young adults with short copies of the gene were about two and a half times more likely than those with long copies to become depressed when faced with severe negative life events.

But of course, lots of people with no known genetic risk also become depressed. Because fewer than half of all cases of depression can be chalked up to genetic factors, it's clear that the environment—that is, all the things we *experience*—also plays a major role.

Child abuse. The experience of severe childhood trauma, for example, has a potentially devastating long-term effect, no matter what sort of genes a person was born with. Children who have suffered physical or sexual abuse are at much greater risk for depression—even later as adults—than those who have not. Tragically, such early trauma can leave an enduring imprint on the brain, placing its stress circuitry on a permanent state of hair-trigger alert, and making it very difficult to shut off once activated.

* Technically, there are not two versions of the gene itself, but of a sequence of molecules (called the *promoter* region) that control the gene's functioning.

Social support. Some forms of experience can also *protect* us against depression. As we've seen, the human species is hard-wired for extensive person-to-person contact, and the supportive presence of loved ones is a powerful signal from the environment that helps keep the brain's stress response in check. Several studies have shown that people with strong social support networks are relatively unlikely to become depressed. In fact, a British team of researchers found that simply having *one supportive confidant*—an emotionally close friend or family member—cut the risk of depression in half following a painful event like separation, divorce, or job loss.

When such support is absent, even owning a pet seems to provide at least some protection, since the comforting experience of close physical contact with any other animal—human or nonhuman—reduces activity in the brain's stress centers.

Not all social contact is beneficial, however. Sometimes, as Sartre complained, "hell is other people." Researchers have found, for example, that the presence of a harshly critical, emotionally abusive spouse renders a person more vulnerable to depression—even more so than if they had no meaningful social connection at all. Some relationships are so psychologically toxic that they can keep the brain's stress response networks in a perpetual state of overdrive, ever teetering on the edge of the depressive abyss.

Thoughts. Another big set of risk factors has to do with the way we *think* about things. That's because the way we react to events often shapes our feelings more than the events themselves. When something upsets us, it's natural to spend at least a little time reflecting on what went wrong, what we might have done differently, and what we could still do to make things better. But some people have an unhealthy tendency to brood on negative events. They spin them around and around in the mind's eye, torturing themselves for days on end with endless thoughts of "woulda, coulda, shoulda."

This kind of rumination is an effective way to keep the brain's stress circuits revved up, and people who dwell on their negative thoughts like this are especially prone to depression. On the other hand, learning how to short-circuit rumination—redirecting attention away from such thoughts so we can engage in more rewarding activities—is a highly effective tool for keeping the illness at bay.

Gender. Women get depressed about twice as often as men do. This is perplexing, and nobody knows for sure what makes women so much more vulnerable. But consider this: Boys and girls get depressed at roughly the same rate during childhood, and men and women also have about the same rate of depression in late adulthood. In other words, the gender gap is there only during the prime reproductive years, when sex hormone levels are at their highest.

Researchers have found that estrogen and progesterone, major female reproductive hormones, have a large effect on mood and other depressive symptoms. Specifically, when estrogen and progesterone levels drop suddenly—as they do during the premenstrual period and also right after childbirth—mood and energy are also liable to plummet. Estrogen levels also swing wildly (with many sudden drops) during the years leading up to menopause, and this is a time of particularly high depression vulnerability for women.

Women with the highest overall estrogen levels also seem to be more vulnerable to the experience of anxiety,* and under some conditions, estrogen even helps prime the brain's stress response.

*At first blush, this might seem at odds with information in the preceding paragraph, but it's not: *sudden drops* in estrogen levels are linked with depressed mood, but *consistently low* levels of the hormone generally aren't.

Among all known primate species (not just humans), females experience anxious arousal more readily than males do—a finding consistent with the role of estrogen and other female hormones in promoting the stress response.

On the other hand, testosterone has been strongly linked to a sense of well-being and to high levels of activity. In other words, this male reproductive hormone is a natural mood booster. It also tends to suppress feelings of anxiety* and to blunt the perception of stress. It's probably no coincidence, then, that men are less vulnerable to depression than women precisely during those prime years of adolescence and adulthood when testosterone levels are at their highest.†

Lifestyle. As we saw in Chapter 1, people who exercise regularly are at much lower risk of depression than couch potatoes. Exercise changes the brain as powerfully as any medication, and it helps slam the brakes on the depressive stress response. Similar protection is found in other lifestyle factors. People who eat lots of fish and other sources of omega-3 fat have greatly reduced depression vulnerability. Likewise with those who are exposed every day to high levels of natural sunlight, and who get adequate sleep each night. And these four lifestyle factors, together with those we mentioned previously—pursuing social connection and engaging activities—are at the heart of the Therapeutic Lifestyle Change program, which allows us to reclaim key protective elements from the ancestral milieu.

---

* This also helps explain why high-testosterone males are more likely to engage in foolish risk-taking behavior.

† Men produce up to forty times as much testosterone as women, although women's bodies are more sensitive to the hormone. Men's testosterone levels also peak during late adolescence and decline slowly into their thirties and forties—after which the pace of decline for most men picks up considerably.

THE GREATEST CHALLENGE

There's an old adage in psychology: *The best predictor of future behavior is past behavior.* In the case of depression, the saying is particularly apt. Consider this: Among Americans, the risk of future depression now stands at roughly 25%, but it rises to well over 50% among those who have been depressed before. And after three episodes of depression, the lifetime risk of relapse—getting depressed again—rises to a staggering 90%. Clearly, the best predictor of future depression is past depression.

But why should this be? Sadly, there's evidence that depression can leave a toxic imprint on the brain. It can etch its way into our neural circuitry—including the brain's stress response system—and make it much easier for the brain to fall back into another episode of depression down the road. This helps explain a puzzling fact: It normally takes a high level of life stress to trigger someone's *first* episode of depression, but later relapse episodes sometimes come totally out of the blue. It seems that once the brain has learned how to operate in depression mode, it can find its way back there with much less prompting.

Fortunately, though, we can heal from the damage of depression. All it takes is several months of complete recovery for much of the toxic imprint on the brain to be erased.* And in the chapters ahead, we'll address the many things you can do to promote such a healing process.

But first we need to consider the most important reason why the rate of depression relapse is so high: Our risk factors tend to remain

* Technically, the toxic imprint on the brain is not actually erased—more like overwritten.

stable over time. For example, with few exceptions,* our genes and our gender don't change. And while you might think that behavior can change like the wind, it actually stays surprisingly consistent for most people. Those who avoid exercise today will probably still be sedentary tomorrow—and next week, and next month, and next year, and the year after that, and so on. Likewise are those who tend to ruminate, those who stay chronically sleep-deprived, those who fail to invest in social relationships, and those who eat too few omega-3 fats. Without a high level of motivation and commitment—and (in many cases) a little outside help†—most of us simply keep repeating the same unhelpful patterns of behavior, despite our good intentions to the contrary.

Over the past few years, I've had the privilege of working with many depressed patients who knew they needed to change the way they were living, but didn't know how to do so on their own. Helping them in that process—and watching them find their way back to lasting health—has been one of the most satisfying, joyful experiences of my life.

None of us gets to choose our genes or our gender or our parents or our underlying brain chemistry: Many risk factors for depression are out of our hands. But no matter what life may have handed us, there's abundant evidence that *what we do today* can profoundly lower our vulnerability in the here and now, and in all the days ahead. It's my hope that in the pages that follow you'll encounter just the catalyst you need to reclaim the many powerfully protective lifestyle features from our ancestral past.

---

* These exceptions include gender reassignment surgery, environmentally triggered changes in gene activity, or radiation-induced genetic mutation.

† As in the case of those who hire a therapist, a personal trainer, or a "life coach."

3

Treating Depression: The State of the Art (and Science)

What's the most effective treatment for depression? When I posed this question to my Abnormal Psychology students, they shot back quizzical stares. They always do. You can see the confusion in their eyes, the wheels spinning: *Is this some kind of trick question? The answer has to be "antidepressant medication," but why would he even ask something so obvious—unless there's a catch?*

I repeated the question, and eventually a thoughtful young man called out from the back of the room, "Dr. Ilardi, I'm pretty sure it's some kind of medication. So are you asking us *which* drug is the most effective?" I shook my head and smiled, and then pointed to a senior in the front row who had her hand raised.

"Okay, even if drugs usually clear up people's depression," she said, "I know this girl who had to quit taking her meds because of all the side effects. So maybe sometimes drugs aren't the best treatment?"

"That's an important point about side effects," I agreed. "And it's something we definitely have to come back to. But right now I'm interested in the first thing you said: 'Drugs usually clear up people's depression.'" Looking out across the room full of three hundred students, I asked, "How many of you believe this? How many of you think antidepressants usually cure depression?" Nearly every hand in the room went up. They always do.

THE EFFECTIVENESS OF DEPRESSION MEDICATIONS: WEIGHING THE EVIDENCE

Virtually everyone now accepts the premise that antidepressants are a potent treatment option for depression. And it's not just because we've all heard the message on a relentless parade of TV ads and public service announcements. Most of us *know* people who've been helped by these meds. Even clinicians who used to treat depression with therapy have jumped on the medication bandwagon. I recently heard a famous psychotherapist claim it would be unethical if he failed to recommend medication for any of his depressed patients.

Besides, with over one hundred fifty million antidepressant prescriptions written in the United States each year—a 400% increase since 1990—it seems obvious that these drugs must be providing at least some benefit. Otherwise, people simply would have stopped taking them long ago.

But exactly how much benefit do these medications provide? Of all the depressed patients who take an antidepressant, how many experience a complete and lasting recovery? It turns out to be a surprisingly low percentage—much lower than I would have guessed before I took the time to wade through the hundreds of studies that address this question.

Consider, for example, the landmark 2004 study that followed several hundred patients treated with one of three popular antidepressants: Lustral, Seroxat, or Prozac. Among those who took the drugs as prescribed, *only 23% were depression-free after six months of treatment.* (As you might expect, patients who failed to take their meds did even worse.) And all three medications yielded roughly the same dismal results.

A fluke result, perhaps? It's actually pretty typical. The recovery rate with antidepressants in similar studies usually falls somewhere between 20% and 35%. Clinical researchers at forty-one treatment sites across the country have just completed the largest real-world study of antidepressants ever conducted, and the results fit the same overall pattern. This multimillion dollar project, sponsored by the National Institutes of Mental Health, followed about three thousand depressed patients who initially took the drug citalopram (marketed under the trade name Cipramil) for about twelve weeks. By the end of that short-term treatment period, *only 28% of study patients had fully recovered.*

The study's 28% response rate might even be an overestimate of the medication's true effectiveness, because patients received higher drug doses and had more frequent doctor's visits than people do in everyday clinical practice. (In real life, insurance companies sharply restrict the frequency of "med check" follow-up appointments).

Remarkably, the study's authors—a veritable All-Star team of clinical researchers—noted that the observed 28% recovery rate was about what they had expected to see based on comparable studies. That's right: They weren't surprised to find that the majority of study patients failed to recover on an antidepressant. In the study's published write-up, the researchers also raised a provocative question: What percentage of their patients might have recovered if they had received a sugar pill—a *placebo*—instead of the medication? Could it possibly have been as high as 28%?

Better Than a Sugar Pill?

It's hard to believe that anyone with a disabling illness like depression could get better simply by taking a sugar pill—which is medically inert—but the placebo response rate in depression is not trivial. In fact, the U.S. Food and Drug Administration (FDA) won't approve any new depression medication until the drug's manufacturers can provide compelling evidence that the medicine outperforms a placebo.

Although this sounds like a ridiculously easy standard for a new drug to meet, it's not. Irving Kirsch, a clinical researcher at the University of Connecticut, recently showed just how tough it can be. Under the Freedom of Information Act, he petitioned the FDA for the results of every drug-company study submitted over a thirteen-year period (1987–1999) for six commonly used antidepressant medications: Lustral, Efexor, Prozac, Cipramil, and Seroxat. Incredibly, he found that *in 56% of these studies, depressed patients taking an antidepressant drug fared no better than those who took a placebo.* Not surprisingly, the drug companies have never published most of these studies.

When Kirsch combined the results of the FDA's antidepressant studies into one huge analysis, he did find some evidence that the drugs worked better than a placebo—but only slightly better. Overall, the placebo effect was 80% as large as that of the medications—equal to a difference of 2 points on the studies' 50-point depression rating scale. This difference was, as Kirsch put it, "very small and of questionable clinical significance." And this shocking result isn't just the handiwork of a single investigator; it's now been replicated by others who have taken an independent look at the FDA database and arrived at the same basic conclusions.

So, what are we to make of all this? Are antidepressants just placebos with nasty side effects? Before we jump to such a radical conclusion, we need to take into consideration an important twist to the story. Among *severely* depressed patients—those whose symptoms are so profoundly disabling that they can no longer function at all—depression drugs have been found to work much better than placebos. Although most severely depressed patients aren't completely cured by antidepressants, at least half of them will experience meaningful improvement within a month or two. By comparison, few such patients ever improve while taking a dummy pill.

But the great majority of people with diagnosable depression don't have such severe disability. They're still able—with some difficulty—to keep working and interacting with family and friends. And among these less severely depressed individuals, antidepressants and placebos work about equally well. This means that most people on antidepressants are receiving no more benefit than they would from a bottle of sugar pills.

And yet if doctors started handing out sham pills—labeled as such—their patients would experience little improvement. Why? Because the placebo effect hinges on an important element of deception: *The person taking the pill has to believe it's an active medication.* They have to believe it's going to help. That's what allows the dummy pills to work their healing magic. Placebo-induced positive expectancies can exert a powerful effect on the brain, increasing activity in circuits of the frontal cortex that are otherwise dormant in depression. Such changes in brain function are sometimes capable of sparking impressive reductions in depressive symptoms.

But it would be unethical for a doctor to deceive patients by giving them sugar pills labeled, say, "Lustral." That's why no one ever takes a placebo for depression in the real world. It happens only in research studies, where patients can consent to being randomly given either antidepressants or sham pills that look and taste just like medication, but that are medically inert. Surprisingly, most study patients believe they're receiving an active medication, regardless of whether they're taking a real drug or a fake one, and this explains why the placebo can work about as well as an antidepressant under such conditions.

Remember, though, neither placebos nor antidepressants are particularly effective. As we've seen, antidepressants lead to complete short-term recovery for about a quarter of the depressed patients who take them. Another 25% or so will experience significant improvement within a couple months, but will still have some lingering symptoms. And *roughly half of all depressed patients won't improve meaningfully on meds at all.* These numbers appear to be about the same for every major antidepressant medication; there's no conclusive evidence that any particular depression drug works much better, on average, than any other.

Even when antidepressants *are* effective in the short run, their healing effects don't always endure. Over time, the drugs may simply stop working—a phenomenon the experts colorfully refer to as drug "poop out." I've worked with many patients who've experienced it firsthand, and they usually describe it as coming more or less out of the blue. In the typical scenario, they've been taking their meds faithfully for months—sometimes for years—and then simply wake up one day to find their old symptoms returning with full force. Often they can't even point to an obvious stressful event as a trigger. According to the best research, up to 50% of those who respond favorably to antidepressant medications will become depressed again at some point. And because most depressed patients fail to fully recover on their meds in the first place, we know that far fewer than one in four are fortunate enough both to get well and to stay well on antidepressants.

These are sobering numbers. Sometimes when I bring them to people's attention they assume I must be "anti-medication." I'm not.

I'm immensely grateful for the relief these medications sometimes provide. I just wish the meds lived up to the immense hype that surrounds them. How wonderful it would be if antidepressants provided a genuine cure for the devastating scourge of depression—if they led to lasting recovery for the vast majority of people who take them. But they don't, and I believe it's important to face the facts head on, especially when other treatment options are available.

Side Effects

There's yet another potential downside to antidepressants: Many people quit taking them because of the unpleasant side effects. According to a recent study, the typical patient goes off his or her prescribed medications after just eight weeks. And of course, when people stop taking their meds, they're much less likely to experience any lasting benefit.

But what are the major antidepressant side effects, and how often do they occur? Although the answers can vary a bit from one medication to another, many adverse effects apply to depression drugs across the board. We'll review the most important of these in this section.

Suicidality. Of all the potential downsides to antidepressant use, none is more troubling than the drugs' reported tendency to cause suicidal thinking and behavior in children and adolescents. It's hard to believe that any drug—let alone one designed to combat depression—could have such a sinister effect. But as the data have accumulated in recent years, it's become clear that these medications pose a genuine risk of increased suicidality in this age group. The evidence on this point is so compelling that the U.S. Food and Drug Administration now requires all antidepressants to carry a "black box" warning label.

This warning, issued in late 2004, came after FDA researchers—under intense public pressure—combed through their database of twenty-four antidepressant studies involving four thousand four hundred adolescents and children. Incredibly, they found that suicidal thoughts and behavior were *twice as likely* among young people on antidepressants compared with those taking a placebo. The risk looks to be particularly high during the first few weeks of treatment, when close monitoring is usually advised.

Although the overall med-related risk of increased suicidality appears to be relatively small—affecting just 4% of the young people in the FDA database—the potential consequences are so disastrous that the finding has to be taken seriously. After all, how many parents would give their child an antibiotic if they knew the drug carried a 4% risk of suicidal thinking or behavior? I believe most people would look hard for other viable treatment options.

And it's not just children and adolescents who face increased suicidality with antidepressant use. A more recent FDA analysis also found a substantially elevated risk among young adults up to the age of twenty-five.*

Emotional numbing. A much more common side effect of medication concerns *emotional numbing,* a decrease in the intensity of emotions—both positive and negative. Although this phenomenon hasn't been widely publicized, there's some evidence that it may afflict the majority of those taking antidepressants. When a person first starts on meds, this emotional blunting can be a welcome experience—providing relief from the wrenching pain of depression. But many people later discover they can no longer feel positive emo-

* Interestingly, no such risk was observed among adults older than twenty-five. The reasons for this discrepancy remain unknown.

tions like joy and excitement and romantic love as intensely as they used to.

Interestingly, some patients with this kind of numbness are oblivious to it. It tends to come on so gradually that it just becomes the "new normal." One of my patients said to me last year, after she tapered off Efexor, "It's so amazing just to be able to *feel* again. But how come I never even noticed how numb I was until I came off the meds?" The answer is paradoxical: Emotional numbing blunts a person's ability to notice (and care about) their emotional numbing.

Sexual dysfunction. Some of the most widely prescribed antidepressants belong to a class of drugs known as SSRIs (selective serotonin reuptake inhibitors), including Lustral, Cipramil, Prozac, and Seroxat. These drugs all influence the function of a chemical messenger in the brain called serotonin.

Because serotonin circuits help regulate the brain's pleasure centers, many people taking SSRIs experience sexual side effects—usually in the form of reduced sexual pleasure or desire. Some people completely lose their ability to have an orgasm, and others experience the blunting of *all* romantic feelings, not just their sex drive.

And these problems don't just afflict those on SSRIs. They're common with other drugs that affect the brain's use of serotonin, such as Efexor and Cymbalta.

Weight gain. Although it's rarely reported in the media, weight gain is a possible side effect of most antidepressant medications (especially with long-term use). Since many depressed patients—like the majority of Americans—are already over their ideal weight, the added pounds are almost always unwelcome.

Insomnia. Most SSRIs and similar medications also carry the potential to cause insomnia for a subset of patients. Such drugs sometimes cause people to become physically active while they're asleep—with periodic limb movements and *bruxism* (teeth grinding)—and this can lead to frequent awakenings. The resulting poor sleep may, in turn, cause other depressive symptoms to get worse.

AS GOOD AS IT GETS?

In the signature line from the classic film about obsessive-compulsive disorder, Jack Nicholson (as Melvin Udall) turns to a group of fellow patients—all still suffering the pain of mental illness despite taking their meds—and asks, "What if this is *as good as it gets*?" It's a poignant question, and one of great relevance. For we've seen that antidepressants, by far the most commonly used treatment option for depression, provide a complete and lasting cure for only a small subset of the people who take them. And this sporadic benefit comes at a high cost—an array of potential side effects that range from the merely annoying (weight gain) to the disturbing (loss of sexual function) to the downright terrifying (increased suicidality).

Yet virtually everyone regards these medications as the treatment of choice. Is this because there's truly nothing better? As disappointing as medication outcomes may be, isn't it possible that depression drugs are still as good as it gets? After all, aren't the antidepressants still better than the other options people have at their disposal—things such as traditional psychotherapy or shock therapy?

ON THE COUCH AND BEYOND

Sigmund Freud, the man who put psychotherapy on the map a century ago, was never optimistic about his ability to cure depression. He thought the only possible remedy would require the depressed patient to spend years on the therapy couch delving into the deep, dark, long-forgotten pains of childhood. And, said Freud, they might need to do this painful psychic excavation work at least four times a week.

Why such drastic measures? Freud viewed depression as a break with reality—a form of *psychosis*. Few think of depression this way today, and for good reason: It's just not true. Those suffering from depression are still very much in touch with reality. And most have no deep, dark, painful secrets from their childhood to explore. Even those who do are usually made worse, not better, by dwelling on such painful events while they're still depressed. (After they've recovered, however, it can sometimes be helpful for them to look carefully at past hurts, and to examine how they still influence the present—a topic we'll cover in Chapter 11.)

Simply put, Freudian therapy for depression isn't particularly effective. In the short term, it often makes people feel worse. But because of Freud's towering legacy—and his lasting influence on the public's perception of what psychotherapy is all about—many people just assume that all forms of therapy for depression must be just as ineffective as the Freudian version. They're not.

The Cognitive Revolution

In the early 1960s, a brilliant young psychiatrist named Aaron Beck challenged the Freudian orthodoxy. In the process, he ended up turning the field's view of psychotherapy on its head.

Beck noticed that most of his depressed patients didn't have the deep repressed childhood traumas Freud said they would. Instead, they spent much of their time thinking about things they felt bad about in the present. They tended to dwell—to *ruminate*—on their negative thoughts, which often seemed to reflect a starkly pessimistic interpretation of the world around them.

As Beck observed, even innocuous events could trigger a cascade of negative thoughts. For example, one of my patients last year saw the cashier at the grocery store smiling warmly at the customer in front of him, and he immediately started thinking, "How come people never smile at me like that? That cashier definitely didn't smile at me the last time I was here. She can probably tell there's something wrong with me. I'm sure she doesn't like me. Nobody does."

Beck was convinced that such negative thoughts cause people to feel more depressed. (Makes sense, doesn't it?) So he decided to start urging his patients to do something about it. He had them write down their thoughts and examine them through the objective lens of reason. Patients started disputing their negative interpretations of things, replacing them with less biased perceptions. This new form of treatment, *cognitive-behavior therapy* (CBT), led some patients to start feeling better fairly quickly, often within a matter of weeks. So Beck decided to jettison the Freudian dogma that therapy should last for years or even decades: A full course of CBT takes only three to four months to complete.

And Beck didn't just develop this novel form of treatment; he set out to prove its effectiveness in carefully controlled studies. He also encouraged others to do the same. Over the past three decades, CBT has been evaluated in dozens of carefully controlled research studies. It's now the most thoroughly researched form of psychotherapy in history. And here's the basic gist of the evidence: CBT is every bit as effective as medication in the short term. It leads to complete recovery—that is, the full disappearance of symptoms—for 30% to 40% of patients who start treatment, and it brings about substantial symptom reduction for another 25% or so.

That's not great, but it still compares favorably with antidepressants. And CBT has two big advantages over medications: There are no noxious side effects, and the benefits of treatment usually last for years after therapy is completed.

Despite this important treatment edge, only a small percentage of depressed patients ever try CBT. Most never even hear of it. How would they? There's no big marketing budget available to inform the public about psychotherapy. Even insurance companies and HMOs—who could conceivably help get the word out—often steer people toward medication, which is cheaper than CBT in the short term (although this cost advantage disappears in the long term).

Do Thoughts Really Matter?

As we've seen, many depressed patients who try CBT—just like many who take antidepressants—find little meaningful improvement. However, clinical researchers in recent years have been searching for ways to make therapy even better. A group of clinicians at the University of Washington appears to have achieved just that. Surprisingly, they did it by taking one small piece of the CBT protocol and expanding it into an entire treatment package.

Although Beck believed it was crucial to help depressed patients stop thinking negatively, he also recognized that *what we do* often determines how we feel. Ever the pragmatist, Beck even outlined a brief set of strategies for changing behavior in order to reduce symptoms of depression. But these behavioral strategies were never the focus of CBT—at least, not until Dr. Neil Jacobson and his research team at the University of Washington decided to see how much therapeutic mileage they could get out of simply changing what people do.

What would happen, Jacobson asked, if depressed patients quit trying to change their thoughts and worked instead on the goal of *doing* things again? How much would patients improve if therapists just helped them become more active and engaged—getting out and socializing and playing and accomplishing things? The answer: They would improve *a lot.* In a recent study, Jacobson's *behavioral activation* approach was more effective than either antidepressant medication or traditional CBT. An impressive 56% of severely depressed patients recovered with behavioral activation, compared with only 36% in CBT and 23% on medication (Seroxat). No traditional form of psychotherapy has ever performed better in a published head-to-head comparison against antidepressant medication.

Ironically, behavioral activation even helps people stop their negative thinking. It's not that patients are ever asked to change their negative thoughts (that is, to think more positively about things). They aren't. But they *are* taught to interrupt the toxic process of rumination by turning to rewarding activities instead. And this strategy works surprisingly well. According to the latest published evidence, antiruminative activity may be the single most effective antidepressant psychotherapy technique ever devised.

Psychotherapy in the Real World

During their medical school training, aspiring doctors are taught to base every treatment decision on an up-to-date knowledge of the relevant research literature, and they generally carry this scientific sensibility with them throughout their careers. So when physicians encounter, say, a patient with a clogged coronary artery, they should automatically begin generating a set of scientifically informed questions: What are the available treatment options? Which option—bypass surgery, angioplasty, medication, and so on—is likely to prove the most effective for *this* patient, given the location and extent of the blockage? What does the research say?

We take it as a given that a doctor's decisions will be guided by the best available scientific evidence, and most of us would be appalled to find a physician who simply ignored or neglected the latest research findings in the field. Surely the same holds true for psychotherapists, doesn't it? After all, just like medical doctors, therapists deal with an array of life-threatening conditions—disorders such as anorexia nervosa and substance abuse and depression. Aren't psychotherapists, like physicians, trained to base their treatment decisions on the best and most relevant research evidence? Sadly, the majority are not.

The problem traces back to the enduring influence of Sigmund Freud, who launched the institution of psychotherapy over a century ago. Despite his superb scientific training as a research neurologist, Freud never felt the need to conduct careful scientific studies on the effectiveness of the psychotherapy techniques he developed. Indeed, Freud was so convinced that his treatment method just *had* to be effective, he asked the world to rely on the "evidence" of mere anecdotes and a smattering of published case studies—some of which were later shown by historians to have been fabricated. Likewise, his followers were encouraged to accept the effectiveness of Freudian therapy as an article of faith, rather than subjecting the therapy to rigorous scientific scrutiny. And for over a century Freud's legacy has persisted: Many practicing psychotherapists still fail to base their clinical practice on sound scientific research.

After decades of tinkering and creative innovation, there are now over four hundred distinct varieties of psychotherapy being practiced by clinicians (with dozens of allegedly new techniques appearing each year), and *the vast majority of these treatments have never been tested scientifically.* Even when it comes to the treatment of depressive illness, many practicing therapists are still using techniques for which there is absolutely no supportive scientific evidence. This is not to say that all of these untested techniques are ineffective. They might work. But then again they might not. The point is that we simply have no way of knowing, and in the absence of solid research evidence we will never know for sure. Freudian therapy was practiced for nearly eighty years before a definitive set of studies showed that it's often ineffective in treating depression.

How many other psychotherapy techniques in widespread use today will prove similarly unhelpful once they're finally subjected to the clear light of scientific scrutiny? Although we have no way of knowing for certain, I believe it is now difficult for any therapist to justify using unproven techniques for treating depression when we have good research evidence that approaches like CBT and behavioral activation—when skillfully implemented—are reasonably effective, with a long-term efficacy at least equivalent to that of antidepressant medication.

THE DESPERATE CURE

Long before the first depression drug was introduced in the 1950s, psychiatrists had a much more radical treatment strategy at their disposal: shock therapy. True to its name, shock therapy entails the conduction of strong electrical currents through the brain. The goal is to induce violent convulsive seizures; if all goes well, they last for about a minute. And for reasons still shrouded in mystery, such seizures can have a profoundly antidepressant effect.

Most people assume shock therapy disappeared from the psychiatric landscape decades ago, a barbaric practice—not unlike the frontal lobotomy—that hasn't been seen since the days of *One Flew Over the Cuckoo's Nest.* But the procedure is still very much with us, albeit under a slightly different name. It's now called *electroconvulsive therapy* (to avoid any lingering negative associations to the word *shock*), and it's been rendered into a somewhat kinder, gentler intervention—with paralyzing muscle relaxants used before each convulsion to make sure the patient doesn't inadvertently break any bones or teeth (as used to happen with some regularity).

In its modern incarnation, electroconvulsive therapy, or ECT, is now used with over one hundred thousand patients every year in the United States and Europe. Most major psychiatric units provide ECT for a subset of their depressed patients—a last resort for those who haven't responded to meds, as well as elderly patients whose bodies can't tolerate the side effects of medication. The typical treatment involves ten to twelve shock sessions in all, scheduled at a pace of three per week.

In the short term, at least, ECT produces much better results than antidepressant medication, with an estimated recovery rate as high as 65%. But there's a big catch: The recovery usually doesn't last long. Most ECT patients, even those who start taking depression meds right after they finish a round of ECT, become depressed again within six months. A recent study found that only about 20% of patients treated with ECT got well and stayed well for a full year.

There's another catch: Patients usually have severe memory disturbance for days after each ECT session. Back when I was still an intern at Duke Medical Center, I would be asked every now and then to do psychotherapy with an ECT patient. It was an exercise in futility. Often, I'd walk into the patient's hospital room for a scheduled therapy session, only to have the patient look up at me quizzically and ask, "Who are you again?" This could happen even if we'd already been meeting regularly for days! A patient might tell me the most intimate details of his or her life during a productive session, and then the following day—after undergoing another round of ECT—the patient would stare at me blankly, as if I were a complete stranger.

Some studies suggest that ECT can even cause permanent brain damage. A few investigations, for example, have observed a clear link between ECT and *cerebral atrophy*—the shrinkage of brain tissue caused by the widespread death of brain cells. ECT can lead to permanent impairment of mental function as well. Up to 70% of ECT patients complain that they can't remember things like they used to—they fumble over the names of people they've known for years, struggle to pull up the right words in a conversation, and lose everyday objects with startling regularity. There's even evidence that ECT can cause a permanent drop in IQ.

I have a strong feeling that future generations will look back on our modern practice of ECT with horror—the psychiatric equivalent of slapping the side of the TV set in a desperate and improbable attempt to render the picture forever clear again.

THE CASE FOR THERAPEUTIC LIFESTYLE CHANGE

As we've seen, the public has been tragically misinformed about treatment options for depression. Sales of antidepressant drugs now exceed $20 billion a year, despite low rates of recovery, high rates of relapse, and an astonishing array of serious side effects. Remarkably, most people still blithely accept the false premise that antidepressants usually offer a lasting cure. They don't.

Traditional psychotherapy isn't much better, at least not as it's currently practiced. Freud-inspired therapy, which involves digging around the patient's psyche for long-repressed childhood traumas, is often of little help when it comes to treating depression. It sometimes even makes matters worse.

Short-term CBT is more promising: It works about as well as medication, but it yields longer-lasting benefits and has none of the noxious side effects. And there's evidence that CBT can be improved by shifting the focus of treatment to a change in lifestyle—helping the depressed patient become more active, thereby breaking the toxic cycle of rumination. This behavioral activation approach, which builds on one of the key principles of Therapeutic Lifestyle Change, has yielded some of the most promising results of any form of psychotherapy studied to date. In a recent study, it was found to be considerably superior to antidepressant medication.

But behavioral activation alone doesn't work for everyone. About 35–40% of depressed patients may not respond favorably to this approach. Why? *When it comes to treating depression, there is no one-size-fits-all cure.* Behavioral activation is a powerful technique, but many people with depression need something more. That's why we now turn to the six steps of Therapeutic Lifestyle Change.

PART TWO

THERAPEUTIC LIFESTYLE CHANGE

The Six Steps

4
Brain Food

If you can picture a lab rat in your mind's eye, it probably looks a lot like one of these little guys: sleek white fur, long twitchy whiskers, tiny pink ears and feet, and beady black eyes with a reddish cast around the edges. They're called *Wistar rats*, and for many years they've been providing researchers with a useful animal model of depression.

We don't normally think of rats as creatures that get depressed, but they do. Sort of. Actually, when researchers treat them badly, the rats start to shut down in ways that resemble depression in humans. Fortunately for the rats, however, they bounce right back to their former perky selves—usually within a day or two.*

The most widely used technique for depressing a rat these days is the *forced swim test.* It basically involves dropping the animal in a tall cylindrical tub of lukewarm water and watching as it tries to claw its way up the impossibly slippery sides to escape. After about ten minutes of frenetic—and ultimately futile—activity, the rat will just give up and go limp, barely managing to keep even its head above water. When it's plopped back in the tank the next day, the poor creature will be lucky to last two minutes in the water before falling into a depressive stupor.

But scientists have discovered some techniques that can keep this rodent version of depression at bay. For example, feeding the rats

* But they won't bounce back until the researchers stop mistreating them.

insanely high doses* of drugs like Prozac will do the trick. So will hitting them with the rat version of shock therapy. Recently, however, a group of Harvard researchers discovered a kinder, gentler way to keep the rats from getting depressed: supplementing their diets with *omega-3 fats*.

FAT HEADS

Fat is a fearsome word to most Americans. For several decades, nutritionists and medical professionals have warned us that fats are bad for us: They raise our cholesterol, clog our arteries, and tend to make us . . . fat. But then researchers discovered that this conventional wisdom was, in many respects, just plain wrong.†

We need fats. We'd all be dead without them. They're critical to the well-being of every cell in our bodies, and they're crucial building blocks for the construction of every neuron in our brains. As we saw in Chapter 1, the human brain is mostly made up of fats.

But all fats are not created equal. For example, the body can manufacture most of the fats it needs, but there are some that we can get only from our diets. The essential dietary fats come in two versions—*omega-3* and *omega-6***—and they play complementary roles in the brain and the rest of the body. When all goes well,

* It sometimes requires doses up to one hundred times higher than those administered to humans (adjusting for body weight).

† It's now known, for example, that most of the fats we eat have no effect on our cholesterol levels. (And some varieties of fat might actually lower cholesterol.) Likewise, the best evidence suggests that reduced-fat diets don't always promote weight loss.

** The names refer to how far from the end (i.e., *omega*) of each fatty molecule you have to go to find the first carbon double-bond: it's three carbon atoms away for omega-3s and six atoms away for omega-6s.

omega-3s and omega-6s work in harmony to keep us firing on all cylinders. But when our dietary fats fall out of balance, we become vulnerable to many forms of illness. Depression is one of the most common.

According to recent studies, our hunter-gatherer ancestors maintained a superb balance of omega-6s and omega-3s in their diets, usually about a 1:1 ratio. The typical American, on the other hand, has a radically imbalanced fat intake—heavily slanted in favor of omega-6s. The ratio of omega-6 to omega-3 in the modern American diet now stands at a staggering 16:1. To understand how our diets fell so badly out of balance (and to figure out how to remedy the situation), we need to briefly review where these fats come from.

LEAVES VERSUS SEEDS

Omega-3 fats are made in the leaves of plants, grasses*, and algae. Any animal that eats one of these omega-3 plant sources quickly absorbs the essential fats directly into its own body. So, for example, we find high levels of omega-3 fats in wild game, which feed on grasses and leaves, and in the many species of wild fish that eat algae.

Omega-6 fats, on the other hand, are usually concentrated in plant seeds. These fats are also abundant in nuts and grains, which are technically seeds, as well. Few untamed animals feed on seeds, so our hunter-gatherer ancestors got little in the way of omega-6 fats from their meat supply. (After all, who ever heard of grain-fed wild game?) But ancient humans still picked up plenty of omega-6s in their diets

* Grasses are technically leaves, as well.

from seeds and nuts. Likewise, our foraging ancestors had little trouble getting enough omega-3s: Wild fish and game generally made up a large part of the hunter-gatherer diet, along with some other plant-based omega-3 sources.

The ancestral 1:1 balance of fatty acids started to shift a bit, though, with the invention of farming around twelve thousand years ago. All of a sudden, grains became the biggest part of everyone's diet—wheat, corn, rice, barley, sorghum, oats, rye, and so on. Omega-6 intake soared. And even though people still got some omega-3s from grass-fed livestock and a few plant sources, the ratio of omega-6s to omega-3s skyrocketed to about 5:1.

Remarkably, people all over the globe—in Mesopotamia, east Asia, north Africa, and central America—started suffering ill effects immediately after shifting to the new grain-based diet. According to the fossil record, these more "civilized" early farmers were, on average, considerably shorter and more disease-ridden than their hunter-gatherer forebears. *Their brains even grew smaller.* (We'll see why in just a moment.)

But even as they became less healthy and less brainy than their Pleistocene ancestors, most people stuck with the impressive new technologies of farming and herding livestock. The promise of a steadier food supply was apparently just too good a bargain to pass up.

Fortunately, over the centuries, humans all across the planet slowly adapted to the new farm-based diet. And, over time, cultures in different parts of the world often incorporated a good deal of seafood and other omega-3 food sources into their traditional diets, as if they intuitively realized something crucial was missing. A few agrarian societies—such as the traditional cultures of Crete (Greece) and Japan—even got close to the balanced fatty acid ratio of their hunter-gatherer ancestors, and they benefitted from increased overall health and longevity as a result.

But then in the twentieth century another radical dietary change took place—one without precedent in human history. Throughout most of the industrialized world, consumption of omega-6 fats went through the roof. It's not as if anyone was *trying* to eat more of these fats: It just turned out that way, as traditional farming steadily gave way to the more efficient practice of modern agriculture.

One of the biggest changes involved the shift from leaves to seeds in the diet of livestock. In the nineteenth century, beef cattle would roam on a free range, where they ate grasses and leafy plants and insects. As a result, beef was a rich source of omega-3 fats: hamburgers and steaks were, in effect, health foods. But as the price of corn steadily plummeted in the twentieth century,* grain-feeding livestock became the new norm: Animals grow considerably larger when they're herded onto feed lots and pumped full of corn—a prime source of omega-6 fats. This widespread practice of grain-feeding livestock—especially cattle, chickens, pigs, and fish—is why, in a nutshell, our meat supply today provides us with far too much omega-6 fat.

In a similar vein, the twentieth century saw an explosion in the consumption of seed oils—corn oil, canola oil, soybean oil, sunflower oil, peanut oil, palm oil, safflower oil, and so on—and derivative products like margarine and Crisco. Not only do people cook with these oils at home, but they also consume them in nearly every fast food meal (in fries, shakes, nuggets, patties, buns, cheeses, and more) and in most of the processed foods sold at the local supermarket.

So, we're all now swimming in a sea of omega-6 fats. That's why the American diet clocks in at an astonishing 16:1 ratio of omega-6s to omega-3s. This unprecedented dietary shift has taken a dramatic

* This price drop is largely due to innovations like the use of petroleum-based fertilizers, motorized combines, pesticides, and genetic selection of higher-yield seed corn.

toll on people's brains, which won't work as designed unless the omega fats are reasonably in balance.

CHEMICAL IMBALANCE

The extraordinary rise in depression rates over the last century has closely mirrored the disappearance of omega-3 fats from the Western diet. Similarly, in countries where people still get a better dietary balance of omega-6s and omega-3s, depression tends to be less common. And even in the Western world, people who become depressed have lower omega-3 blood levels than those who don't.

But how, exactly, does an imbalance of the fats we eat make us more vulnerable to depression? Neuroscientists have identified three different mechanisms that play a role.

Serotonin. In Chapter 2, we saw that serotonin is a chemical that helps turn off the brain's stress response. When serotonin function shuts down, the stress response system can go ballistic.

Like all neurotransmitters, serotonin is a chemical messenger. It does its job by hopping from one brain cell (neuron) to the next, relaying its signal in an elegant chemical code. Yet when brain cells don't have enough omega-3 fats, they have trouble understanding the message of serotonin, and they start to misfire. This leads to a massive loss of serotonin function throughout the brain, increasing a person's vulnerability to the sort of out-of-control stress response that triggers the onset of depression.

Dopamine. It's much the same story with dopamine, another chemical messenger in the brain. Neurons tend to scramble dopamine signals—just as they do with those of serotonin—when omega-3 levels get too low.

One of dopamine's big jobs is to activate the frontal cortex. People with poor dopamine function may have especially low activity in the *left* frontal cortex—the part of the brain that helps put us in a good mood and pushes us to go after the things we want. And as we've seen, when the left frontal cortex goes off-line, this can lead directly to depressive illness.

Inflammation. Throughout the body, omega-6s promote *inflammation*—the blood vessel reactions that make up the body's first line of defense against infection. You can see the body's inflammation response kick into high gear whenever you get a splinter. The surrounding area gets red and swollen as more blood—rich with immune cells poised to attack any offending intruders—is rushed to the site of injury. Without the body's ability to mount a vigorous inflammation response, every cut, scrape, or nick could easily turn into a lethal infection.

Although inflammation is healthy as a local, short-term reaction to a specific injury, the process can also spin dangerously out of control. When inflammation becomes chronic—when it fails to shut down after several days—it starts to affect the entire body. Such runaway inflammation actually causes the body to turn on itself, as if there were treacherous intruders to be attacked in every single one of its cells.

This is not good. In fact, researchers have recently identified chronic inflammation as the common denominator underlying many widespread diseases in the industrialized world: diabetes, atherosclerosis, Alzheimer's disease, heart disease, allergies, asthma, stroke, metabolic syndrome, and even many types of cancer.

Inflammation is also one of the big culprits behind the depression epidemic. Over time, it interferes with the brain's ability to manufacture and use serotonin,* and it can lead to reduced activity in the

* Specifically, inflammation triggers a reduction in blood levels of *tryptophan*, the primary building block of serotonin molecules. The result: less serotonin synthesized in the brain's neural circuits.

frontal cortex. It also impairs the function of brain regions such as the *hippocampus*—critical for memory function—that have been implicated in the onset of depression. Finally, chronic inflammation causes the brain to ramp up its stress response in an attempt to put things back in balance, since the stress hormone *cortisol* has powerful anti-inflammatory properties. Unfortunately, cortisol has its own set of depressive effects on the brain.

Tens of millions of people throughout the industrialized world suffer from chronic inflammation, and the major cause is now clear: a radical imbalance in dietary fats. The specialized hormones* that trigger inflammation throughout the body are actually made out of omega-6s. On the other hand, omega-3s stimulate production of the body's anti-inflammatory hormones. These two essential fats work in tandem to keep the inflammation response in proper balance—available when you need it for a short-term immune boost at the site of an injury, and yet held in check so it's not able to run roughshod over the entire body for months on end. But with the superabundance of omega-6s and the scarcity of omega-3s in the Western diet, all balance has been lost: inflammatory hormones rule, and chronic inflammation runs rampant.

RESTORING THE BALANCE

In his brilliant book *In Defense of Food*, Michael Pollan tells the story of ten middle-aged Australian Aborigines who abandoned their traditional hunter-gatherer lifestyle in favor of modernity. Per-

* These specialized hormones are known as *eicosanoids*.

haps not surprisingly, the adoption of a Western diet took a big toll on their bodies, and they all soon developed adult-onset diabetes and a host of other inflammation-linked disorders like *metabolic syndrome*.* This unhappy turn of events led a clever nutrition researcher to issue the group a provocative invitation: Let's see what would happen to your health if you left civilization and went back to living in the bush. Intrigued, the Aborigines agreed to try the experiment for seven weeks. They returned to their erstwhile hunter-gatherer ways and began roaming the Western Australian coast and inland rivers, subsisting on seafood and kangaroos and insect larvae and wild plants.

When the Aborigines returned to civilization less than two months later, researchers were amazed to discover every one of them in remarkably better health, with major improvement of their diabetes. Their blood work revealed why: All had undergone a dramatic increase in circulating omega-3 fats (and decreased omega-6s).

Most of us, of course, are not about to make such a trek into the wild, no matter what it might do for our health.† Fortunately, though, we can still reclaim from our collective hunter-gatherer past the many benefits of a balanced fat intake, and we can do so from the comfort of home.

To restore your dietary balance of omega-6 and omega-3 fats, there are really only two major possibilities to consider. You can either:

* Metabolic syndrome is a complex condition that typically involves obesity, high-blood pressure, and disordered carbohydrate and fat metabolism throughout the body.

† And I'm definitely not recommending that you try it. Remember, the Aborigines had already spent years living as hunter-gatherers, learning how to survive under such harsh, challenging conditions.

- Increase your intake of omega-3s
- Decrease your intake of omega-6s

Most of the published research has focused on the first option—consuming more omega-3s. In fact, during the past decade, *lots* of different depression researchers from all over the world—Britain, Australia, Israel, Japan, Brazil, Taiwan, India, and the United States—have studied the effects of omega-3 supplementation. More than a dozen clinical trials have even met the "gold standard" of high-quality drug study design—the inclusion of patients randomly assigned to receive placebo capsules instead of the omega-3 supplement. (The placebo is there for the sake of comparison, to make sure any observed improvement isn't due simply to the positive expectancies that arise from being in a treatment setting, seeing a doctor, swallowing pills, and so on.)

This impressive body of research now makes one thing clear: *omega-3 fats have a potent antidepressant effect.**

Of the six major elements in the Therapeutic Lifestyle Change (TLC) treatment protocol, the omega-3 supplement is the one my patients most consistently rave about. I've even had several tell me they started feeling better—noticing clear improvement in mood and energy and sleep and appetite and concentration and mental clarity—within a few days of beginning the omega-3 regimen. However, like most depression drugs, the omega-3s usually take at least a week or two—and sometimes up to four weeks—for their antidepressant effect to kick in.

---

* Even though antidepressant medications often fail to outperform placebos in head-to-head comparison studies (as we reviewed in Chapter 3), omega-3 supplementation has proven superior to placebos in most published studies from around the world.

To make sure you get the maximum benefit of adding such a supplement to your diet, we need to dive (briefly) into a few gory details of omega-3 chemistry.

THE LONG AND SHORT OF OMEGA-3

Omega-3 molecules come in three varieties, and they vary in length: there's DHA (long), EPA (medium), and ALA (short). These three major forms of omega-3 play different roles in the body and brain.

The long one, DHA (*docosahexaenoic acid*), is the only omega-3 molecule that's abundant in the brain. And when brain cells don't have enough DHA, their membranes tend to get rigid and inflexible. This makes it hard for them to transmit their signals effectively. Not surprisingly, depressed patients often lack enough DHA in their brains—especially in the critical neurons of the brain's frontal cortex. So it makes sense that a DHA supplement could be helpful.

EPA (*eicosopentaenoic acid*), the medium-length omega-3 molecule, is also crucial for proper brain function. There's little EPA in the brain itself, but the molecule is able to flit in and out of neurons to help them use brain chemicals like serotonin and dopamine more effectively. EPA is also the key building block for many anti-inflammatory hormones, so it can have an additional antidepressant effect by turning off the body's chronic inflammation response.

The short version of omega-3, ALA (*alpha linolenic acid*), doesn't actually affect brain function directly. Instead, it influences cells in other parts of the body. Some studies, for example, suggest that it may help stabilize heart rhythm. But there's no good evidence that it helps with depression.

Since DHA and EPA are the two omega-3 molecules that play an important role in the brain, depression researchers have carefully studied the effects of supplementing with each one. And based on the available evidence, EPA looks like the more potent of the two—by far. Clinicians have also experimented with a wide range of EPA doses, and the best supported daily dosage, used across a number of different studies, is 1000 to 2000 milligrams (mg) of EPA per day.

There's some indication that DHA supplements can be useful, as well. But the optimal dose is just not clear yet. More studies are required before we'll know for sure. In the meantime, I believe it's important to act on the best evidence we have, and here's what the research says so far: DHA is not very effective as a treatment for depression when used on its own, but it does seem to *add* to the beneficial effect of EPA. In particular, every published study that's combined EPA and DHA in a roughly 2:1 ratio has seen an impressive antidepressant effect. In other words, there appears to be a benefit in getting *both* EPA and DHA, as long as there's about twice as much EPA. (Interestingly, this same 2:1 ratio is found naturally in many varieties of seafood, and in many fish oil supplements).

THE OMEGA PRESCRIPTION

I recommend a starting omega-3 dose of *1000 mg of EPA and 500 mg of DHA* each day to all of my patients. If you currently have symptoms of depression, or if you want to help prevent the onset of illness in the future, this is the dose I suggest you begin with, as well. Depending on how you respond after a few weeks on this regimen, you might need to tweak the dosage a bit, and we'll discuss that possibility in the next section.

Fish Oil

What's the best way to get your daily dose of omega-3 (EPA and DHA)? By far the most convenient approach—and the one used in all the best research studies—is to obtain it in the form of fish oil, the richest natural source of both EPA and DHA. Just a few daily capsules (or teaspoons) of high-quality fish oil will do the job. It's such an easy lifestyle change—requiring less than a minute each day—that most people have no trouble making it part of their daily routine.

I have to admit, though—fish oil can be unappealing. For one thing, it smells bad. It tastes bad, too. The first time I ever took the plunge and tried fish oil capsules (about eight years ago), I was plagued by a common, nasty side effect: fishy burps. Soon after swallowing the pills, I found myself involuntarily belching up the foul taste of rancid fish every few minutes, and this went on for hours. Not good. It was years before I worked up the courage to try it again.

At that point, I was still ignorant of a crucial fact: All fish oil pills are not created equal. Some are fine, and some are downright awful. The thing is, fish oil rots quickly in the open air. So if your supplement wasn't processed properly, you'll wind up with rancid oil encased inside a gel cap. Because the capsule is airtight, you won't even know there's anything amiss until your digestive juices release the spoiled oil into your stomach.

Thank goodness this problem can be avoided. Many superb fish oil supplements are now available—most health food stores and many drug stores carry several varieties—and some of the best supplements are also highly affordable.

Here's the biggest thing you'll want to keep in mind when looking at fish oil products: The oil should be *molecularly distilled*, and it should say so right on the label. This designation simply means the manufacturer has refined the oil by taking out the contaminants and impurities all the way down to the molecular level. If the company has taken the trouble (and expense) of going through this refinement process, it's a safe bet that the fish has also been handled and processed properly. In other words, you don't have to worry about the oil being rancid. Equally important, some commercial fisheries are now exposed to dangerous pollutants such as mercury, arsenic, dioxins, and PCBs, and the distillation process helps keep these toxins from making their way into your supplement.

In many cases, the label will also say that the product is *pharmaceutical grade,* which means it meets purity and dosage accuracy standards similar to those used for prescription drugs.

Labels and Such. The EPA and DHA content of each fish oil capsule (or teaspoon, in the case of a liquid) should be clearly stated right on the bottle, as depicted on the sample label in Figure 4-1.

Please keep in mind that sometimes—as in the example in Figure 4-1—stated omega-3 amounts are based on a serving size of *two capsules*. So, in this example, each softgel capsule would contain only 250 mg of EPA and 125 mg of DHA; it would thus take four such capsules to make up the recommended starting dose of omega-3s.

Other Important Considerations

To make sure you get the greatest possible benefit from your fish oil supplement, we need to briefly address a few other important points.

FIGURE 4-1.

Nutritional Information from a Typical Bottle of Fish Oil Capsules

Nutrition Info		
Serving Size: 2 Softgels		
	Amount Per Serving	% Daily Value
Calories	20	
Calories from Fat	20	
Total Fat	2 g	2%*
Saturated Fat	<0.5 g	2%*
Trans Fat	0 g	†
Polyunsaturated Fat	1.0 g	†
Vitamin E (as natural d-alpha Tocopherol with Mixed Tocopherols)	0.5 mg	70%
Natural Fish Oil Concentrate	**2,000 mg**	†
Omega-3 Fatty Acids	**1,000 mg**	†
Elcosapentaenoic Acid (EPA)**	**500 mg**	†
Docosahexaenoic Acid (DHA)**	**250 mg**	†
Other Omega-3 Fatty Acids	**250 mg**	†

* Percent Daily Values are based on 2,000 calorie diet.
† Daily Value not established.

Antioxidants. As mentioned, fish oil and oxygen don't mix: the oxygen spoils it. And we all have some harmful forms of oxygen in our bodies, carried around by dangerous molecules called *free radicals*. These molecules can damage any fish oil you consume just as soon as it hits the bloodstream, making the omega-3s less useful to your brain. Luckily, *antioxidants*—nutrients like Vitamin C—can protect omega-3s from such damage.

To ensure that you have enough antioxidants in your system, it's advisable to *take a daily multivitamin, in addition to a vitamin C supplement at a daily dose of 500 mg*. Or, if you're willing to eat five servings of fruit and vegetables each day—as nutritionists recommend—you'll get plenty of natural antioxidants in your diet (more than enough to reap the full benefit of the omega-3s you consume, even without taking a vitamin supplement).

GLA. Even though we eat far too many omega-6 fats—which are turned into inflammatory hormones that ravage the body—one type of omega-6 is an exception. It's called GLA (*gamma linolenic acid*), and it's a building block for fats that act a lot like omega-3s—they make hormones with a nice anti-inflammatory effect.

When we take a good fish oil supplement, the large amount of EPA we ingest can cause the body to cut back its production of GLA. Low levels of GLA can, in turn, trigger unwanted inflammation. So just to be on the safe side, it's best to make sure you're getting a little GLA in your diet. Luckily, only a small amount is required: 5 to 10 milligrams (mg) per week.

Not many foods have GLA, but oatmeal turns out to be a decent source. It has to be slow cooked oatmeal, though, not the instant kind. Eating two big bowls a week should give your body all the GLA it needs. Another option is to take a supplement of *evening primrose oil,* which you can get at most drug stores or health food stores. However, this oil contains a remarkably high concentration of GLA, so only one capsule each week is necessary. (Some nutritionists explicitly advise against taking it any more frequently than that.)

The freezer trick. Even when using a high-quality fish oil supplement, a few people still experience a bit of burping afterwards. This problem usually can be eliminated, however, by storing the supplement in the freezer and taking it within an hour of bedtime. The frozen capsule will pass through the stomach and on to the small intestine before it fully dissolves—effectively getting rid of the burping.

(Remembering to take the capsule on a full stomach is another trick that's worked for some of our TLC patients.)

Tweaking the Dose

Even though our foraging ancestors kept a nicely balanced 1:1 ratio of omega-6 and omega-3 fats in their diets, our "design specs" as a species also leave some margin for error (thank goodness). Most of us can do just fine with an omega-6 to omega-3 ratio as high as 3:1.

If you take a high-quality omega-3 supplement at the starting dosage I've recommended—1000 mg EPA and 500 mg DHA each day—there's a good chance you'll shift your dietary fat ratio down below 3:1 and into the healthy range. But some people don't. If you eat *lots* of omega-6 fats—fried foods, grain-fed beef and pork (and chicken and fish), vegetable oils, junk food, and so on—you may need a higher dose of omega-3s to balance things out. Likewise, as we've seen, if you don't have enough antioxidants in your system, it may be difficult to keep enough omega-3s available in your body to do the job.

How can you tell if you have a healthy ratio of omega-6 to omega-3? One approach is simply to make an educated guess based on how your body functions. If your ratio of omega-6 to omega-3 is still way too high, you'll probably have some of the following common symptoms:

Fatigue
Poor concentration
Sluggishness (especially upon awakening)
Sinus congestion

Carbohydrate craving
Dry skin
Dry eyes
Dense stool or constipation
Brittle nails and hair

Most of my patients have reported improvement in several of these symptoms within a few weeks of starting their omega-3 supplement. Many have also noticed similar symptom relief with other chronic inflammatory conditions. Some, for example, have said their achy knees started to improve within a week or so of starting the omega-3 regimen. And last year, two patients even told me the fish oil capsules had helped clear up their seasonal allergies. (I have to confess, this last claim sounded pretty far-fetched at first, but I later found research evidence that omega-3s actually help suppress some allergic reactions.)

But for our purposes, the best indicator of your omega-6 to omega-3 ratio is your depression itself. If you don't see some improvement in depressive symptoms within four weeks of taking an omega-3 supplement, it's likely you need a higher dose to get into a healthier range. In that case, I'd recommend doubling your initial dose, bumping it up to *2000 mg of EPA and 1000 mg of DHA each day.* If that doesn't lead to any obvious results within four more weeks, I'd suggest getting a more intensive—and more accurate—reading of your omega fat profile.

With a simple blood test, it's possible to find your exact omega-6 to omega-3 ratio. The test measures both EPA and a key omega-6 fat—called *arachidonic acid* (AA)—and it gives you the precise ratio of AA/EPA (omega-6/omega-3).

The ideal ratio on this blood test is believed to be about 2.0 (not 1.0, as you might have guessed, since the ratio is a little higher in the blood than it is in the brain). But if you're reasonably close to 2.0—anywhere between 1.0 and 3.0—you're probably in a healthy range. And you never want to take so much omega-3 that the ratio gets *too* low, because there's an increased risk of infections when the ratio falls below about 0.7. There's even a risk for some types of stroke if it gets below 0.5.

You should consult your doctor for options for testing omega-3 and omega-6 fatty acid levels.

FREQUENTLY ASKED QUESTIONS

Now that we've covered the basics of omega-3 supplementation, we'll turn our attention to some related questions that come up from time to time.

1. I'm a vegetarian. Is it possible to get enough EPA and DHA from plant-based sources? Every time I give a talk on fatty acids and depression, someone will ask about vegetarian omega-3 sources—flaxseed oil, canola oil, walnuts, and so on. It's true that these are all good ways to get ALA (the short molecule of omega-3), but you'll recall that this is the one form of omega-3 that doesn't help with depression. And unfortunately, our bodies can convert only a small percentage of the ALA we get in our diet to the longer molecular forms of omega-3 we need (EPA and DHA). One recent study looked at people who started taking high doses of ALA-rich flaxseed oil, and their key omega-6/omega-3 ratios barely budged.*

---

* Out of roughly 8000 mg of ALA in a tablespoon of flaxseed oil, most people will convert less than 400 mg to EPA.

I know of only one good vegetarian source of antidepressant omega-3 fats: algae. But most algae-based supplements have very little EPA (despite high levels of DHA). Fortunately, however, a Swiss company called *V-Pure* has figured out how to get more EPA into an algae supplement. Their product still has a lot more DHA than EPA (with a 4:1 ratio), but at least it's now possible to get enough EPA from this vegetarian source. I'll warn you, though: It's very expensive. At the time of this writing, it costs about thirty times more than high-quality fish oil.

(If you go this route, keep in mind—when calculating your daily dose—that your body can also convert about 10% of the algae-derived DHA to EPA. As a result, you could get your target level of 1000 mg of EPA with only about 700 mg of EPA coming directly from the supplement: With every 700 mg of EPA from this algae source, you'd also get a whopping 2800 mg of DHA—of which an additional 280 mg would be converted to EPA.)

2. I'm not sure I want to take fish oil pills every day. Is it possible to get enough omega-3s naturally, by incorporating the right kinds of meat and other foods into my daily diet? Yes, it's possible, but it's fairly difficult. Fatty fish—especially salmon, tuna, mackerel, sardines, anchovies, herring, whitefish, and shad—are by far the richest natural source of EPA and DHA, so the obvious strategy is to start adding plenty of these fish into your daily diet. But it takes a lot of fish to get an antidepressant dose of omega-3s. On average, you'll need two to three servings each day.

The Japanese make up one of the few large populations in the world that eats this much fish. They have an impressive average omega-6 to omega-3 ratio of just under 2:1, and their rates of depression are extremely low. In addition, they're healthier than we are overall, and they enjoy a longer life expectancy.

As we've seen, however, fish are sometimes tainted by toxins such as mercury and pesticides, so you'll want to take some precautions if you choose to add seafood to your diet on a daily basis. In general, ocean-caught fish are safer than farm-raised fish, many of which are imported from countries that don't always make sure they're free of contaminants. Also, large fish at the top of the food chain—tuna and swordfish, for example—normally have higher toxin levels than small fish like sardines and anchovies.

Although it's certainly possible to get adequate EPA and DHA without a supplement—if you're highly motivated and willing to change your entire diet—such an approach is much harder than simply taking a few fish oil pills every day. Most of us won't stick with something if it takes too much time, energy, and effort—and that's doubly true for anyone fighting depression, which robs us of initiative. That's why I recommend a high-quality fish oil supplement as the best omega-3 source in treating depression. It's something just about everyone can do.

3. What's the difference between fish oil capsules and liquid supplements? Is one better than the other? They're just different ways of taking the same oil. No one likes the taste of fish oil (even the high-quality stuff), so most people prefer taking the oil in capsule form, which prevents us from having to taste the oil itself.

On the other hand, some of us don't like swallowing big pills. That's why I'm among the brave souls who take the fish oil "straight-up," right out of the bottle. Luckily, most liquid products now have a lemon flavoring to help mask the fishy taste, and I've found that chasing the oil with a shot of grapefruit juice works wonders to cover up the aftertaste. Still, you'll probably want to have your toothbrush close at hand just to make sure.

4. Is it possible to get my omega-6 to omega-3 ratio in balance simply by cutting out the omega-6s from my diet, instead of adding all those omega-3s? It makes perfect sense. We get way too many omega-6s in the Western diet, so why not just cut most of them out? We can, and we should.

However, omega-6s stay in the body a long time, so even if you managed to get rid of the omega-6s from your diet, it would take months before your omega-6/omega-3 ratio dropped in a big way. When someone is depressed, they don't have months to wait: They want relief as soon as possible. And omega-3 supplements provide quick relief, because they start improving the omega-6 to omega-3 ratio within days.

Certainly, though, as a long-term strategy to prevent future depression, cutting out omega-6s is a great idea. Here are some simple things you can do to get started:

- Switch to grass-fed beef, or simply drop beef from your diet altogether
- Stick mostly with lean meats like chicken breast and fish
- Stay away from fried foods (and most fast food in general)
- Cook with olive oil or coconut oil (fruit-based oils), and avoid seed-based oils like soybean oil, corn oil, canola oil, and sunflower oil; use the same principle when it comes to salad dressing
- Use butter instead of margarine
- Avoid snack chips and baked goods
- Start reading product labels, and stay away from foods that contain lots of seed-based oils (there are thousands of them)

5. I'm not sure I can afford a molecularly distilled fish oil supplement. Can't I just take the cheaper kind they sell down at the drugstore? Believe it or not, some high-quality (molecularly distilled) fish oils are available online for about the same price you'd pay for a lower-grade supplement at your local drugstore. Sometimes the good stuff can even be cheaper. For example, I recently went online and found a molecularly distilled supplement that costs only $6.87 for a month's supply. Then I checked at a few local discount stores, and the best comparable price I could find was over $8.00 for the same quantity of *low-quality* pills.

However, if you do happen to find a great deal on a lower-quality supplement—that is, one that's *not* molecularly distilled—I can pass along some reassuring news. A recent study by ConsumerLab.com looked at forty-four brands of fish oil (mostly the lower-quality variety) and found that none had dangerous levels of mercury or PCBs. But they didn't test for every possible toxin, so I'd still recommend that you stick with a pharmaceutical-grade supplement just to be on the safe side.

6. I understand how important the fish oil supplement can be, but I just can't remember to take it. What should I do? This is a common problem, but it's usually easy to overcome. It simply requires the use of a memory aid. Over the years, my patients have shared with me several clever remedies they've discovered:

- Store the bottle next to your toothbrush or something else you use every day. (If you need to keep your capsules in the freezer to prevent burping, you can put them in a different container and still keep the empty bottle by your toothbrush as a memory cue.)
- Store the bottle on your pillow or bedside stand.
- Program your cell phone or PDA to ring you every day at a certain time; this will be your "wake-up call" that it's time to take the fish oil.

- Find a friend or family member who's willing to give you a gentle, friendly reminder each day.
- Buy a daily pill box—the kind sold for a dollar or so at any drugstore—and store the capsules in that.

OMEGA-3S: A CLOSING THOUGHT

Change is hard. Yet some new habits are a lot easier to pick up than others. Luckily, the simplest change in the entire Therapeutic Lifestyle Change program—adding a daily fish oil supplement—is also one of the most potent in its ability to fight depression and keep it from coming back. It's a change that takes only a minute of your day, but it can change your life immeasurably for the better.

5
Don't Think, Do

Brenda had been an A student in my Abnormal Psychology class a few years earlier, and had since graduated and begun working in the area. Soon afterward, however, she found herself battling several symptoms of depression, so she decided to drop by my office for some advice.

She told me that right after she'd started feeling depressed, she pulled out her old lecture notes and began reviewing the things I'd mentioned in class about the antidepressant effects of exercise, fish oil, sunlight, and so on. Then, completely on her own, Brenda started putting the Therapeutic Lifestyle Change (TLC) program into practice.

"But I must be doing something wrong," she said, "since I'm not getting better at all. I mean, it's not as bad as it was back in college—when they put me on Lustral—but I can't let it get to that point again." She sighed. "I was really hoping the TLC stuff would work for me."

"Well," I offered, "why don't we take a look at the things you've been doing, and maybe we'll get some ideas about why they haven't helped."

She quickly ran through an impressive litany of lifestyle changes. In recent weeks, she had started walking about forty-five minutes a day;

getting plenty of sunlight exposure; taking a high-quality fish oil supplement at the recommended omega-3 dose; averaging a good eight hours of sleep a night (although she still had occasional trouble falling asleep); and increasing her social connectedness, not only by seeing her boyfriend every day, but also by meeting with a few old friends on a regular basis. She even was taking steps to get closer to her new coworkers.

It was puzzling that none of this had made much of a difference. "Maybe," I thought, "She's the exception that proves the rule." I had never seen someone put the entire TLC protocol into practice and remain depressed, but I certainly couldn't rule out the possibility. On the other hand, one stone still remained unturned. I hadn't asked Brenda yet about rumination.

"Do you remember," I asked, "what we covered in class about rumination?"

She shrugged. "Isn't that just, like, thinking about things?"

"Yes, thinking about them over and over and over. When we're depressed, we tend to dwell on things—especially negative things—replaying them again and again in our minds. And for many depressed patients, that kind of negative thinking can go on for hours."

"Yeah," she offered, "I definitely do that sometimes. A lot, actually. Like when I'm working out or doing the dishes or something, all these thoughts will just be going through my head. 'What if things don't work out with my boyfriend?' or 'Why can't I get closer to people at work?' or 'I can't believe my dad forgot to call me on my birthday' or 'How come I'm getting depressed again?' And then I'll just sit there thinking about things."

"And when you let yourself brood over things like that, does it change the way you feel?"

"Um," she looked down at the floor as she pondered the question for a moment. "It makes me feel worse. Definitely."

"Well, if you're spending a lot of time dwelling on these negative thoughts, it might explain why your depression hasn't cleared up yet."

Brenda shifted in her seat uncomfortably. "But I don't know how to just stop thinking about things. I mean, it's not like you can really control what you think about."

"That's true—we can't always control where our thoughts might lead. But once a thought has popped into our heads, we can decide whether or not we're going to *keep* thinking about it; we can shift our focus onto some other activity instead."

She looked skeptical. "It's not like I haven't tried to get my mind off all this stuff already."

I nodded. "I know. Rumination has become a habit for you—like it is for most people with depression. And habits are tough to break. But I've worked with hundreds of patients who've learned how to stop ruminating, and many of them were more severely depressed than you are right now. Mostly, it just takes a commitment—and some practice."

"Well," Brenda said weakly, "I *want* to stop thinking about all these things all the time . . ." Her voice trailed off. "I'm willing to try, anyway." She smiled wryly, "Even though none of your other TLC stuff has helped."

Brenda worked hard over the next month to break her rumination habit, using each of the major strategies described in the pages ahead. Perhaps because she had already put so many other parts of the treatment protocol into practice, her depressive symptoms cleared up in just a few weeks once she brought her rumination under control.

Even though my parents grew up in rural Maine, I was raised in the suburbs. In fact, I was a teenager before I even saw any farm animals up close—on a visit to a relative's cattle ranch in north Georgia. And one of the first things that caught my attention—aside from the pungent smell—was the cows' limited behavioral repertoire: lots of standing around and lots of chewing. I guess there was also a bit of grazing mixed in there, but after just a short while, the cows would stop eating to regurgitate all the grass (and some unlucky insects) back up in the form of cud—a bolus of semidigested food. And then they just stood there chomping away for hours, slowly and methodically breaking the cud down into smaller and smaller pieces, until it was ground down enough to fully digest.

The cows' digestive process is known as *rumination.** And it provides a rich metaphor for something we do—not with food, but with our deepest thoughts. It seems that we, too, sometimes need to chew things over for a while before we can actually stomach them.

MULLING THINGS OVER

Rumination appears to be an instinctive human response when something goes wrong. It's as if we're hardwired to replay our recent trials and tribulations over and over again in the mind's eye—to mull things over for a while before we're ready to move on. And a little such dwelling can be helpful, since it often leads to valuable insights—providing greater clarity about what just went wrong, what can be done to correct things, and what might help us prevent similar negative outcomes in the future.

* Derived from the word *rumen*—the part of the bovine stomach where cud is formed.

But after just a brief period of intense pondering, we've usually extracted all the useful bits of meaning from the situation that we're ever likely to find. We soon hit the point of diminishing returns, when any more dwelling is simply a waste of time. But some people stay at it long past the point when enough is enough. And, unfortunately, extended rumination can have several damaging effects.

For one thing, it tends to amplify negative emotions. If you spend some time mulling over very sad events, for example, you'll soon find yourself feeling morose (certainly much more so than when you started). Likewise, when your thoughts become fixated on a potential threat, this process will inevitably start ramping up your feelings of anxiety.

Rumination also makes people less active. It's an inert, inward-focused process that keeps us locked more or less inside our heads. When we're brooding, we're especially inclined to avoid activity, as it would force us to shift attention away from our internal machinations and out onto the world around us instead.

In a nutshell, when we ruminate, we withdraw. That's especially true on the social front. When someone is locked in a bout of rumination during a social encounter, they're simply not all there mentally. When spoken to, they may nod politely and say "uh huh," but they won't register anything that's being said. In other words, they'll go through the motions on the outside, while still spinning the ruminative wheels inside their own private little world. When this process becomes a habit, it takes a huge toll on their ability to stay connected with others.

Finally, because it has such a potent ability to turn up the volume on our emotions, rumination sends the brain's stress response circuits into a flurry of sustained activity. And that, in turn, can trigger a full-blown episode of depression.

As it turns out, the link between depression and rumination is a particularly strong one. Through its powerful effects on emotions, behavior, social connection, and brain function, rumination renders us much more vulnerable to depressive illness. It also plays a key role in *maintaining* an episode of depression once it's begun. That's why—as we saw in the case of Brenda at the beginning of the chapter—*when someone continues ruminating on a regular basis, they'll find it extremely difficult to overcome their depression, no matter what else they do in an attempt to get better.*

If you find yourself locked in the vise grip of rumination, however, I can offer some words of reassurance—breaking the habit may sound difficult, but the process is surprisingly straightforward. It only involves two major steps: learning to notice when it's happening (increasing awareness), and learning how to redirect your focus to some other activity.

BREAK THE HABIT: AWARENESS

What is it about depression that causes us to dwell at length on negative thoughts? The answer has a lot to do with human memory.

Although it's miraculous that the brain—a three-pound lump of neural tissue—can store any memories at all, the human memory system has some surprising quirks. Most notably: We forget things. The forgotten information is still there in our brains somewhere; it's just that it's difficult for the brain to put its (metaphorical) hands on any one specific memory when it's needed. There's so much other competing information in there.

To solve this problem, the brain often has to rely on memory *cues*—bits of information related to the thing we're trying to recall—to jog our memories. Pretty much anything can serve as such a cue, as long as it's associated somehow with the information we're looking for. For example, researchers have shown that when people learn a list of words in a particular room, they'll do a better job recalling the words the next day if they're taken back to the same room (as opposed to, say, the one next door). The room setting becomes a cue that helps trigger the words in memory. Likewise, students who study for an exam while drinking coffee will perform better if they consume a similar amount on the day of the test.

As it turns out, *the brain uses our mood state as its single most important memory cue.* Believe it or not, the brain tags every one of our memories according to the emotional state we're in when the event occurs. And whenever we're in that same mood down the road, this can serve as a powerful retrieval cue.

When you're sad, for example, that despondent mood starts lighting up all sorts of memories from other moments when you were in similarly low spirits: previous experiences of failure and loneliness and rejection and similar unhappiness. However, when people are sad, they generally find it difficult to recall any of the specific times in the past when things were going well.

I saw this principle in action a few months ago when my eleven-year-old daughter Abby—a bubbly, upbeat child—was upset about a friend who had hurt her feelings. As I tried to console her, Abby assured me—through many heartfelt sobs—"Things *never* work out right. *Everything* is *always* bad. *Always.*" The next day, after she had regained her emotional equilibrium, I asked my daughter about her starkly negative assessment of life the day before. She just shrugged as she smiled blithely and said, "I don't know. It really *seemed* like that yesterday." Exactly—because memory is such a slave to mood.

So, when people are depressed, their intensely sad mood will cause sad memories to percolate—unbidden—up to the surface of their conscious awareness. Such upsetting memories, in turn, will cause them to form negative judgments—to infer that horrible outcomes are pretty much the norm. And as all of these upsetting memories and judgments are unleashed, they'll quickly serve to intensify the despondent mood, which in turn primes even more negative thoughts, turning the mood even more negative, and so on. It's a vicious cycle of rumination that can go on more or less indefinitely—until something comes along to interrupt it.

Whenever I bring up the topic of rumination in one of our TLC groups, most patients readily acknowledge that it's something they do. But here's the curious thing: They've often said that until I brought the issue to their attention, they had never even noticed they were doing it.

During an episode of depression, dwelling on negative thoughts is so effortless and automatic—it's possible to spend long stretches of time doing so without any awareness of what's happening.

Think of when you're driving a very familiar route home. If you're like most people, you've probably pulled into your driveway at some point with the jarring realization, "I have no idea how I just got here." You know that somehow you've managed to make a bunch of correct turns and navigate successfully past other cars, but because you've also made the same drive so many times before, you were able to let your attention lapse while doing so.

In similar fashion, people who've battled depression know the well-worn path of rumination by heart; they can navigate it on autopilot. Long stretches of time—sometimes even hours—can pass without their ever once noticing, "Hey, I'm just sitting here ruminating again, and I've been at it for a *long* time already."

That's why the first step in breaking the rumination habit is simply to increase awareness, to *notice* when it's happening. Once you learn to pay attention—moment by moment—to when you're ruminating and when you're not, you'll be well on your way to breaking free. Until then, however, you'll remain at the mercy of a thought process that can hold you in its paralyzing grip more or less indefinitely, with or without your active consent.

Take a Mental Inventory

How do you go about increasing your awareness of rumination? One helpful strategy is to start deliberately monitoring your thought process every hour or so, just to see what you've been paying attention to—and to make a note of any rumination that's occurred since the last time you checked.

Simply remembering to monitor your thoughts on a regular basis can pose a challenge, however, especially at first. If you find this task difficult, try tying it to a specific prompt. For example, many cellphones and PDAs can be programmed to beep every hour or so. Likewise, if you happen to own a clock with a chime setting, its hourly clang can provide an effective cue for taking a mental inventory. Or, if you lack any such gadgets, even a periodic, everyday activity like getting a drink or going to the restroom can serve as a memory prompt.

But the single most helpful thing you can do in monitoring your rumination is to keep an hour-by-hour log of your day. Table 5-1 provides an example of what this log might look like.

As you can see, it's just a matter of writing down what you were doing each hour, how much time you spent ruminating, and how intense your negative mood was at the time. This may sound like a lot of work, but it doesn't take more than about five minutes a day to complete. You'll probably find it easiest if you keep such a log with you

TABLE 5-1. *Sample Rumination Log*

Time	*Activity*	*Rumination (minutes)*	*Negative Mood (0–10)*
6:00	Sleep, then lying in bed awake	25	7
7:00	Breakfast, shower, and so on	20	6
8:00	Drop off kids, commute	15	6
9:00	Work	2	4
10:00	Work—boring staff meeting	30	6
11:00	Work	5	5
12:00	Lunch with coworkers	2	3
1:00	Work	0	4
2:00	Work	0	3
3:00	Work—told about upcoming deadline	30	7
4:00	Work	10	5
5:00	Commute, picked up kids	15	6
6:00	Made dinner, ate with family	0	5
7:00	Helped with homework	0	4
8:00	Watched TV	30	7
9:00	Got kids ready for bed, watched TV	15	7
10:00	Watched TV	40	8
11:00	Bedtime routine, sleep	10	7
12:00	Sleep		
1:00	Sleep		
2:00	Sleep		
3:00	Woke up for 45 minutes	40	8
4:00	Sleep		
5:00	Sleep		

throughout the day and pull it out briefly every hour or so to fill in your most recent activities. Not only will this provide a useful prompt for periodic self-monitoring, but it will also serve as a superb source of information about which activities tend to make you feel the best (and worst), and which are the most and least effective in preventing rumination.

During the first week or two of monitoring your rumination on a regular basis, you should gradually become more skillful at catching yourself in the act. And the more you practice it, the more the self-monitoring process becomes a habit—something that begins to happen more or less automatically. In other words, with enough repetition, you'll eventually develop your own spontaneous mental alarm to alert you anytime your thoughts take a ruminative turn. As one patient put it recently, "Before I was in treatment, I was ruminating constantly, but I hardly ever noticed it. Now I'm catching myself all the time. As soon as it starts up, it's like there's this still small voice in my head saying, 'There you go again. You're doing it, and it's time to stop.'"

Watch Out for High-Risk Situations

As you become increasingly tuned in to your mental life, you'll notice that some situations are particularly hazardous to your emotional well-being. The research on this point is clear: *People typically ruminate—and feel the worst—when they have nothing else to occupy their attention.*

And, given the depressed mind's inexorable drift inward upon itself, the single biggest risk factor for rumination is simply spending time alone. This is particularly unfortunate because, as we've seen, depression involves a strong tendency to withdraw from others. In other words, depressed individuals usually seek out alone time, which leads to rumination, which leads to greater withdrawal, and so on—a vicious cycle.

Spending time with others usually helps counteract brooding, unless the person you're with is also depressed. A recent study of depressed teenagers, for example, found that adolescent girls often *ruminate together* in their conversations—a process that brings mood down for both parties. So, if you're spending time with someone who's also prone to dwelling on negative thoughts, it will probably be helpful to discuss the dangers of joint rumination with that person in advance, and for both of you to agree to avoid giving voice to any ruminative thoughts.

Watching television is another high-risk situation. This might seem counterintuitive, since people often look to TV as an escape—something to take their mind off things. But here's the problem: Most programs are simply not interesting or engaging enough to fully occupy the mind, so it's all too easy for our thoughts to wander off when we're sitting in front of the tube. Add to this the fact that depression impairs our ability to concentrate—including the ability to stay focused on a TV program—and it's no surprise that watching television is often a recipe for disaster. It's one of the most effective ways to usher in an extended bout of rumination.

The same basic principle applies to any situation that fails to fully engage your attention. Over the years, my patients have clued me in to numerous potential high-risk scenarios to watch out for, among them: sitting in traffic, listening to sad music, driving, doing mindless chores, daydreaming, and lying around the house. (Later in the chapter we'll look at what you can do to minimize the risk when such situations can't be avoided.)

BREAK THE HABIT: REDIRECTING

Once you've learned how to catch yourself ruminating, you're still left with the challenge of stopping it. The solution involves learning to redirect your attention, to turn away from the inner world of thoughts and memories to the outer world of other people and activities. Simply put, it means more doing and less thinking.

In Chapter 2, we saw how depression shuts people down, squelching brain circuits in the left frontal cortex that allow us to translate our thoughts into action. And when that key part of the brain goes dormant, we find it enormously difficult to initiate activity.

So what happens? We start doing less and less. And the less we do, the more we just sit and brood. That only serves to make the depression worse, which then renders the left frontal cortex even less active, which makes it even harder to do things, and so on.

But the vicious cycle can also run in reverse. We can nudge ourselves to do something—or even just to respond to the gentle prompting of someone else—even though we feel like just sitting there instead. This temporary increase in activity helps stimulate the left frontal cortex, which in turn boosts mood and leads to a bit of reduction in depressive symptoms, which then makes it a little easier to initiate more activity, and so on. In other words, by simply engaging in activity—*any* activity—we can change the brain in a way that helps reverse depression.

Find the Motivation to Let Go

Before we examine the redirection process in detail, it's a good idea to address up front a potential obstacle to kicking the rumination habit: lack of motivation. I've learned over the years that sometimes people don't *want* to let go of the habit. Even though they realize how harmful it can be, they still want to hold on.

One of my patients a few years ago explained a big reason why: Rumination can be seductive. It promises to deliver the goods, but it rarely, if ever, delivers. Here's how she put it, "You know you need to stop, but it's like, 'if only I spend a little more time thinking about this, *then* I'll figure things out, and I'll feel so much better.' Now, deep down you know that's not really true, but it feels true while you're ruminating. So it's easy just to give in and keep at it. And then before you know it, an hour has passed and you're still spinning your wheels—and nothing has changed."

To help combat the seductive quality of rumination—the enticing idea that it will usher in an array of life-altering insights—I usually ask my patients to consider the following question: When you're ruminating, how long does it take to hit the point of diminishing returns, when any more fresh insights are unlikely to emerge? The consensus answer: five to ten minutes.

So, I make a deal with them: When you catch yourself ruminating, give yourself permission to continue thinking about things for a *maximum* of ten minutes. But be sure to set a timer, and then resolve to shut the process down as soon as the timer goes off (if not sooner). It's proven to be a remarkably helpful strategy—making it much easier for them to let go of the toxic thoughts that would otherwise linger indefinitely.

Many patients have even decided to take this last step a bit further. They've begun *writing down* their ruminative thoughts as a prelude to walking away from them. Simply putting our thoughts down on paper actually makes it easier to stop thinking about them. You may have seen this principle at work, say, the last time you found yourself writing out a shopping list or a to-do list: once you've transferred the information to a sheet of paper, you generally feel less need to keep rehashing it over and over in your mind. You can write it down and then promptly turn your thoughts elsewhere.

Find Activities

Whenever you catch yourself ruminating, it's important to have on hand a list of activities engaging enough to capture your attention. As a rule, we can put an end to brooding only when we're caught up in something else—something absorbing. And in most cases, it just takes a few minutes of immersion in a good alternative activity before the spell is broken.

But finding the activities that work for *you*—the ones that do a great job of grabbing your attention—will involve some trial and error. Individual results may vary. Some of the things I find riveting—for example, reading dense academic journals and watching college basketball—might seem utterly boring to you.

Fortunately, although there's no one-size-fits-all formula when it comes to finding the right activities, some things turn out to be anti-ruminative for just about everybody:

Engage in conversation. Carrying on a two-way conversation takes a surprising amount of mental focus—so much so that it's virtually impossible to ruminate while also keeping a decent dialogue afloat. (Of course, the verbal exchange has to be reciprocal. If you're unlucky enough to find yourself talking with someone who likes to dominate the conversation, you can easily start brooding as your companion drones on and on.)

In TLC, we ask patients to make a list of all their potential conversation partners, all the people they could conceivably talk with—either

TABLE 5-2. *Conversation Partners*

Contact	*How Comfortable? (1–10)*	*How Available? (1–10)*
Mom	8	10
Dad	4	9
Sally (best friend)	9	5
Jill (sister)	5	3
Danny (brother)	7	5
Bob & Joanie (neighbors)	4	2
Jessie (boss)	3	5
Sandy (friend from high school)	8	?

by phone or in person—during a bout of rumination. That includes not just members of their immediate and extended family, but also friends, coworkers, neighbors, and anyone else they can think of—even old acquaintances who've moved halfway across the country.

I invite you take a moment to make such a list (as shown in Table 5-2, above). As you do so, it may be helpful to rate each person according to how comfortable you'd be contacting them (on a 10-point scale), and their availability to talk when needed.

The next time you're in need of a conversation partner, it's best to begin by contacting the people you feel particularly comfortable with, especially if they're also likely to be available when you most need them. The idea is simply to initiate a conversation—or some other form of engaging activity—*the moment you notice yourself dwelling on negative thoughts.*

You may be able to increase your comfort level with some people on your list—and perhaps even their availability—simply by telling them about your plan to use conversation as a tool to interrupt the toxic rumination process. There are no guarantees, of course, but I've observed that friends and loved ones often react with surprising grace and compassion when they're confided in like that. Probably the most frequent response my patients have received is, "Thank you for trusting me enough to tell me about this, and feel free to call anytime you need me."

Pursue shared activities. Many of the most effective anti-ruminative activities are the ones we can share with others. There's something about the mere presence of another person that helps keep our thoughts from drifting inward.

For example, a few years ago I treated a lonely, depressed housewife who began volunteering with Habitat for Humanity after her youngest child went off to college. The first time she told me about how much better this activity made her feel, I assumed it was because she had made new friends while volunteering. But I was wrong. She was still very socially withdrawn, and she hadn't really connected with anyone there. Instead, what had helped her was simply having specific tasks to do—pounding nails, moving boards, sanding sheetrock—things she could focus on with others. "If I had done any of those things by myself, at home," she said, "I wouldn't have enjoyed it, and I probably would have ruminated the entire time. But just having someone else there with me made all the difference. I'm not sure *how*, exactly, but it kept me from getting lost in my own thoughts—even though we never really did much talking while we worked."

I've certainly found this principle to be true in my own life. (And it's been observed that men are often more comfortable connecting around shared activities than around intimate conversations.) For example, back when I was in graduate school, I sometimes struggled with ruminative, stress-filled thoughts about my yet-to-be-completed dissertation (which ran into some serious snags along the way). The most effective remedy, by far, involved simply leaving my books and jumping into a game of full-court basketball down at the local playground. Within a few minutes of running up and down the court (often with a group of complete strangers), I became swept up in the challenge of the game as it unfolded in front of me, and my mind soon became a worry-free zone.

Play. Interactive games represent a particularly effective way to end rumination. This is especially true if you can take part in a game that involves physical activity—tennis, golf, softball, racquetball, volleyball, basketball, bowling, and so on—because the mere act of coordinating your body's movement requires a great deal of focus from one moment to the next. (Such active games also provide the antidepressant benefit of physical exercise and—often—enhanced social connection.)

An interesting new option on this front has emerged with the advent of the wildly popular Nintendo Wii gaming system, which uses a wireless controller to simulate active sports and games. Surprisingly, the Wii has become a huge hit even among people who normally avoid vigorous activity—nursing home residents, for example—because it allows them to savor the taste of otherwise inaccessible experiences (like tennis and golf and baseball) through the magic of a wireless remote linked to on-screen simulations.

But even card games and sedentary board games can serve a similar anti-ruminative purpose, especially when they bring us into contact with other people. And, again, technology can make such gaming experiences available in a way that would have been unimaginable a few decades ago. Specifically, there are Web sites that can connect you in an instant to thousands of potential online gaming partners eager to join you in play anytime, anywhere in the world. In literally less than a minute, you can find yourself caught up with others in a game of online Scrabble, Monopoly, checkers, bridge, chess, backgammon, spades, or any number of other engaging distractions from your rumination.

Listen to music. Although sad music can serve as a trigger for rumination—as can music that we merely *associate* with upsetting events—most people find at least some types of music absorbing enough to interrupt a bout of brooding. If this is the case for you, it will open up a wide range of anti-ruminative possibilities. Most importantly, you'll be able to listen to music to prevent dwelling on negative thoughts during otherwise high-risk activities: driving, resting, performing mundane chores around the house, doing yard work, and so on. (As we'll see in Chapter 6, many forms of exercise also lend themselves to rumination especially when you work out alone but engaging music can serve as a wonderful antidote.)

Listen to books on tape. Depression can temporarily rob us of our ability to concentrate, which makes reading very difficult. Many patients have told me, however, that listening to a book on tape (or CD) is a much more realistic possibility. And audiobooks can even serve a function similar to that of listening to music—especially useful during those times when you're alone and engaged in a mindless activity that would otherwise lend itself to rumination.

Watch videos. Spending time passively in front of a screen—watching TV or movies—is usually something depressed patients should avoid, since it can so easily lead to rumination. (It can also decrease activity in the left frontal cortex, making depressive symptoms even worse.) However, in a pinch—when no other effective alternatives are available—you'll likely find that some movies and TV programs are absorbing enough to help break an episode of rumination. For this reason, it's probably not a bad idea to have a few compelling DVDs or tapes around to pop in when you're alone and in need of a quick, easy distraction.

Brainstorm. We've barely scratched the surface of activities you can use to help end a bout of rumination. Over the years, my patients have mentioned dozens of other options, including gardening, playing an instrument, cooking, shopping, listening to talk radio, playing with a dog or cat, visiting an animal shelter, going to a karaoke bar, volunteering at a museum, watching children play in the park, writing a letter, needlepoint, and hiking.

With a little brainstorming, you'll doubtless be able to come up with additional activities to add to your own list. I encourage you to take a moment now to compile a list of at least ten things you can turn to when you next find yourself ruminating. It can include options we've already covered, as well as some others that you've come up with on your own. Please note: If you've been depressed for some time, it may help to think back to things you used to enjoy before the illness struck. You can still reclaim many of them as anti-ruminative activities in the present.

Take charge. Earlier we discussed the importance of identifying the high-risk situations in your life—times when you're most likely to get stuck in an extended bout of brooding. The most effective way to address such situations is by taking an active approach: map out each day's schedule in advance and fill in any times of potential inactivity or social isolation with engaging activities.

For example, if you look at my patient's sample rumination log, shown in Table 5-1, you'll see that much of her brooding took place during two high-risk activities: commuting and watching TV. How might she improve things? First, the big block of time devoted to TV viewing after work could be targeted directly—circled on her calendar as a vulnerable period each day, and then filled in with alternative activities (any of the dozens described in this chapter). Likewise, the time spent commuting—while probably not avoidable—could still be rendered less toxic through such simple strategies as listening to engaging music or audiobooks on the drive (or, alternatively, through finding someone to carpool with—which would provide a conversation partner).

If you haven't done so already, I encourage you again to begin keeping an hour-by-hour log to track your own rumination (and the activities that promote it and prevent it, respectively). This exercise will not only help you identify and address the troublesome spots in your calendar (when rumination is the most likely), but will also serve as a catalyst to increase your overall activity level.

ACHIEVE BALANCE

Some of the effective anti-rumination strategies we've looked at—socializing and exercising, for example, are intrinsically antidepressant in nature, and most people would benefit from devoting more time to them. On the other hand, some of the activities we've covered—like playing games and watching videos—are valuable mostly because they happen to provide a momentary distraction from upsetting thoughts.

As we've seen, bit of distraction can be enormously helpful. But when the strategy is used too often, it can turn into full-blown avoidance—serving as an escape, not just from negative thoughts, but from the rest of life, as well.

That was the case for Julie, a patient in one of our TLC groups last year. She discovered that she could effectively divert attention from her rumination by spending time on her computer—playing video games, surfing Web sites, and so on—but before long she was spending most of her day glued to the screen. And that led her to avoid many other important—but less enjoyable—activities: paying bills, doing laundry, grocery shopping, balancing her checkbook, and cleaning her apartment. The nagging sense of guilt over such neglect, in turn, began to overtake her whenever she took a break from the computer. Paradoxically, her chronic avoidance led to an *increase* in ruminative thoughts (e.g., *I really need to pay that bill before it's overdue*) during every unguarded moment of downtime, which in turn led her to spend even more time on the computer as an escape.

When she brought up her dilemma in our group, there were knowing, sympathetic nods all around the table. Depression can so completely rob a person of their energy that even simple tasks start to feel overwhelming; it becomes all too tempting to avoid them. And that avoidance eventually becomes a habit, one that can linger long after depressive symptoms begin receding. Fortunately for Julie, however, her fellow patients gently pushed her on the point, helping her recognize the dangerous trap she'd fallen into and her need to bring the pattern of avoidance to an end.

When the use of distraction morphs into a habitual avoidance of things that need our attention, the process can still be turned around fairly quickly. But there are a few important principles worth bearing in mind.

First, when an avoided task feels overwhelming, it can usually be broken down into smaller, less daunting steps. If, say, cleaning the entire kitchen feels like it's too much to handle right now, you can divide the project into simpler tasks: unloading the dishwasher, putting a new load in, wiping down the counters, washing the pots and pans, sweeping the floor, and so on. These subtasks can then be taken on one by one, for as long as your energy holds out.

It's also helpful to make a list of all tasks that you've been avoiding, and to start with the easiest ones first. Simply completing any task—

even a short, straightforward one like paying a bill—often brings a nice feeling of accomplishment. And for most of us, merely crossing something off a to-do list is an innately rewarding experience. It helps create a sense of momentum we can build on.

However, in taking up long-neglected tasks, it's important to *set realistic goals for how much you can accomplish at any one time*. As a general rule, it's good to start with modest goals, especially if you've been using avoidance a great deal, or if your depressive symptoms are still severe. A realistic starting goal for some of my patients has been to spend just ten minutes a day on previously avoided tasks like paying bills or doing housework. But they've usually been able to increase that time by a few minutes a day as their stamina grew.

Finally, keep in mind the ageless principle: *everything in moderation*. In overcoming rumination, and in healing from depression itself, maintaining a sense of balance is crucial. Spending some time on long-neglected tasks is beneficial (and it can be anti-ruminative), but devoting too much time to chores can itself be overwhelming—and can make things worse. Likewise, a moderate use of distraction—playing video games and watching movies and surfing the Internet—is just fine, especially when it serves to end a bout of rumination, but excessive distraction can easily turn into a perilous avoidance of responsibility.

Similarly, as we've seen, even a moderate amount of rumination can serve a constructive purpose when it leads to important insights into our situation. But a little bit of dwelling on our problems goes a long way. For most people with depression, the balance between thinking and doing is easily lost, and rumination becomes a persistent habit that borders on addiction—amplifying depressive symptoms and standing as a formidable roadblock on the path to recovery.

But by putting into practice the strategies and principles covered in this chapter, you'll find the rumination habit is one that can, indeed, be broken. In so doing, you'll make the all-important journey from the inner prison of your own thoughts to the vastly more rewarding world you were designed for—that of other people and activities.

6
Antidepressant Exercise

Like most of the patients who enter our treatment program, Alice had been clinically depressed for a long time—in her case, about twelve years. And nothing had ever helped. Not meds. Not therapy. Not even the passage of time. At sixty-one, she had pretty much given up hope of ever making a full recovery. But then she saw a story about our Therapeutic Lifestyle Change approach in the local paper and decided it might be worth a try.

Even before contacting us, Alice had noticed that going for a stroll often made her feel a little better. So, when we told her about the antidepressant benefit of regular exercise, it struck a resonant chord. She asked if walking was an intense enough activity to make a difference, and we assured her that it could be, if she were willing to start walking faster, longer, and more regularly. To help her with this, we asked one of our personal trainers to begin meeting with Alice each week for brisk hikes together. Not only did Alice enjoy the invigoration of these outings, but she also valued the companionship, which made the time pass by much more quickly. She also timed her outings to take full advantage of the mood-elevating effect of sunlight exposure. Before long she was taking brisk walks several times a week, often in the company of her husband or a friend. To her surprise, she started noticing a gradual improvement in her sleep, energy level, mood, and ability to think clearly.

Within three months, Alice was, as she put it, "99% depression free." She felt better than she had in years. And while she credited each part of our treatment program with helping her recover, she was convinced that exercise made by far the biggest difference.

THE EXERCISE DILEMMA

According to the latest fitness research, the majority of Americans get no regular exercise at all. It's not a surprising finding, but it does raise an interesting question: Since just about everyone *wants* to be in good shape—wants to be exercising on a regular basis—why are so few of us doing it? Well, for one thing, we all have a litany of excuses. We're too busy, too tired, too overworked, too sore, too unmotivated, too strapped for cash, too burdened with responsibilities, too intimidated—maybe even too embarrassed to be seen exercising in public. But such excuses often serve to mask a deeper truth: Working out is just plain *hard*.

If you're like most people, you've probably even vowed at some point to start an ambitious new exercise routine, only to find your resolve crumbling in a matter of days. Unless you're one of the lucky ones—someone who actually enjoys working out for its own sake—you may even approach the topic of exercise with a vague feeling of dread.

I'm with you. In fact, I believe there's something about trying to exercise that's downright *unnatural*. To understand why, we need to return to the fact that our bodies and brains are still largely designed for life in the Stone Age, for the hunter-gatherer conditions that existed for most of human history. And here's the thing: hunter-gatherers never work out. They don't need to. They get so much physical activity in the flow of daily life—several hours each day—that they actually avoid extra exertion whenever possible.

Why? Imagine if one of your hunter-gatherer ancestors had decided to start working out. On top of the ten miles he already traveled each day while hunting, hauling water, and scouting out campsites, perhaps he went off and decided to run a few extra miles a day just for fun. Not a very wise choice, I'm afraid, since all that extra running would have burned off thousands of precious calories—calories that could have been stored as body fat, reserve fuel during the next inevitable food shortage. Frankly, given the ever-present risk of starvation in the ancestral environment, it's a safe bet that few Stone Age runners ever survived long enough to pass on their "working-out genes" to future generations.

So our wisest ancestors were the ones who followed a simple rule: *spend your energy only on activities that have a clear purpose.* This rule was so important to people's survival that it ultimately became part of our genetic legacy, part of the brain's built-in programming. It's a rule that's still with us. Many people discover this the hard way when they try to work up the willpower to work out. As they approach the dreaded treadmill or stationary bike, it's as if a part of their brain is screaming out, "Don't do it! You're not actually *going* anywhere on that thing. You need to conserve the calories!"

We can even observe this same principle—the same built-in programming to avoid needless activity—in laboratory rats. Exercise researchers have a devil of a time trying to get the little guys to run on a treadmill. The rats will go to incredible lengths to avoid running, even to the point of just squatting down on their haunches until the machine starts to wear the fur and skin off their backsides. When it comes to forced exercise, they feel our pain. But unlike the rats, we have a nagging feeling that we *should* be working out more.

THE BENEFITS OF EXERCISE

Doctors have been telling us for years that we need to get more exercise. Most of us can even recite a long list of health benefits that accompany physical activity: lower blood pressure, boosted immune function, greater bone density, and a reduced risk of diabetes, obesity, and heart disease. Regular exercise even helps our bodies remain youthful. (Think about legendary fitness guru Jack LaLanne, who looks better in his nineties than many people half his age.)

But even though everyone knows that exercise is a key to maintaining physical health, few realize that it's equally important for preserving *mental* health. The latest research shows that exercise can even stop depression in its tracks.

When I was a graduate student at Duke University in the early 1990s, one of my professors, Dr. Jim Blumenthal, was beginning to study exercise as a treatment for depression. It's embarrassing to admit now, but when I first heard about Blumenthal's research I thought the idea was kind of nutty. I can still remember talking with one of my classmates about it. "Sure," I said, "you might feel better for a few minutes after working out, but how in the world is that supposed to help you if you're seriously depressed? I just don't see it."

But Blumenthal knew the powerful antidepressant effect of exercise from firsthand clinical experience. At the time, he was carrying out the most ambitious study of exercise and depression the world had ever seen. The study involved 156 depressed patients—mostly middle-aged and pitifully out of shape—who were randomly assigned to treatment with either Lustral (a commonly prescribed antidepressant medicine) or exercise.

You might imagine that an exercise regimen would have to be pretty grueling to be effective against depression. Maybe hours of running every day? Or some kind of strenuous weight lifting—the kind that makes people's neck veins bulge? Incredibly, however, Blumenthal simply had his patients take *a brisk half-hour walk three times a week*. That's it. And yet this remarkably low "dose" of exercise proved to be more effective than the Lustral. The two treatments worked about equally well for the first few months, but by ten months into the study, the exercisers were much more likely than those taking Lustral to remain depression-free.

And this study wasn't just a fluke: Over a dozen clinical trials now show that exercise can effectively treat depression. How does it work? As we saw in Chapter 1, *exercise actually changes the brain*. Like an antidepressant medication, it increases the activity of important brain chemicals like serotonin and dopamine. It also stimulates the brain's release of a key growth hormone (BDNF), which in turn helps reverse the toxic, brain-damaging effects of depression. It even sharpens memory and concentration, and helps us think more clearly. Simply put, *exercise is medicine*—one that affects the brain more powerfully than any drug.

THERE HAS TO BE A BETTER WAY

Yet, at this point it's fair to ask: What good is it to know about all the benefits of exercise if we still can't bring ourselves to do it? After all, we've seen that we're designed to *avoid* extra physical activity. So how can we possibly find a way to make regular exercise a reality?

Fortunately, there's a way out of the dilemma. Yes, we're wired to avoid extra physical activity—but what about *necessary* activity? Have you ever noticed how much easier it is to be physically active when you're caught up in something that has a clear goal or purpose?

This point hit home for me recently when my wife, Maria, told me about her Grandma Peterson. Well into her eighties and hampered by arthritic knees, Grandma had taken to spending the better part of each day with her pet Chihuahua on a recliner in the living room. She was almost completely inert. Her doctors got on her about it, of course. They told her if she would just get a little exercise, she'd probably notice an improvement in her arthritis. But it didn't matter; she couldn't get motivated. Family members would beg and plead for Grandma to join them for a walk around the neighborhood, but she wasn't having any of it. "It's too *hard* for me now," she'd say. "You go on ahead while I finish watching my show."

Then one day the family hit on a different tactic. They invited Grandma to join them on a trip to the local shopping mall. After all, she used to love shopping, but she hadn't been to the mall in years. Fortunately, she found their offer too tempting to pass up, so off they went. Maria estimated—charitably—that her grandmother might last about ten minutes before pooping out. But to everyone's surprise, Grandma was still going strong after three solid hours. She got caught up in the fun of a day out with the girls, and simply forgot all about her sore knees. Somehow she was able to keep on "hunting and gathering" right there with the best of them.

As it turns out, *whenever we're caught up in enjoyable, meaningful activity, our tolerance for exercise goes up dramatically*. Tim McCord is a man who puts this principle to better use than anyone I know. An unassuming junior high teacher from Titusville, Pennsylvania, Tim has been in the national spotlight for chasing an outrageous goal: to get every student in his school district involved in an intensive daily exercise program. Through years of heroic effort, he's managed to get Titusville's students working out—vigorously—more than forty minutes a day. Many kids even make their way to school voluntarily over the summer vacation to get a workout in.

In one of life's wonderful coincidences, I found myself seated next to Tim on a cross-country flight a few years ago. The more we talked, the more I was blown away by what he's accomplished with his students. I don't know about you, but I used to dread going to gym class, and I certainly don't remember anyone getting in great shape there (rope burns, yes; great physical conditioning, not so much). How in the world, then, did Tim get so many kids on board with his fitness program?

"The most important thing," he said, "is to make the workouts as engaging as possible. When the kids are really into it, they don't notice how hard they're working. Take the exercise bike. It's a boring piece of equipment, right? Put most kids on that bike, and they'll give it a little half-hearted effort and then hop off after a few minutes. But a couple of years ago we hooked some of our bikes up to a video game interface—it's called *Game Riders*—where the kids have to pedal to play. Now they're so caught up in it, they sit there and pedal like crazy. You can't get 'em off the darn things!" He laughed and went on to give one example after another of students getting absorbed in their workouts: The kids were able to get caught up in activities ranging from dance contests to virtual reality games to team sports to old-school playground games like tag and keep-away.

It makes perfect sense, doesn't it? Time really does fly when we're caught up in something enjoyable, even when there's physical exercise involved. It's a principle that worked beautifully for Tim McCord's students—and for Maria's grandmother. It's the same principle we're going to keep clearly in view as we begin to outline an antidepressant workout routine you'll actually be able to stick with.

FIRST: MAKE IT AEROBIC

How hard do you have to work out to see an antidepressant effect? Researchers have looked at the question extensively, and they've consistently observed a powerful therapeutic benefit from *aerobic* exercise—the kind of workout that causes your heart rate to stay elevated for several minutes at a time. Common aerobic activities include jogging, brisk walking, swimming, cycling, racquetball, team sports, hiking, dancing, and climbing stairs.

Technically speaking, a workout is aerobic whenever it gets your pulse between 60%–90% of your maximum heart rate. You can estimate this maximum—the greatest number of times your heart can possibly beat in a minute—with a simple formula: It's just 220 minus your age. But you won't have to do any math on this one. Instead, Table 6-1 displays your estimated maximum heart rate, along with the aerobic values that range from 60%–90% of this maximum number. (These values are listed for every adult age group.) We'll return to these numbers shortly.

Before you can exercise aerobically, you'll also need to have a reliable way of measuring your heart rate, or pulse. Chances are, you've had your pulse taken at the doctor's office many times, so you probably remember the basics: They hold your wrist, look at a watch, do a little counting and some quick math, and that's about it. Not much to it, right? But it turns out to be a little trickier than it looks (especially in the middle of a workout).

Although taking your pulse seems easy enough, most people need a little coaching and some practice to get it right. If you feel up to the challenge, many nurses and doctors are happy to walk you through the basic steps during a routine office visit.

Ultimately, though, I think you'll find it more convenient to buy a portable heart rate monitor. This is a little watch-like device (used

TABLE 6-1. *Maximum Heart Rate by Age*

	Aerobic Range			
Age	*60% Maximum Heart Rate*	*75% Maximum Heart Rate*	*90% Maximum Heart Rate*	*100% Maximum Heart Rate*
20–24	120	150	180	200
25–29	117	147	176	195
30–34	114	143	171	190
35–39	111	139	166	185
40–44	108	135	162	180
45–49	104	131	156	174
50–54	102	127	153	170
55–59	99	123	149	165
60–64	96	120	144	160
65–69	93	116	140	155
70+	90	113	135	150

with a chest strap) that gives an accurate, continuous readout of your pulse. High-quality monitors are now available through sporting goods and electronics retailers (as well as online vendors) for as little as $40. That's not inexpensive, I know, but it's an investment that will pay big dividends, helping you stay within your target aerobic range during every workout.

However, even if you never buy a pulse monitor or learn how to take your pulse, you can still use some low-tech rules of thumb to get a rough idea of whether or not your heart rate is in the optimal range. For example, if you're able to effortlessly carry on a conversation during your workout, it's probably not aerobic. Making conversation is always a bit tougher when you're in the aerobic range; your sentences become choppier because you're breathing so hard. Likewise, if you're able to *sing* while working out, you're definitely not in the aerobic range! On the other hand, if you ever find yourself gasping for breath, you've likely gone *above* your aerobic range, and need to slow down.

Having covered these important basics, we're now ready to move on to the process of choosing an aerobic activity.

SECOND: CHOOSE AN ACTIVITY

Engineers who study the human body—its structure, joints, musculature, and so on—marvel at how exquisitely well-designed it is for walking. It's an activity that comes to people so naturally, so effortlessly, that even babies who receive no prompting will eventually just start to walk on their own, as if propelled by instinct. Walking is something we're truly born to do.

And for the vast majority of human history—until the advent of the automobile a few generations ago—people walked a lot. Our remote ancestors walked an estimated ten miles a day. For them, "a day at the office" often meant a day spent tracking down dinner. Even as recently as the nineteenth century, when most Americans still made their living on the farm, people spent the better part of each day working and traveling on foot. Before car ownership became the norm in the 1940s, most people continued to walk several miles every day. But things are different now. Each day, the average American travels over forty miles in a car, and less than one mile on foot.

Because our bodies are designed for it—and because it's something just about everyone can do—walking is an ideal antidepressant exercise. Sometimes when I tell this to my patients, however, they ask, "Is walking really intense enough to make a difference?" It really doesn't seem like it should be, does it? And yet walking had a surprisingly potent effect in Jim Blumenthal's famous exercise study (the one in which exercise beat Lustral). The key: Blumenthal's patients walked briskly enough to get their heart rates up into the aerobic range, and long enough to allow that aerobic activity to work its healing magic on the brain.

In light of its many advantages, I suggest that you consider walking as the place to begin your antidepressant workout routine. But this is not a one-size-fits-all recommendation. For example, some people can't walk due to injury or illness. If that's the case for you, you'll need to consult with your doctor to find an aerobic alternative your body can tolerate. (I have a paraplegic friend, for example, whose workouts include kayaking and wheelchair racing.) Likewise, some people already have another favorite aerobic activity, something they know they'll want to do on a regular basis. If that's true for you, then by all means, go with it.

The most important thing is to find an activity you'll be able to stick with. Although my clinical experience suggests that brisk walking usually fits the bill, individual results may vary. Because finding the right workout routine sometimes involves a little trial-and-error, it actually will be useful for you to identify *three* aerobic activities you might enjoy. This will give you plenty of options to work with as we outline an exercise program in the remainder of the chapter. And to help get your creative juices flowing, I've listed several aerobic possibilities in Table 6-2.

THIRD: DETERMINE HOW MUCH, HOW LONG, AND HOW OFTEN

How much time will you need to invest in all this? The best research suggests that it takes only *ninety minutes of aerobic activity each week*

TABLE 6-2. *Some Aerobic Possibilities*

Outdoor Activities	*Competitive Sports*	*Activities in a Gym*
Brisk walking	Basketball	Treadmill (jog/walk)
Jogging	Soccer	Aerobics class
Swimming	Tennis	Weight lifting (circuit)
Cycling	Racquetball	Dance class
Cross-country skiing	Handball	Jumping rope
Inline skating/ice skating	Flag football	Row machine
Hiking	Volleyball	Water aerobics
Rock climbing	Squash	Elliptical trainer
Heavy yard work	Badminton	Spinning (cycling) class

to provide an antidepressant effect. That's the weekly target I'm asking you to aim for. (It's much less time than the average American spends watching TV in a single *day*.) Here are some related points you'll also need to keep in mind:

It takes about five minutes of working out before most people get their pulse into the aerobic range. So, it's best if you consider the first five minutes of each workout as warm-up time. This brief warm-up period will not count toward your weekly ninety-minute target.

Plan on splitting your ninety minutes of exercise each week into at least three shorter workouts. If you're in reasonably good physical health and at least somewhat active already, it's ideal to plan for three workouts of thirty minutes each. (If you add five minutes of warm-up time, the workouts will each take thirty-five minutes). Why split things up like that? Because unless you're already in exceptional shape, your body just won't have the stamina to last more than about thirty minutes in the aerobic range. It's truly best not to overdo it.

In fact, if you've been completely sedentary over the past several months, I suggest starting with an even briefer workout time, and gradually building up to that thirty-five-minute target. You might, for example, begin by walking only five or ten minutes a day for the first week, and then add five minutes to your daily walk time every few days—until you've increased your stamina enough to last for thirty-five minutes without becoming physically exhausted.

Although you're technically in the aerobic range at 60% of your maximum pulse rate, the best research studies have asked people to work out somewhat harder—usually in the middle-to-high end of their aerobic range. Therefore, I suggest that you set your target pulse at 75% of your maximum. (You can refer to the corresponding heart rate value for your age group in Table 6-1.) During each workout, try to keep your pulse reasonably close to this 75% target.

FOURTH: MAKE IT ENJOYABLE

We've already talked about how important it is for each workout to be as enjoyable as possible. But how can you make this ideal a reality? Following are some discoveries we've made along the way with the Therapeutic Lifestyle Change program:

Make it social. Whenever possible, it's best to work out with someone else—especially someone whose company you enjoy. Because spending time with others tends to be highly absorbing, it makes the workout pass more quickly; it also gives you the mood-elevating benefit of social support. The latest research suggests that exercising with others may be even more effective in fighting depression than working out alone.

So, the next time you're planning a brisk walk, consider inviting a friend or loved one to join you. Or, if you own a dog, you might try having a regular canine workout companion. (Dogs, like us, are built for much more physical activity than they usually get.)

Another option—one that many of my patients highly recommend—is to meet regularly with a personal trainer. Not only can they provide important companionship during your workouts, but most trainers will also give expert coaching and timely pointers along the way. Any local gym or health club should have a list of personal trainers in your area.

Of course, some aerobic activities already have a built-in social component. Sports such as basketball, racquetball, and tennis are fantastic in this respect (Table 6-2 lists several others), and many communities now offer year-round recreational sports leagues for men and women of all ages and skill levels.

Make it absorbing. Sometimes it's just not possible to exercise with someone else. But there are other ways to make your workout absorbing.

Most of us, for example, find it easy to get caught up in our favorite music. This is true for many of the patients I've worked with. Swept up in the rhythm of a great song, they find themselves carried along by the music—with a level of stamina and vigor they'd never achieve when working out in silence. So the next time you're exercising by yourself, you might consider taking along a portable music player and a playlist of up-tempo songs.

Listening to audiobooks is another great possibility. Melanie, a friend of mine who overcame her depression using the TLC approach, struggled for months to work up the willpower to use her home treadmill. It mostly just sat in her basement gathering dust. And no matter how hard she tried, she couldn't make herself stay on the thing for more than a few minutes before the sheer drudgery wore her out. But then she took a long road trip, and happened to bring along some books on tape. Remarkably, the hours on the road simply *flew* by. And that's when it hit her—maybe the tapes would help her on the treadmill, too. So she went and checked out a few audiobooks at the local public library, and made a deal with herself: She was allowed to listen to the tapes *only* while she was on the treadmill. It worked beautifully. Melanie soon found herself putting in more workout time than she had imagined possible (over two hours a week). Remarkably, she even started looking forward to the time on the treadmill as one of the highlights of her day.

Games also tend to be good at capturing our attention, so any workout that has a game-like quality to it will be especially engaging. Stan, one of the patients in a recent TLC group, told us that when he's out on the racquetball court, an hour will go by in what seems like the blink of an eye. I've heard the same thing from others about sports as varied as basketball, squash, tennis, soccer, ultimate Frisbee, and volleyball. Several active video games on the market can also provide a surprisingly good aerobic workout; these are especially popular with kids and teens, of course, but many grown-ups find them great fun as well. One of our patients last year, for example, loved to work up a sweat playing *Dance Dance Revolution* (a fast-paced dance contest) on the Sony PlayStation with her teenage daughter.

One more thing about absorbing activity: *Nature itself has an uncanny ability to capture our attention.* We're all hardwired to enjoy the beauty of natural settings, and there's something almost transcendent about being immersed in the sights and sounds and smells of the great outdoors. Most of us will find hiking in nature to be among the more absorbing (and peaceful) workout activities in our repertoire.

Make it purposeful. As we saw earlier, exercise is easier and more enjoyable when it incorporates a goal or purpose. For example, the average visitor to Walt Disney World walks about seven miles—nearly on par with the daily workout of hunter-gatherers. But how many of these visitors will ever work out like that again after leaving the park? Without all the built-in purposeful activity—checking out the next cool ride or exhibit around the bend—they just won't have the motivation.

As a rule, people are usually willing to walk much farther when they're doing it for a specific reason; it can even be an indirect reason—enjoying the beauty of nature, the companionship of a friend, or the satisfaction of giving a dog some badly needed exercise. But the most obvious reason for walking is simply to *get* somewhere.

So the next time you go for an aerobic walk, you may want to choose a destination that matters to you. It could be a friend's house, an ice-cream shop, a record store, a scenic waterfall, a restaurant—anyplace at all, as long as it's someplace you want to be, and someplace you can walk to safely and comfortably.

You can also put the principle of purposeful activity to work for you right in your own backyard: mowing, raking, shoveling, mulching, hauling, or gardening. Because yard work is so goal-oriented, many people find it highly energizing—which allows them to stay at it for long stretches of time. And believe it or not, this sort of activity is usually aerobic. (You can test this by taking your pulse the next time you're out working in the yard.)

One more thing about purpose before we move on: Over the years, many of my patients have reminded me that exercise already carries an intrinsic sense of meaning for them—the goal of fighting depression. In other words, the quest to overcome depression can itself become the purpose sufficient to motivate and energize each workout. When viewed in this light, each stride you take can literally be seen as another step on the path to recovery.

FIFTH: CREATE A SCHEDULE

One of the most important things I've learned about antidepressant exercise is how helpful it is to write out a workout schedule. When we set aside space in our calendars for working out in the week ahead, we're much more likely to reach our exercise goals. Following are some key principles to keep in mind.

Set aside an hour. Even though you only need about thirty-five minutes to get in an antidepressant workout, you'll want to set aside at least a full hour to give yourself enough time to change into comfortable clothes and shoes beforehand and to clean up afterwards. You'll also want to build in ample additional time if you need to travel to your workout destination.

Create a routine. Whenever possible, set aside the same blocks of time every week. Habits are hard to break—even a seemingly arbitrary habit like working out the same time every Tuesday. See if you can identify at least three openings in your schedule that are guaranteed to be free from week to week.

Space things out. It's best to space out the exercise evenly over the week (as opposed to working out three days in a row and then taking the next four days off). That usually means taking a day off in between each workout, a practice that has the added benefit of giving your body plenty of time to recover each time.

Avoid ending late. When we work out aerobically, our bodies experience a powerful adrenaline rush. Although this can be invigorating, it can also lead to insomnia if we don't allow enough time to cool down before bedtime. As a rule of thumb, you'll want to finish your workout at least two hours before you turn in for the night.

Bearing all this in mind, please take a moment now to schedule three blocks of time—each one at least an hour long—for working out in the week ahead.

SIXTH: MAKE YOUR WORKOUT SPECIFIC BUT FLEXIBLE

After you've completed your first three workouts, take a few minutes to reflect on how things went. Remember, your goal is for each exercise period to be at least somewhat enjoyable. So even though the pleasure of exercising tends to increase for most people over time (especially during the first several weeks), you should find at least *some* enjoyment in your workouts from the outset. If you don't, it's important to incorporate one (or more) of the strategies we covered earlier, such as exercising to music or books on tape, or including a workout partner. You can also shift to one of the other workout activities on your list.

SEVENTH: BE ACCOUNTABLE

The biggest single obstacle to working out—especially for those battling depression—is simply to overcome the profound sense of inertia that sets in when we're inactive. Virtually every patient I've ever worked with has told me they enjoy exercising once they're doing it, but they often lack the motivation and energy to get started.

Reduced initiative is a hallmark of depression. The depressed brain actually has an impaired ability to initiate activities, so those battling depression usually have a difficult time starting anything new. But they typically do just fine with a new activity if someone else can help them get going.

That's why it's so important to have someone who can give you the nudge you may need to get off the couch and into your exercise routine. One obvious possibility is a workout partner—someone committed to joining you at a specific time and place. The sense of accountability that comes with this arrangement—the fact that you won't want to disappoint your workout companion—is usually enough to get you started, and your partner's presence and encouragement can help you stay with it. As a bonus, you'll feel good about providing the same incentive and encouragement for your companion.

But if you don't have someone in your life right now to work out with, a personal trainer can play this role. Or, if need be, your accountability could come from someone who doesn't even work out with you. It just has to be someone who's willing to check in with you (even if only by phone) at the beginning of each workout to hold you accountable for getting started, and to provide gentle encouragement to stick with it.

A good friend or trusted family member can often play this role. But so can a therapist, a nurse, or a coworker. And even though it may be a little scary to think about asking for help, it can be well worth it. In fact, our TLC patients have been consistently and pleasantly surprised at how willing other people usually are to provide such accountability. In most cases, others will be profoundly impressed with your commitment to the recovery process and honored to support you. They may even be inspired to start working out themselves.

As we've seen, our bodies are designed for a high level of physical activity. And exercise is extraordinarily important for maintaining both physical and mental health. Aerobic exercise is the most potent antidepressant activity ever discovered, with the ability to reverse the toxic effects of depression on the brain. Physical activity even has mood-elevating effects that can usually be felt in a matter of minutes. As one personal trainer told me recently, "I don't think I've ever seen someone leave the gym in a worse mood than when they arrived."

And, despite the fact that most vigorous physical activity has been engineered right out of our twenty-first-century lives, it's still possible to recapture the benefits of regular exercise. The key steps laid out in this chapter provide a clear sense of what this process looks like, and I've watched patient after patient make it happen. They always do so by simply taking it one step at a time. *Anything more can be overwhelming; anything less can lead to inertia.*

I invite you to take that first step. Remember, you were designed to be physically active, free of depression, and surrounded by people who can support and encourage you along the way.

7
Let There Be Light

This was unexpected. Callie had been symptom-free for nearly a month, and yet there she was in my office, a complete wreck. I could tell she was starting to get depressed again the minute she walked in. It was as if the light had gone out of her eyes.

Plopping down in the chair next to my desk, Callie—a tall, athletic preschool teacher in her mid-twenties—stared absently out the window, as if trying to gather her thoughts. "I don't know what went wrong," she said softly. "I thought I was better, but I guess I'm not. The depression is back." Her voice rose in desperation. "It's like I'm right back to square one."

I tried to reassure her that we'd get to the bottom of things—figure out what had caused her setback—and turn things back around. But I have to confess: I was a little rattled.

Callie had first come to see me three months earlier for help with her depression. Hearing about my research in the local newspaper, she said she'd felt some rekindling of hope. And her motivation in treatment was exceptional. Week after week, she pushed herself to add exercise, fish oil, engaging activity, and social interaction to her daily routine. Within eight weeks, she said she was feeling "pretty much back to normal."

But that was before the setback.

"So," I asked, "did anything happen? Anything unusual or upsetting you can think of?"

"No. It's not like anything happened. I just started feeling run-down all the time. And it's taking me forever to fall asleep; then once I finally do, I can't wake up. It's like I could sleep in until noon, but even that's not enough. And it affects everything else, you know? I feel like crap, dragging around all day. I'm eating all the time, my mood's awful, I can't focus at work . . . it's just like it was before."

This was puzzling. And there were dozens of possibilities we might have to explore in sorting it all out. But I had a hunch about where to begin. "Remind me again: You first started getting depressed back in December, right?"

"Uh, it was right after Thanksgiving last year. Yeah, I think it was maybe early December."

"And you told me you'd been depressed three times before that—once in high school and twice in college?" She nodded. "Can you remember when those episodes started? What month of the year?"

She glanced up at the ceiling. "Uh, well, back in high school I was depressed for two years. It started sophomore year. I guess it got bad after Christmas break, maybe January. And then in college . . . my freshman year it was at the end of fall semester, so probably December. And then junior year—I think it was pretty much the same thing."

Bingo. Four episodes of depression, and each one started in December or January. It was the classic seasonal onset pattern: depression triggered by a lack of sunlight during the short, cold, dreary days of winter. I floated the idea past Callie.

"But it's only October," she said. "Isn't that too early?"

"Maybe. But think about what it's been like out lately." It had rained for several straight days, and had been unseasonably cold and cloudy, to boot. "You usually spend a lot of time outside with your job, right? What about this week?"

She shook her head. "I normally have the kids outside for a few hours every day, so sunlight is never really an issue for me. But it's been so gross out lately; it was indoor play every day. I haven't been out in a week." She leaned forward. There was a little more life in her eyes. "Do you really think that's the problem?"

"I don't know. It could be, but there's only one way to find out for sure." I asked Callie to sit tight while I ran down the hall and grabbed a light box from my lab. We set it up right next to her, and she spent the final thirty minutes of our session basking in light as bright as the morning sun. There was no immediate effect, though she said her mood was maybe a little better by the session's end.

Since it was Friday afternoon, I sent her home with the box to try over the weekend, a half hour after getting up each day. And then on Monday morning I got a call at the office. "Dr. Ilardi? It's Callie. You're not going to believe this, but my sleep's getting better, and I'm kind of starting to feel like myself again. Thank you so much for the light box! Oh, and I just ordered one for myself online; FedEx should have it here by tomorrow."

For my ninth birthday, my parents got me a Polaroid camera. It was one of my favorite gifts of all time. I can still remember the thrill of hitting the shutter and watching as it spit out one of those humble little blank prints, promissory notes that could morph magically into true-to-life images in a matter of minutes. It was like instant gratification in slow motion.

One of the things I always wondered about that camera, though, was why I always had to use a flashbulb inside, but never outside, even on the dreariest, cloudiest day. Sure, it might be a *little* brighter out there, but it didn't seem like that much of a difference. After all, I could see just fine indoors, so why couldn't the camera? I even tried taking pictures inside without a flash, but they always came out a dark, muddled mess.

What I didn't realize at the time was just how *much* brighter it is in broad daylight. As shown in Figure 7-1, *the natural light of a sunny day is over one hundred times brighter than typical indoor lighting*. That's a huge contrast. We don't notice it only because our eyes and brains are so cleverly designed—adjusting effortlessly to nearly any change in lighting conditions, and hardly ever missing a beat.

FIGURE 7-1. *Brightness in Lux*

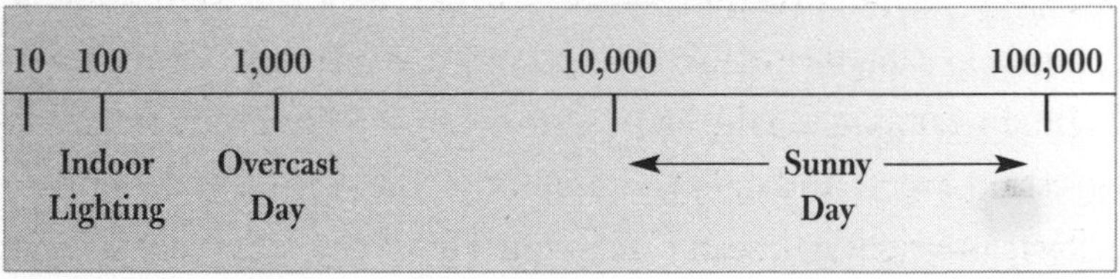

10 100 1,000 10,000 100,000

Indoor Lighting

Overcast Day

← Sunny Day →

But here's the thing: Even though our eyes *can* work okay inside, they're designed for the great outdoors. Our hunter-gatherer ancestors were outside all day, every day. Even as recently as a century ago, most people spent the majority of their waking time in natural daylight.

So it makes sense that our eyes are engineered for the lighting conditions outside. They even have special light receptors, hardwired straight to the middle of the brain, that respond only to the brightness of outdoor lighting. Why don't they work inside? Because they're looking for light at least as luminous as a gray, overcast day outside—which is over three times brighter than your living room with all the lights on.

If you spend most of your time inside—as people generally do these days—your eyes' light receptors simply aren't getting the stimulation they need. And that, in turn, can have a major effect on both your brain chemistry and your body clock.

THE SEROTONIN CONNECTION

Bright light stimulates the brain's production of serotonin, that crucial chemical emissary. And making sure we have adequate serotonin function is a big deal: It's a neurotransmitter with widespread effects on mood and behavior.

Stress and depression. As we saw in Chapter 2, serotonin circuits help calm the brain's depressive stress response. Thus, bright light, by ramping up the brain's serotonin activity, exerts an antidepressant effect. And unlike traditional medications, the therapeutic effects of bright light can kick in quickly, often in less than a week. (In contrast, the typical lag time with drugs like Prozac and Efexor is two to four weeks.)

Well-being. Bright light doesn't just suppress stress-related emotions; it also boosts feelings of well-being. That's another nice benefit of increased serotonin activity. According to the latest research, people usually feel some elevation of mood within an hour of two of exposure to bright light. I've even had patients tell me they could sense their mood beginning to lift within *minutes* of basking in the sun.

Social activity. When your mood is upbeat, you're also more inclined to socialize. According to the latest research, bright light propels us to seek out more social contact, and to find it more appealing. A recent study also showed that people under the influence of bright light are less likely to argue or fight with others. These effects, too, are due in part to a light-based serotonin boost, which can even stimulate positive social interactions in rodents and monkeys.

ON THE CLOCK

The brain works hard to keep the body running like clockwork. And buried deep inside the cranium is a nifty little chronometer—the so-called *body-clock**—that stays remarkably accurate, *as long as we get enough light each day.*

When we're deprived of ample light, however, the body clock falters, our one hundred trillion cells quickly fall out of step with each other, and all hell breaks loose: Hormone levels get out of whack, sleep grows erratic, and energy ebbs and flows at all the wrong times. For some individuals, these effects actually can usher in a full-blown episode of depression.†

Here's the thing: The body's built-in timepiece is *pretty* accurate, but it's not exactly a Rolex. (It's more like the wind-up job you'd buy from some guy in a trench coat.) If it doesn't get reset regularly, the body clock starts to drift—losing or gaining up to an hour a day. And a week or two of drifting is all it takes to send the body into a tailspin.

---

* The body clock is a cluster of neurons in a region of the brain called the *suprachiasmic nucleus*

† Among those who are less genetically vulnerable, the effects of prolonged light deprivation usually aren't as catastrophic: They may range from mere sluggishness to feeling blah (or, on occasion, agitated).

So resetting the clock each day is an important priority, and it all hinges on those specialized light sensors at the back of the eyes, which are exquisitely sensitive to minute-by-minute changes in brightness. They send continuous input back to the brain, which uses all that lighting information to lock in on the timing of sunrise and sunset each day. (Since these events take place at the same time every day, they can be used like beacons to keep our internal clocks in sync.)*

How much bright light exposure is required? Luckily, it's not that much. For most people, fifteen to thirty minutes each morning† is enough to keep the body clock reasonably on track.

Despite our penchant for staying indoors, most North Americans and Europeans still get enough light in the summertime, when the days are sunny and warm and it's bright outside from early morning until late in the evening.

It's a different story in the winter, though, when the days are dark, dreary, cold, and short. Across much of the industrialized world, people spend virtually all day, every day cooped up inside. Not surprisingly, the typical American is dangerously light-deficient from November through March. (And in more northern locales, the light deficit can last from October through April.)

---

* Although the timing of both sunrise and sunset always varies by a minute or two each day, such small, *gradual* changes are easy for the body clock to account for.

† The body clock is especially tuned in to the timing of sunrise each day. To figure out when sunrise has occurred, it looks for a telltale lighting pattern that goes from very dark (nighttime) to semibright (at sunrise) to very bright (about a half-hour after sunrise). Even inside our modern houses, the first two steps of the sunrise pattern hold: It goes from dark at night to semibright inside when we turn the lights on after waking up. But the brain also needs to see that third step of the pattern—the much greater brightness that quickly follows sunrise. When we're missing that part, the body clock doesn't get reset accurately.

SEASONAL AFFECTIVE DISORDER (SAD)

According to researchers, the average American is less happy (and more sluggish) during the winter. The rate of clinical depression goes up, as well—and the more northern the latitude, the greater the increase. An estimated 20% of the population battles the "winter blues," with at least some clinically significant depressive symptoms between November and March.

And, as we've seen, this pattern can be explained by a lack of light exposure, which disrupts the body clock and depletes the brain's serotonin circuits—leading to social withdrawal, depressed mood, and an elevated stress response.

Clinicians refer to the winter-onset pattern of depression as *seasonal affective disorder*,* or SAD. Diagnostically, it's simply a subtype of depressive illness. But SAD does have a few distinctive clinical features.

For example, while most people with depression struggle with insomnia, those with SAD tend to sleep too much—often up to twelve hours or more each day. And even after they finally wake up, they usually feel extremely groggy and sluggish.

SAD sufferers also frequently find themselves gaining weight—with a voracious appetite for sweets and other simple carbohydrates† that the body can convert directly to sugar. Many researchers now believe this sugar craving represents an attempt to "self-medicate," since surging blood glucose can trigger more serotonin activity in the brain, temporarily lifting mood. But there's a big downside: eating sugar (and other simple carbs) promotes inflammation—and as we saw in

---

* The DSM-IV doesn't actually use this term, however. Instead, it notes some major depressive episodes follow a "seasonal onset pattern."

† Simple carbohydrates are starchy foods like snack chips, white bread, noodles, pasta, and fries.

Chapter 2, chronic inflammation is a major culprit in promoting depression. So, the sugar-based self-medication strategy ultimately fails—in a big way.

Those with SAD also tend to be extremely sensitive to light deprivation year-round. This means they can develop depressive symptoms any time of year—whenever there's a long stretch of gloomy weather that keeps them from getting enough bright light.

BRIGHT LIGHT THERAPY

The clear treatment of choice for SAD is bright light therapy. It's now been evaluated in over seventy research studies, and often yields even better results for SAD patients than medication (with far fewer side effects).

But bright light therapy turns out to be useful in treating *all* forms of depression. It's not just for those whose symptoms follow the winter onset pattern, or for those who have the distinctive symptoms we usually see in SAD (things like sleeping too much, weight gain, and sugar craving).

Remember, we were all designed to get bright light on a regular basis. That's why it has such widespread beneficial effects: boosting mood, turning down the brain's stress response, keeping the body clock in sync, and even making us more likely to socialize.

Nature versus the Light Box

For most people suffering from depression, thirty minutes of light exposure each day is all it takes to provide an antidepressant effect.

However, as we've seen, the light needs to match the brightness of a sunny day—an intensity of at least 10,000 lux—in order for that thirty minutes' worth of exposure to do the trick. (On an overcast day, it's much less bright out—often only about 1000 lux—so you'd need at least a few hours of exposure to such dim lighting to achieve the same clinical effect.)

Getting your bright light exposure the natural way (that is, by spending time outside) has some clear advantages. For example, we're all hardwired to find outdoor settings appealing, since our bodies and brains are still adapted to the Stone Age—a time when people were immersed in nature 24/7. Researchers have discovered that people all over the world generally prefer the beauty of nature to any man-made creations. And mere exposure to a natural setting—especially the sights and sounds of the great outdoors—can lower stress hormone levels and reduce feelings of anxiety. This holds true even when we're only enjoying the "natural setting" of an urban park or a suburban backyard.

An additional advantage of light exposure outside: We can easily combine it with other antidepressant lifestyle elements like exercise and social interaction. Some of my patients, for example, have scheduled weekly meetings with their friends at restaurants that offer outdoor seating. Likewise, others now combine their bright light exposure and aerobic exercise by taking a brisk thirty-minute walk each morning.

The light box, on the other hand, has two clear advantages of its own: It's reliable and it's convenient. As long as you have access to a power supply, it will give you all the bright light you need at the flick of a switch.

Of course, if you're lucky enough to live in a sun-drenched locale—someplace where you can count on access to sunlight year round—

you can probably do without a light box. Simply going outside each day will be the best way to get your bright light fix.

Many of us, though, don't have that luxury: We live in places where sunny days are sometimes few and far between. Here in Kansas,* for example, my wife and daughter and I endure long stretches of overcast weather each winter. There are some weeks when we might not see the sun at all!

If you live in such a less-than-hospitable clime, you have three options for making sure you can always get an antidepressant dose of light, especially during the harshest months of the year. You can move someplace sunnier; you can spend at least two hours outside on every dim, overcast day (no matter how cold or rainy it might be out); or you can buy a light box. Since most people will find the first two options undesirable or impractical (or both), a light box can be essential to have on hand for those days when we lack access to natural sunlight.

Thinking Inside the Box

A few different light box technologies are now available. In this section we review the two most promising.

10,000 lux box. By far the most widely researched type of light box for depression—and the one I've employed in my studies—involves the use of *fluorescent* bulbs to provide 10,000 lux of white light.† In essence, this simulates the brightness of a sunny morning. Because

* We live in the college town of Lawrence, just outside Kansas City.

† It's also known as *broad-spectrum* light, since white light includes all the colors of the visible light spectrum.

we know this technology works—numerous studies back it up—it's the one I recommend.

Even if you go this route, you'll still have an important choice to make because there are dozens of different fluorescent light boxes on the market. They vary quite a bit by size, weight, design quality, and price.

As you might imagine, these boxes can be expensive—ranging from $100 to well over $500, so cost can be a big consideration. But as we saw in the case of fish oil supplements, some of the least expensive products are also among the best.

One of the most important features to look for in a light box is an adjustable stand, which allows you to position the box slightly overhead, with the light shining down on your eyes from above—just as the sun does when you're outside. This positioning provides the best possible angle for stimulating the eyes' specialized light sensors.

It's also helpful to keep in mind that some fluorescent lights flicker, causing potential eyestrain and headache. I recommend looking for a box that uses flicker-free technology. (One adjustable, flicker-free light box that my patients rave about is the *Day-Light DL930* by Uplift Technologies, which at the time of this writing is available from Amazon.com for less than $150.)

Blue-spectrum box. A hot new entry onto the light therapy scene is the *blue-spectrum* box. Because the eyes' light sensors respond best to light on the blue end of the spectrum, it doesn't take a lot of blue light to reset the body clock: About 400 lux seems to be enough to get the job done. That's twenty-five times less light than you need with a fluorescent (white light) box, which allows manufacturers to put out a much smaller, lighter box.

But researchers have only recently begun to test the effectiveness of blue light boxes in treating depression. Although the evidence so far is promising, at this point the jury's still out. And there's also a potential health concern to keep in mind. Blue light turns out to be hard on the retina,* and there's evidence that it might not be good for that part of the eye. (Since pure blue light doesn't occur in nature, it's not far-fetched to think the eyes might have trouble with it.) So, until this safety concern is adequately addressed—and until there's more solid evidence that blue light boxes truly work in treating depression—I suggest you stick with the tried-and-true fluorescent light box technology for the time being.

Light box tips. Here are a few additional points to keep in mind for getting the most out of your light box:

- It's best if you can set the box up about six inches or so *above eye level.*
- If possible, position the box so it's centered in front of you, not off to one side.
- Light boxes usually work best when they're positioned about eighteen to twenty-four inches from your eyes. But there's an interesting tradeoff when it comes to distance. The farther away the box is, the more it will reach every part of your eyes (a good thing) but the lower the number of lux it will deliver (not so good). Most high-quality boxes can deliver 10,000 lux at a distance of at least eighteen inches, but some boxes need to be a bit closer. (The product insert will tell you just how close you need to be to receive 10,000 lux.) However, positioning the box any closer than twelve inches can cause uncomfortable eyestrain.
- Never stare directly at the box itself. It will be far too bright, and very hard on the eyes. Instead, fix your gaze on something

* The retina contains the light-sensitive cells lining the back of the eye.

in front of you—a computer screen, a book, a newspaper, a conversation partner—with the light shining down into your eyes from above.

- If you can't position the box above you for some reason, it will still work okay if you locate it slightly off to your side—as long as it's still facing you from the front. But make sure to keep things balanced by switching sides (from your left to right or vice versa) halfway through the exposure period.

BRIGHT LIGHT EXPOSURE: TIMING

The single most important thing to keep in mind with bright light exposure is that *it has to happen at the right time of day.* Although that "right time" will be in the morning for most people, some will benefit more from light exposure in the afternoon or evening. More than anything, finding the ideal time depends on your current sleep habits. Please take a moment to see which one of the following four sleep patterns most closely matches your own:

- *Late shift:* You experience morning sluggishness, with difficulty waking up on time; you usually have trouble falling asleep at night as well. People with this pattern often find their bedtime drifting later and later, as they stay up to the point of exhaustion so they can fall asleep. They're sometimes able to sleep ten or more hours and still feel tired.
- *Early shift:* You have little trouble falling asleep, but have a tendency to wake up way too early in the morning. Often, people with this pattern are awake at least two hours before their desired wake-up time, but are unable to go back to sleep.

- *Fragmented sleep:* You wake up frequently throughout the night, with no obvious time pattern to the awakenings.
- *Healthy sleep:* You have little trouble falling asleep, staying asleep, or getting up in the morning.

In this section we describe light exposure guidelines for each of these basic sleep patterns.

Late Shift

About 80% of people with the winter blues experience a *late shift* sleep pattern: Their body clock has slowed down and needs to be reset to an earlier time. All it usually takes is thirty minutes of bright light exposure soon after waking up each morning—ideally, within the first hour upon waking. But it's important for the light exposure to occur at about the same time every day, which means you'll need to keep roughly the same wake-up time each morning, even on the weekends.

Let's say, for example, that you normally stumble out of bed at 7:30 on weekdays (after hitting the snooze button on your alarm clock several times). On the weekends, however, you sleep in past noon. In this scenario, you'd have to begin your light exposure each morning by no later than 8:30—even on Saturday and Sunday—because that's one hour after your usual wake-up time.

Most of my patients with this late shift pattern have opted to sit in front of a light box at home for a half hour soon after getting up, usually while eating breakfast or reading the newspaper. Others have enjoyed sitting outside on a patio or deck in the morning when it's nice and sunny out.

Of course, you may have to start waking up a little earlier to make room for a thirty-minute block of light exposure in your morning routine. Then again, you might have a work setting that allows you to sit in front of a light box at your desk. (Many people like to set up the light box right next to their computer monitor.) In that case, you could keep your normal wake-up time, as long as you're able to begin the light exposure at work within an hour or so of getting up.

Within a week, most people start noticing at least some benefit from the light exposure. They often experience less trouble falling asleep at night, an easier time waking up in the morning, and an improvement in mood and energy throughout the day. Some people, however, need more than thirty minutes of light exposure to get good results. If you don't notice any improvement within the first week, I recommend extending the exposure time to one hour.

You may also find it helpful to get another half-hour of bright light exposure in the late afternoon, especially if you're usually dragging later in the day. However, please note that this afternoon light exposure *can't be as bright as the light you get in the morning*, or you could throw your body clock off even more. The safest approach is simply to sit twice as far away from the light box for your second exposure. Or, if you want to get that afternoon light exposure outside, you can wait until about thirty minutes before sunset to make sure it's not too bright out.

Most people with the late shift pattern gradually find their sleep returning to a regular schedule—and other depressive symptoms improving—within two to six weeks of the bright light therapy we've outlined. If you have this sort of favorable response, you can eventually cut back on the amount of bright light exposure you need each day. I'd suggest dropping the exposure time by five minutes every day until you're down to fifteen minutes—an ideal maintenance dose. (However, you may still want to get additional natural light exposure throughout the day to take advantage of its mood-boosting effect.)

Early Shift

Early shift is the most common pattern in clinical depression. If you have this problem, you probably have no trouble falling asleep at night, but you wake up far too early in the morning and find it difficult to get back to sleep. This pattern is a sign that your internal clock thinks it's much later than it really is: It needs to be reset to an earlier time.

The most effective approach is to get thirty minutes of bright light exposure in the early evening. For the first week, it's best to start the exposure five hours before your usual bedtime. So, for example, if you normally go to bed at 11:00 pm, you would begin getting bright light at 6:00 pm. Also, while you're resetting your internal clock like this, you'll need to avoid getting any bright light exposure in the morning, because such exposure can actually shift the clock in the wrong direction. This means you'll have to wear sunglasses whenever you're outside in the morning, at least until your sleep is back to normal.

After a week on this exposure schedule, some people find their sleep greatly improved. But if you're still not able to sleep through the night by then, it's best to shift your light exposure a half hour later. (In the preceding example, you'd slide the starting time from 6:00 to 6:30 pm.) Keep the new exposure time for three days, and then keep pushing the time back another half-hour later every three days until you're no longer waking up too early.

There's an important limit to bear in mind, however: Bright light exposure can't occur within two hours of bedtime, or you'll likely have trouble falling asleep at night. But what if you've pushed your light exposure time all the way back to that two-hour threshold and you're still not sleeping through the night (or seeing improvement in other depressive symptoms)? If that's the case, you can try extending your exposure time from thirty minutes to sixty minutes for a few additional weeks. There's a good chance that will help.

After you've reestablished a healthy pattern of sleep and maintained it for a month, you can start slowly cutting back the late light exposure. But it's best not to quit cold turkey, or you could end up with a rebound effect that can make your symptoms return. Instead, taper off gradually, reducing the exposure amount by five minutes each day until you're down to a duration of fifteen minutes. You can then shift to a maintenance schedule of fifteen minutes of exposure in the morning.

Fragmented Sleep

Some people have fragmented sleep—waking up frequently throughout the night—but they have no obvious pattern to the wakenings that could indicate a major shift in their body clock.* If you're in this category, you may still benefit from bright light exposure. It can actually strengthen activity in the brain circuits that signal a need for sleep, which can in turn make your sleep deeper and more restful through-

* In other words, they're neither waking up way too early nor finding it impossible to fall asleep at a regular time each night.

out the night. In addition, the bright light can have an antidepressant effect by boosting serotonin function in the brain.

With a fragmented sleep pattern, it's best to get your bright light exposure in the morning. But you don't want to start too early or you could wind up accidentally shifting your body clock ahead—causing you to start getting drowsy too early at night and waking up too early in the morning. Accordingly, I recommend waiting a half-hour to an hour after your normal wake-up time.

Start with thirty minutes of exposure for two weeks, and then take stock of your sleep quality. If you're still experiencing fragmented sleep, try increasing the duration of morning light exposure to sixty minutes. (After your sleep quality improves, you can then reduce the duration of light exposure by five minutes a day, until you reach a maintenance dose of fifteen minutes.)

Healthy Sleep

If you have a pattern of healthy sleep, fifteen minutes of bright light exposure in the morning can help make sure that it stays that way. It's best to wait at least a half hour after your normal wake-up time, but to get the exposure within two hours of awakening.

There's one exception to this guideline, however. If you have symptoms of depression—which is rare (but not unheard of) among people with healthy sleep—you'll benefit from a full thirty minutes of bright light in the morning for its antidepressant effect. After two weeks, if you're still not seeing any improvement in your depressive symptoms, you can extend the exposure time to sixty minutes. (Some people need a full hour of bright light exposure to trigger an antidepressant increase in serotonin function.)

FREQUENTLY ASKED QUESTIONS

Now that we've covered the basics of bright light exposure, we can address some of the questions people commonly have about it.

1. Should I check with my doctor before using a light box? Researchers have found light boxes to be safe for the vast majority of people who use them.* Nevertheless, it's always a good idea to check with your doctor before starting any new treatment that can affect your body.

A few medical conditions, especially eye problems, can be made worse by a light box. It's definitely *not* recommended for use by anyone with a serious eye disorder such as macular degeneration, retinopathy, or retinitis pigmentosa. Likewise, you should avoid using a light box if you have extreme light sensitivity, even the temporary kind caused by a medication.

In addition, if you have bipolar disorder (formerly known as *manic depression*), you should never start light therapy except under a clinicians direct supervision, because bright light can occasionally trigger an episode of mania† in vulnerable individuals. Similarly, if you have a seizure disorder, there's a very small risk that a light box could cause an epileptic reaction, so you should consult with your doctor before using one.

Finally, many people with diabetes experience eye complications along with the disease itself. So if you're diabetic, it's recommended

---

* These devices have been evaluated with thousands of patients across many different studies.

† Mania is a condition marked by elevated mood, impulsiveness, reckless behavior, racing thoughts (and feeling "sped up"), distractibility, irritability, and a decreased need for sleep.

that you talk with a physician about whether or not a light box would be safe for you.

2. Are there any other possible side effects of using a light box? Most people experience no side effects. Of the many patients we've treated in our TLC research, no one has ever reported any. However, it's possible that you could have some eye irritation (especially burning or itching sensations), headache, or mild nausea the first few times you try a light box. All of these annoyances usually clear up within several days as your eyes adjust to the device, so it's important to stick with it if you can. You can also move the box farther away—double your original distance—to see if that helps, and then gradually move it back toward its original location. If that doesn't work, try reducing your daily exposure to five minutes, and then increase it by a few minutes each day until you get back to the full (original) exposure time.

3. Is there ever a risk of getting too much bright light? As you'll recall, bright light stimulates serotonin activity in the brain. While that's usually a good thing, some people produce too much serotonin after extended light exposure. That can lead to nervousness, jitteriness, or nausea. If this happens to you, it's a good idea to stop the light exposure until you talk with a clinician about how to slowly build back up to a level you can tolerate.

Another possible effect is a shift in your body clock. With excessive morning light, you may find yourself waking up too early and getting drowsy too early at night. If that happens, it's a good idea to cut your light exposure time in half, and to shift it to an hour later, as well.

The same type of problem can be seen in reverse with too much light exposure in the early evening, which can make it harder to fall asleep at night. In that case, you would want to cut your light exposure time and schedule your exposure at least an hour earlier.

4. Can I get enough morning light exposure when I'm driving to work? It's possible, but conditions outside have to be just right. For example, it's not very bright out at sunrise—only 400 lux—and it doesn't usually reach 10,000 lux until about forty minutes later. Even then, it still won't be bright enough inside your vehicle, because the tinted glass cuts your light exposure by about 50%. This means you'd need to wait until the brightness reaches 20,000 lux, and it doesn't get that bright until about an hour after sunrise on a crisp, sunny day.

Similar considerations apply if you're trying to get late afternoon or evening sunlight during your drive home from work: Within an hour or so of sunset, the brightness will dip below 10,000 lux inside your car.

Also, please remember: If you have the late shift sleep pattern, you need to avoid bright light exposure in the late afternoon and early evening, so you should wear sunglasses for your evening commute if it's still very bright out. Likewise, if you have the early shift pattern, you'll need to avoid bright light in the early morning; you may need to wear sunglasses for your drive in to work.

5. I've seen ads for full-spectrum light bulbs that are supposed to mimic sunlight. Will they work just as well as a regular light box? *Full spectrum* simply means the light includes all the colors of the visible spectrum, along with invisible forms of light such as infrared and ultraviolet. But most full-spectrum bulbs fall far below the target brightness level—10,000 lux—that's been shown to have an antidepressant effect in carefully controlled research. And even if you could find a full-spectrum light box that puts out 10,000 lux, there's still no evidence that full-spectrum light is any better than regular white light* (the kind used in most light boxes) when it comes to treating depression.

6. I'm supposed to get light exposure in the morning, but I missed out on it today because I was running late. Is it better to try to make up for it later in the day or just wait until tomorrow? When you miss your scheduled light exposure, it's usually better to make up for it later in the day, as this will still allow you to get the mood-elevating benefit of increased serotonin activity in the brain. However, if you're supposed to get your light exposure in the morning, it's important not to wait too late in the day before you begin. (Evening light exposure can throw off your internal clock and cause you to have trouble falling asleep when you turn in for the night.) If possible, try to complete your light exposure within five hours of your bedtime; if you can't, it's generally better to wait until the next morning instead.

7. I've heard that some people are particularly sensitive to the effects of bright light. Is there any truth to that? Yes. People with fair skin and blue eyes sometimes require less light exposure than others to achieve the same effects. If you have very fair features, you may be able to adjust downward by about 30% all the recommended exposure times in this chapter. For example, where I've suggested thirty minutes of light exposure, you can try it with only twenty minutes. Likewise, instead of a recommended fifteen minutes, try ten. If you don't see adequate results with those briefer exposures, you can always go back to the original suggested times.

---

* Regular white light is sometimes called *broad spectrum light*. (Not surprisingly, people often confuse it with *full spectrum light*.)

8. I like to use a tanning bed in the winter, and I know it makes me feel better. Am I getting enough light exposure just by tanning? No, you can get enough light exposure only when you keep your eyes *open*, and it's definitely advisable to have one's eyes closed inside a tanning bed.

Still, there is something to the claim that tanning boosts mood, despite the fact that dermatologists commonly warn against the practice (and for good reason, because it can age your skin and increase the risk of some forms of cancer). Of course, much of the mood-elevating effect of tanning rests on basic psychology: If you feel better about yourself with a tan, seeing your skin newly aglow might put a bounce in your step. But some people also get a rush of endorphins—the body's natural feel-good chemicals—while tanning, and that can induce a pleasant, relaxed sense of well-being. Finally, tanning increases exposure to ultraviolet light, which causes the skin to start making vitamin D. As we'll review in the chapter's final section, vitamin D can also have a potent antidepressant effect.

THE D PRESCRIPTION

Vitamin D is absolutely essential for life. We'd all be dead without it. It isn't even a proper vitamin at all: Vitamin D is a *hormone*, one of the most important ones ever discovered. A chemical key, it unlocks hundreds of genes that control the day-to-day functioning of your brain, heart, immune cells, bones, skin, nerves, and blood vessels. In fact, a vitamin D deficiency can induce an extraordinary range of health problems. Rickets—a disorder that causes children's bones to grow weak, brittle, and misshapen—is the one most people know about. But scientists have recently linked vitamin D deficits to an array of much more common diseases* ranging from multiple sclerosis to colon cancer to atherosclerosis to Crohn's disease—to depression.

On average, depressed patients have perilously low blood levels of vitamin D. Supplementation, however, has been shown to lift mood among those with deficiencies. In one recent clinical trial, giving SAD patients just a single vitamin D megadose—two hundred fifty times higher than the amount in your multivitamin—was found to have a large antidepressant effect.

How does vitamin D fight depression? In part, the effect follows from the nutrient's role in regulating gene function in the brain and other vital organ systems. But vitamin D also has a powerful anti-inflammatory effect throughout the body. This is important because—as you'll recall from Chapter 5—chronic inflammation is a major culprit in depression; it interferes with serotonin function and shuts down activity in key brain regions. Accordingly, vitamin D's anti-inflammatory properties turn out to be antidepressant, as well.

Because Vitamin D is such a crucial hormone, our bodies are endowed with the ability to make all we need. But it takes a little sunshine to get the process going. Basically, when the sun's ultraviolet (UV) rays† penetrate the skin, they kick off a chain reaction that converts cholesterol (of all things) into vitamin D. It's an efficient procedure, and most of us can get an entire day's supply with a bit of midday sun exposure, except in the winter.

Our hunter-gatherer ancestors never had to worry about getting enough vitamin D, because they spent hours in direct sunlight each day. And those who lived in more northerly climes—where the sun

* Vitamin D deficiency is not the only cause of these diseases, but it contributes to the risk of contracting them.

† These are the same UV rays that stimulate melanin production and cause us to tan.

wasn't strong enough to make vitamin D in the winter—simply stored in their bodies all the excess they made during the summer and fall, so they had enough to last all year.

But vitamin D deficiency is a big problem today throughout the industrialized world. Over half of the U.S. population is now deficient at the end of each winter, and many people have perilously low levels all year long. Interestingly, the well-intentioned, widespread practice of fortifying milk and dairy products with vitamin D hasn't protected us the way it was supposed to. For one thing, people aren't drinking nearly as much milk as they did in the past; and there isn't a great deal of vitamin D in milk to begin with. More importantly, the molecular version that's widely used in milk—vitamin D_2 (*ergocalciferol*)—isn't the same as the version made by our bodies. We need vitamin D_3 (*cholecalciferol*), and much of the D_2 we get from milk (and from some other supplements) is simply unusable.

How, then, can you make sure you're getting enough vitamin D to keep your brain and body in good working order? There are two main possibilities worth exploring: taking a high-dose supplement of vitamin D_3, or spending a little time in the sun on a regular basis. We'll briefly address each option.

Vitamin D Supplement

If you take a multivitamin, the chances are it will contain 10 mcg of vitamin D—the EU RDA (recommended daily allowance). But, as we now know, vitamin D has dozens of other critical roles in the body (beyond ensuring healthy bone development), and it takes a lot more than 10 mcg each day to get the job done on these other fronts.

A group of Canadian medical researchers recently tried to find out just how much more. They recruited volunteers from their own hospital, and measured everyone's blood levels of vitamin D during the dead of winter. Most people, of course, were deficient. So the human guinea pigs were randomly assigned to start taking either 25 mcg or 100 mcg of vitamin D_3 each day. Surprisingly, even after a few months, many people taking 25 mcg a day—two and a half times the recommended amount—still didn't get their blood levels up high enough. It took 100 mcg a day—for a period of up to three months—to bring everyone up into the ideal range.

Doctors can get skittish, though, when you starting talking about such a large daily dose of vitamin D. The biggest worry is that it might throw off your calcium balance, since vitamin D helps regulate the body's ability to use this key mineral. However, no one in the Canadian study had any calcium-related problems (or any other adverse health effects) at the 100 mcg dose. Even more reassuring, a study last year looked at a group of multiple sclerosis patients taking *1000 mcg of vitamin* D_3 *every day* (one hundred times the recommended daily allowance), and none of them had any adverse medical effects, either.

Still, the official medical *tolerable upper intake level* for vitamin D, published by the Institute of Medicine in 1997, is listed at only 50 mcg per day. Anything above this level is considered potentially unsafe. Although numerous researchers in the area say this recommendation is outdated—that the tolerable limit should be raised—doctors are understandably reluctant to practice outside the field's official guidelines.

So what should you do if you want to go the supplement route to make sure you have enough vitamin D? I'm afraid there's no perfect solution, but you at least have some decent options.

The simplest approach is to start by taking 50 mcg of vitamin D_3 in supplement form each day. (You can pick up a couple months' supply at a local health food store for a few dollars.) This dose is high enough to push most people up into the ideal range for vitamin D blood levels. However, because the dose is also right at the tolerable upper intake level, it's important to check with your doctor before starting on such a high-dose regimen. In addition, after a few months of supplementing at this dose, it would be a good idea to have your doctor do a blood test to make sure you're actually getting *enough*. According to the best published evidence, your blood level of vitamin D* should be at least as high as 30 ng/mL (or 75 nmol/L) for optimal health.

A more aggressive approach—but one you should definitely consider if you're currently depressed, or if you have a history of seasonal affective disorder—is to see your doctor right away to have your blood level of vitamin D evaluated. If it's very low (below 15 ng/mL or 37 nmol/L), you can talk with your doctor about taking a high dose of vitamin D_3—up to 250 mcg per day—for several weeks under his or her supervision, with regular monitoring to make sure there are no side effects, and to ensure that your blood levels make it quickly into a healthier range.

Sun Exposure

The other option is to let your body make enough vitamin D on its own, with an assist from the sun. It's an approach that many will still find attractive, and there's even some research evidence that the body

---

* It's measured in a molecular form called 25(OH)D.

can use its own natural vitamin D more effectively than the kind we get from a supplement.

How much sun exposure does your body need each day to make enough vitamin D? The answer depends on several factors: the time of day, the time of year, local weather conditions (how cloudy it is), where you live (how far north or south), and your complexion (how fair or dark-skinned). As a rule of thumb, adequate vitamin D synthesis takes about the same amount of sun exposure that's required to develop the faintest hint of a tan (or to turn your skin ever-so-slightly darker).

Let's start with an optimal exposure scenario, the one that would take the least amount of time. A person with fair skin in a swimsuit would get a full day's supply of vitamin D in about two minutes on a sunny midday in the summertime in Miami. But as we start tweaking parameters (time of day, season, complexion, clothing, and location), the required exposure time changes. Finding the exact time needed on any given day can get complicated, but there are three easy guidelines you can follow:

- In the continental United States and Europe, your body should make enough vitamin D from May through August if you average ten to fifteen minutes a day of sun exposure between 11:00 in the morning and 3:00 in the afternoon. (That's assuming you aren't wearing any sunscreen and that your arms and face are exposed.)
- In March, April, September, and October, it will probably take at least twenty to thirty minutes per day.
- If you have a dark complexion, you may need to double all recommended times.

Even at this low level of recommended sun exposure, you'll likely build up some vitamin D reserves for your body to draw on in the winter. But just to be on the safe side, it's still a good idea to supplement from November through February, as described in the previous section.

Direct sun exposure has obvious benefits, but it also comes with its inherent downsides. Not only can it age skin prematurely, but it can also elevate the risk of skin cancer (a condition that will afflict up to one in five Americans). However, while the link between sun exposure and skin cancer is strong for the experience of sunburn, there's not as much evidence of a link at the relatively low levels of exposure needed for vitamin D synthesis. In fact, the Web site of the National Institutes of Health has recently added a recommendation of ten to fifteen minutes of sun exposure (periodically) as a way most people can avoid vitamin D deficiency. Still, before scheduling any time in the sun, you should weigh the pros and cons of the issue with your doctor. Depending on your skin type, your medical history, and your family history of skin cancer, you may conclude that sun exposure isn't worth the risks—especially since viable alternatives are available. Whichever way you decide, the critical thing is to ensure that you benefit year-round from the healing, antidepressant effects of vitamin D.

8

Get Connected

Some animals are natural-born loners. Parasitic wasps, for example, can live out their entire lives without any meaningful social contact—nothing, at least, beyond a few brief bouts of mating. But we humans find isolation an unnatural state of affairs. Extended seclusion is so uncomfortable that it constitutes a form of criminal punishment.

We are literally born to connect. The drive is etched deeply into our DNA: From the first moments of life, we crave the company of others. And it's not just for the food and protection they provide. Babies even need social contact to help regulate their breathing and heart rate. They're exquisitely attuned to the biological rhythms of those around them—the ebbs and flows of respiration, heart rate, alertness, and so on—and they mimic these natural cadences to keep their own bodies in sync. That's one reason babies howl in protest when they're left alone: They instinctively know it's a recipe for biological disaster.

You might suppose that such abject dependence is something we all eventually outgrow. But we never do—at least, not completely. Even as adults, we still rely on the presence of others. When we're deprived of it for just a few days, our stress hormones escalate, mood and energy plummet, and key biological processes quickly fall out of balance. On the other hand, our bodily rhythms readily synchronize with those of others—even pets—in our immediate vicinity. (The process happens even while we're sleeping.)

Our innate dependence on others is an ancient legacy. For hundreds of thousands of years, our ancestors lived in small, intimate social bands, facing together the relentless threat of predators, the forces of nature, and hostile neighboring clans—a context in which survival was impossible apart from the support and protection of the group. Even brief periods of isolation carried overwhelming risks, to be avoided at all costs.

Such a clannish sensibility is still keenly present among modern-day foraging bands (and other traditional, pre-agrarian societies). According to anthropologists, "alone time" is virtually unknown among such groups. They spend nearly twenty-four hours a day in the company of friends and loved ones: hunting together, walking together, gathering food and water together, eating together, playing together, and sleeping together. Often, they even wander off to relieve themselves together (a smart policy in a world where predators and unfriendly neighbors might be lurking nearby).

Within such traditional societies, isolation is regarded as an obvious hardship, and those who are able to endure a few days of solitude—shamans, for example—are revered for their heroism. In the industrialized West, on the other hand, we've strayed far from this ancient sensibility. Many now find solitude to be the default mode of existence: They work alone, eat alone, recreate alone, and sleep alone. According to the latest research, nearly 25% of Americans have no intimate social connections at all, and countless others spend the bulk of their time by themselves. Because the obvious physical risks of social isolation have receded—most predators now reside on endangered species lists, after all—we've become increasingly oblivious to solitude's equally real *psychological* dangers.

As we saw in Chapter 1, isolation is a major risk factor for depression: Those who lack the benefit of meaningful social connection are highly prone to becoming depressed, especially in the face of severe life stress. And, unfortunately, once a person starts experiencing depressive symptoms, they tend to withdraw even further from the world around them. This, in turn, exacerbates the depression, sparking a vicious downward cycle of illness and seclusion that often proves difficult to break.

But why, exactly, should depression prompt social withdrawal in the first place? In large part, it's because the brain responds to depression as it does to any other serious illness, directing us to avoid activity—especially *social* activity—so the body can focus on simply getting well. This withdrawal response is triggered by a decrease of serotonin activity in the brain, which, as we addressed in Chapter 2, is one of the major features of depression. (Because the brain's serotonin levels plummet when we're fighting a serious infection, some scientists even speculate that the ensuing withdrawal response evolved to help fend off the spread of disease.)

Think about the last time you had the flu. How much did you feel like socializing? When I had a bad case of the illness a few years ago—complete with a 103-degree fever, shakes, chills, and assorted body aches—I just wanted to crawl into a hole and wait for it all to go away. That's a typical reaction. And, interestingly enough, it's similar to the way people react when they're fighting a severe episode of depression.

But there's one crucial difference: With the flu, such withdrawal helps to promote recovery—with depression it only makes things worse. So, even though depressed patients feel—right down to the core of their being—that pulling away from others is going to help, that's only because their brain has been misled. In effect, depression tricks the brain into thinking something akin to an infectious illness needs to be fought.

Tragically, the ensuing social withdrawal amplifies depression. It stands as a major obstacle on the path to recovery. Conversely, anything that enhances social connectedness—increasing either the quantity or the quality of our bonds with others—proves immensely valuable in fighting (and preventing) the disorder.

FINDING CONNECTION

Of course, increasing social connection is easier said than done. And the process raises a host of practical questions. Who's available to connect with? What should I be doing with them? Should I focus more on family or friends? What about coworkers? And what if certain people make me feel worse every time I'm around them? Am I supposed to spend more time with them, as well?

In navigating this tangled maze of questions, it helps at the outset to keep in view one critical fact: There are many varieties of social connection, and all of them are potentially helpful. For example, members of traditional societies like the Kaluli of Papua New Guinea—among whom social support is abundant, and depression virtually unknown—benefit from social ties that span multiple levels of closeness: from the deep intimacy of immediate family and friends to the comforting familiarity of extended family to the profound sense of belonging provided by membership in the clan itself (a hundred or so people linked by a shared identity and a common destiny).

Anyone lucky enough to draw upon such deep, multilayered sources of social support will be unlikely to get depressed. But such fortunate individuals are now the exception, not the rule, throughout the modern industrialized world. Sadly, the past few decades have seen the steady erosion of social bonds across every domain of American life.

Compared with our counterparts from even a generation ago, we're much less likely to know our neighbors, to invite friends over for dinner, to join social clubs, to participate in a local church or synagogue or mosque, or to take part in community sports leagues (bowling, softball, tennis, and so on). We're less likely to get married, and less likely to stay married when we do take the plunge. We also spend less time developing and maintaining friendships. According to a recent landmark study of American social life, half of all adults lack even a single close friend they can rely on.

What's happened? I believe many of us now live as if we value things more than people. In America, we spend more time than ever at work, and we earn more money than any generation in history, but we spend less and less time with our loved ones as a result. Likewise, many of us barely think twice about severing close ties with friends and family to move halfway across the country in pursuit of career advancement. We buy exorbitant houses—the square footage of the average American home has more than doubled in the past generation—but increasingly we use them only to retreat from the world. And even within the home-as-refuge, sealed off from the broader community "out there," each member of the household can often be found sitting alone in front of his or her own private screen—exchanging time with loved ones for time with a bright, shiny object instead.

Now, I'm not saying that any of us—if asked—would claim to value things more than people. Nor would we say that our loved ones aren't important to us. Of course they are. But many people now live *as if* achievement, career advancement, money, material possessions, entertainment, and status matter more. Unfortunately, such things don't confer lasting happiness, nor do they protect us from depression. Loved ones do.

For most of us in this culture of isolation, there's considerable room for improvement when it comes to enhancing social connectedness. This is especially true for those who've battled depression, because the disorder—with its characteristic pattern of withdrawal and negativity—has a corrosive effect on relationships.

In the pages that follow, we'll outline strategies for improving connections with friends, family members, coworkers, and other members of the community. The ideal, as we saw earlier in the case of the Kaluli people, is to benefit from abundant support across each of these important domains.

Achieving this ideal takes some time, and it may not be a realistic goal for everyone in the short-term, especially for those currently in the midst of a depressive episode. Fortunately, however, any improvement in social connection can be of some immediate benefit in the fight against depression, so the focus of each section ahead will be on those changes that can make a difference right away. (We'll also point out some potential longer-term goals for those who are not depressed, but still want to reduce their risk of illness in the future.)

FRIENDS

Over time, depression can take an enormous toll on friendships. When someone first becomes depressed, there's a natural tendency for friends to rally to their side—to provide increased support, and to try whatever else they can think of to help. But as the weeks pass and the symptoms persist, the illness starts to weave its toxic spell of social isolation, straining even the strongest of bonds.

For those friends who don't understand the seriousness of depression, the disorder's characteristic withdrawal can become a source of great pain and frustration. Simply put: It's hard to watch someone pulling away from you and shutting down, especially when you can't figure out why in the world it's happening.

Even friends who know that social withdrawal is a core symptom of depression may find themselves feeling rejected. After all, it's only human to feel hurt when a friend starts shutting you out—failing to return phone calls, refusing offers to get together, and sending signals about their complete lack of interest in connecting.

Ironically, those suffering from the disorder commonly feel as if they're doing their friends a favor by pulling away. My patients tell me this all the time. Under the influence of depression's starkly negative thinking, they say things like: "My friends are better off without me." "I'm such a downer to be around, no one could possibly want to spend time with me." "They're only calling me out of pity." Even though such thoughts may be wildly distorted and off-the-mark (as they are in the vast majority of cases), such perceptions still feel true to the person in the grip of depressive illness.

It's little wonder, then, that most patients withdraw from even their dearest, closest friends—with predictably tragic results. Fortunately, however, it's almost always possible to turn things around, to renew the bonds of friendship, no matter how much depression may have strained a relationship. In my clinical experience, the following steps usually prove helpful in that respect.

Disclose. Because of the lingering stigma associated with depression, many people are reluctant to let even their closest friends know about their struggle with the illness. It's understandable: No one wants to risk being viewed as "crazy" (or weak, or lazy, or any number of other qualities mistakenly attributed to those suffering from depression). But I believe our friends have a right to know what we're going through, especially when we're facing a treacherous enemy like depression. Honest disclosure about our struggles is essential to maintaining (or reestablishing) the health of any friendship.

Educate. Often, however, mere disclosure is not enough. Many friends need to be educated about depression as well. In particular, they have to understand three things: Depression is an illness—one that robs people of their ability to function; like many other forms of illness, depression typically leads its victims to withdraw from friends and loved ones; nevertheless, social support can play an important role in the recovery process. It's also often useful to ask friends to read a good overview* of the disorder that covers these points in some detail.

Ask. Many of us find it difficult to ask for help, even from our closest friends. But depression is such a serious affliction that most people are eager to do whatever they can for a friend who's been laid low. When I speak about depression in the community, the most common question I get is, "What can I do to help someone who's fighting this illness?"

The most useful thing, by far, is to spend regular time together in shared activities: walking, working out, grabbing a meal, playing games, going to a concert, attending a play, watching a film, and so on. As we saw in Chapter 5, such activities are especially effective in combating depressive rumination. They also help to reactivate

---

* Peter Kramer's *Against Depression* provides a superb comprehensive summary. Chapter 2 of this book also includes a brief overview of the disorder.

the brain's left frontal cortex, which itself provides a direct antidepressant effect. Accordingly, in our Therapeutic Lifestyle Change (TLC) groups, each patient is asked to adopt the goal of scheduling at least three such activities each week with friends or other close acquaintances.

Jamie, a fortyish real estate agent in one of our TLC groups, was intimidated by this goal, but she told us she was willing—despite her fear of rejection—to start by calling her best friend Deb (whom she hadn't seen in weeks) to see if she might want to get together sometime. With trepidation, she began the conversation by telling Deb some of the things she'd learned in treatment: that depression had caused her to withdraw, that her isolation was making the depression worse, and that she needed help from friends and loved ones to break the destructive pattern of withdrawal. To Jamie's immense relief, her friend told her, "Look, I'm here for you—for anything you need, and I'm so glad there's something I can do that might help." Before hanging up, they penciled a weekly lunch date into their calendars, and even made plans to hit a karaoke bar together that weekend.

Jamie also asked Deb for help *initiating* their future get-togethers. As we've seen, depression shuts down activity in those areas of the brain that allow us to initiate things. So, good intentions, including the plan to spend more time with friends, don't always get translated into action. Acknowledging this point openly with her friend, Jamie told her, "I really want us to get together more often, but because of the depression, I might have trouble taking the initiative sometimes. Would you be willing to stay on me about it—to call me anytime you haven't heard from me in a while, and to insist that we set something up?" Predictably, her friend was more than willing to help on this front, as well.

Avoid negativity. Under the bleak spell of depression, people's thoughts often turn starkly negative, even when they're in the company of friends. Although sharing such dark thoughts might seem like a natural thing to do, excessive disclosure on this front can quickly turn counterproductive. Remember, spending time with others is helpful in part because it's a powerful way to interrupt rumination—the depressive habit of dwelling on upsetting thoughts—but it can do so only if the social interaction centers on something other than the depressing thoughts themselves. Unfortunately, the process of sharing negative reflections with friends can easily lead to a full-blown episode of rumination.

Consider the following dialogue, based on a conversation one of my patients, Becky, had while meeting with her friend Joan (after several weeks of self-imposed isolation):

Joan: It's so good to see you. I've really missed you, you know?

Becky: Yeah, I've missed you, too. (*Awkward pause.*) God, I'm such a mess right now—I can't even make small talk. I'm just not much fun to be around.

Joan: Hey, come on. You know that's not true. And besides, we all go through rough patches sometimes. That's when we need our friends the most, right?

Becky: I guess so. But I just hate being such a burden to people all the time . . .

Joan: What are you talking about? Becky, you're not a burden.

Becky: I'd probably say the same thing if I were you. But no one wants to be around someone who's like this. I mean, look at me. I feel like crap, I'm cranky as hell, and my mind doesn't even work right half the time. (*She starts crying softly.*)

Joan: (*Holds her hand reassuringly.*) Look, I'm sorry you're going through such a hard time right now, but I want you to know I'm here for you.

Becky: Even though I'm ruining your whole day?

Joan: Becky, that's crazy! You're not ruining my day.

Becky: (*Sighs*) Well, you sound kind of irritated . . . I guess I don't blame you.

Joan: No, I'm not irritated, I'm just—it's just hard to see you being so tough on yourself.

Becky: I'm sorry. I don't mean to be so hard to be around. That's the only thing I'm really good at right now—making people upset. I knew it was a bad idea for me to come over . . .

Notice that the more Becky gave voice to her negative thoughts, the more she was unable to turn her attention away from them, despite her friend's reassuring attempts to help her see things in a more positive light. Sadly, once a conversation takes this sort of ruminative turn, it can be difficult to prevent the ensuing downward spiral. That's why it's usually a good idea to rein in the impulse to give voice to negative thoughts, and to plan social interactions as much as possible around shared activities instead.

(Becky discovered the wisdom of this approach for herself during her next social get-together with Joan—a night of country line dancing. Even though she told me beforehand how much she had dreaded going out, she later conceded that the outing was more fun than anything she'd done in months.)

Another dangerous trap to avoid with friends and loved ones is excessive *reassurance seeking*. Although the quest for reassurance can sometimes take the form of a direct question ("Do you really want to spend time with me?"), in many cases it's more subtle: putting oneself down in order to hear the reassurance that reliably follows. For example, every time Becky beat herself up—"I'm not much fun to be around"; "I hate being such a burden"; "I'm ruining your day"—her friend responded with words of support and encouragement. Such reassurance can be addictive, especially for someone who's already feeling insecure (as most depressed patients are), and it can "program" people to become even tougher on themselves. (It's not a conscious strategy on their part, by the way; those with depression are not consciously thinking, "I'll criticize myself so people will say nice things about me"—but the reliable connection between self-criticism and reassurance registers with the brain, which often guides future behavior on an unconscious level.)

Sadly, the reassurance of others rarely make things any better: The positive feedback clashes so sharply with the depressed individual's negative self-view that it's dismissed almost immediately. Ironically, the best way to combat depressive feelings of insecurity is often to ignore them, to divert attention instead to more engaging social activities that have the power to lift mood and shift the brain into a less negative mode of thinking.

FRIENDS AT A DISTANCE

During one of our very first Therapeutic Lifestyle Change groups, I asked each patient to write down a list of all the people they felt the closest to, no matter how far away (geographically) they happened to be. Not surprisingly, given our highly transient society, every single patient said some of their dearest friends lived hundreds (or thousands) of miles away.

I also learned that most of them were rarely in touch with their faraway friends, despite the deep feelings of affection that remained. It was as if the imposing physical distance had somehow ruled out the possibility of keeping such relationships alive in the present. But as my patients and I thought this through, we realized that it didn't have to be that way, especially in the age of cheap long-distance phone rates and high-speed Internet connections.

So I asked them to identify at least three people they still felt close to in spite of geographic separation—childhood friends, college buddies, long-lost cousins, old roommates, former coworkers, erstwhile neighbors, and so on—and to schedule time in their calendars to contact them within the following week. There was a surprising amount of enthusiasm for the idea. It did, however, raise some important questions:

- *Should I tell them about my depression?* ("Yes," I said, "by all means.")
- *How much can I talk about my problems before it turns into rumination?* ("It's probably helpful to briefly describe what you've been going through, but then try shifting the focus to the things you're doing to get better. That should serve as a safeguard against excessively dwelling on the negative.")
- *What else should I talk with them about?* (My response was, "Pretty much anything that doesn't lead to rumination. You can reminisce about good times you shared together in the past; ask to hear in detail what they've been up to; talk about common interests; get updates on mutual friends and acquaintances; and so on.")

In most cases, my patients have found it enormously helpful to reconnect with their old friends like this. They've usually been pleased to discover how easily they're able to pick things back up where they'd left off, and how much they enjoyed the process. And many have had old friends open up to them about their own battles with depression and other painful experiences life had thrown their way. As a result, my patients have often been able to provide as much support and encouragement as they've received, and they've experienced the deep satisfaction that comes from helping a loved one in need.

Video chats. With the advent of free computer software like Skype,* the Internet now makes it possible to have virtual face-to-face chats—through videoconferencing—with old friends (and just about anyone else on the planet). All that's needed is a video camera—available for less than $40—and a reasonably fast Internet connection.

Because we humans are such a highly visual species—with much of the brain's cortex devoted to vision—we're designed to get much more out of a conversation when we can see the person we're talking with. Not surprisingly, then, it's even easier to feel close to a friend during a video chat than it is during a regular phone call.

Internet friends. It's also now possible—through Internet chat rooms and forums—to forge meaningful friendships with strangers online. For example, my friend Linda recently endured a painful battle with anorexia, and in her search for friends who could truly understand what she was going through, she stumbled onto several virtual communities on the Internet—forums where hundreds of other women gathered to share their struggles with eating disorders, and to offer one another words of support and encouragement. Linda credits her online friends with playing a major role in her eventual recovery, even though she's never met a single one of them in person.

---

* You can download Skype at www.skype.com.

Dozens of such virtual communities are now available to those suffering from depression—places where fellow-travelers on the path to recovery gather to chat and encourage one another on a 24/7 basis. Some of the more popular sites at the time of this writing are depressionforums.org, healingwell.com, and beatingthebeast.com.

TOXIC RELATIONSHIPS

In my clinical experience, most friends and loved ones are eager to help facilitate healing from depression in any way they can. But there are some important exceptions: toxic relationships that stand as major obstacles on the path to recovery.

In some cases, the harmful influence of others is unintentional. For example, psychologists have documented a powerful effect of emotional contagion: the spreading of our emotional states to others, just as we might transmit a cold or flu bug. When two friends or loved ones are fighting depression at the same time, they can inadvertently ramp up the intensity of each other's sadness just by spending time together. This process is especially common in marriage, and it helps to explain why the risk of getting depressed goes up for anyone whose spouse is fighting the illness.

Please bear in mind, however, that such emotional contagion isn't inevitable. It can be prevented, even when you're spending lots of time with someone who's severely depressed. But both parties have to avoid the temptation of dwelling on their negative thoughts together, since joint rumination is a particularly damaging process in depression. So, you'll probably need to set firm limits in advance when you're talking about one another's problems, sharing disappointments, airing complaints, and so on. I'd suggest a time limit of five minutes of verbal negativity per interaction.

Interestingly, after they learn about the process of emotional contagion, my depressed patients often start to worry about *me*—fearing they'll somehow "infect" me with despair, and cause me to lose my emotional balance. It's a touching concern, but it turns out to be unnecessary. You see, emotional contagion works in both directions: It can spread *positive* moods just as readily as negative ones. So, believe it or not, I always look forward to spending time with my patients, including those still in the depths of despair, because it provides an opportunity to help infect them with an authentic sense of hope about their eventual recovery.

If you're currently struggling with depression, I encourage you to put the power of positive emotional contagion to work for you. You might, for example, write out a list of the people you know—even casual acquaintances—who are consistently upbeat and sunny, and make a deliberate effort to start spending more time in their company. If no one in your life fits the bill right now, a good psychotherapist could even play that role for you on a weekly basis.

Conversely, you may need to limit the amount of time you spend with those whose negativity consistently rubs off on you. Again, it's not that you should avoid interacting with others just because they happen to be depressed. But it *will* be important, if you do spend time with someone who's blue, to steer most of your time with them toward upbeat activities and conversations.

Toxic Beyond Repair

Although many unhealthy relationships can be improved with some effort, others are so destructive they make recovery impossible. For example, I have a friend, Karen, who found herself in a horrifically abusive relationship while she was struggling to heal from severe depression some years ago. Although she had already put many of the principles of Therapeutic Lifestyle Change into practice, the toxic impact of her boyfriend's relentless emotional and physical abuse kept her brain locked in a depressive runaway stress response. Yet, because she loved him, she found it impossible to simply let go and walk away. She hung on for months—telling herself that he would change, that she couldn't live without him, that things weren't really that bad—until her growing desperation finally brought about an epiphany: The relationship, by perpetuating her depression, was slowly killing her. In a genuine act of courage, with the support and encouragement of her therapist, pastor, and loved ones, she cut off all contact with him and—despite the searing pain of separation—gradually found her way back to health. (She's now happily raising boisterous twin boys, and working to help others combat the depressive illness that almost took her own life.)

Likewise, I worked a few years ago with a twenty-one-year-old college student, Annie, who hung out with a clique in her sorority that could have come straight out of the movie *Mean Girls*—a group of snobbish, hypercritical elitists who tortured one another with impossibly high standards of physical beauty, status, wealth, and style. Although Annie was a sweet young woman, her deep insecurity caused her to find these girls irresistible, as she desperately wanted to win their acceptance and approval—which, of course, never came. Week after week, she told me how everyone in the clique made her "feel like crap," and yet she continued spending all her free time with them. She also wondered why her depressive symptoms—while greatly improved since she began treatment—never completely cleared up.

So I asked her a simple question. "Annie, are there any other girls in your sorority who make you feel good about yourself when you're around them—people who accept you for who you are?"

"I guess so," she said. Then she rattled off a list of a half-dozen names.

"And how much time do you spend with these girls, the ones who make you feel good about yourself?"

Annie started laughing. "Pretty much none."

"Does that make sense to you?" I asked. "I mean, does it make sense that you'd spend all your time with girls who criticize you, who don't even seem to care about you, and then ignore these other girls who actually like you? Can you help me understand that?"

"It sounds crazy when you put it like that. But it's like I just don't care as much what people think about me when they're really nice to everyone. It's like it doesn't count then, or something."

"Okay, that makes sense," I reassured her. "But I wonder what would happen to your mood if you started limiting your time with these 'toxic friends' of yours, and started spending time instead with girls who accept you for who you are. Do you think it would make a difference with your depression?"

She shrugged, and then did her best to change the subject. Clearly, she didn't want to go there. I wasn't at all surprised, since toxic relationships are usually hard to let go of, no matter how destructive they might be. They hold out the tantalizing promise of something desirable—love, acceptance, approval, protection—even though they never really deliver. In Annie's case, it took her two full months to finally admit to herself that the "mean girls" were the main source of depressive stress in her life, and to recognize that she would never gain their approval, no matter how hard she tried. Following this tearful revelation, she was finally ready to start limiting her contact with these girls. And that, in turn, freed her to begin connecting with others who genuinely appreciated her, to start forming a new set of healthy, authentic friendships that laid the groundwork for a full and lasting recovery.

When to Let Go

But how can you tell if a relationship is so harmful to your psychological well being that it needs to be limited or cut off altogether? Unfortunately, there is no simple set of rules that applies to every case. I can, however, offer a few time-tested principles that may prove useful as you evaluate the troublesome relationships in your life.

First, it's important to ask yourself: "Do I usually feel worse when I spend time with this person?" If so, you'll need to identify: (a) what it is about the interaction that's the source of distress, and (b) whether or not it's something that can be improved. For example, as we've seen in the case of relationships that drift toward joint rumination and negative emotional contagion, it's often possible to redirect the focus of interaction toward something less toxic (e.g., shared activity or non-ruminative conversation). But, if you have a friend or loved one who is unwilling or unable to make such a shift, it might be helpful to limit the time you spend with them—at least until you've made a full recovery.

Sometimes, of course, people find themselves in relationships that are clearly toxic beyond the point of repair. That was the case with Karen and her abusive boyfriend, just as it was with Annie and her malicious sorority "sisters." Such harmful relationships are pretty easy to spot, since the offending party is typically abusive: harshly critical, demeaning, demanding, hostile, and controlling. And because depression causes its victims to "beat themselves up" anyway, such abusive partners only serve to strengthen the depressive sense of self-loathing—a process that makes full recovery impossible.

SPOUSES

Although the principles we've covered so far can be applied to virtually any relationship, in this section we'll address some specific ways they're relevant in marriage and other romantic partnerships. (Much of the content can also be applied to any emotionally intimate relationship, romantic or otherwise.)

Whenever a person is caught in the grip of depressive illness, the situation is agonizing for their spouse, as well: It's horrible to see someone you love in pain. Almost invariably, the spouse winds up feeling powerless. After all, they know they can't just encourage their partner to "snap out of it." (Or else they learn the hard way that this only makes the situation worse.) And in many cases they're even told by clinicians there's nothing much they can do to help—that they simply need to stand by and wait for the effects of treatment (usually medication) to kick in.

But in most cases, this is utterly wrong. Spouses can be an invaluable resource in the recovery process. They can do so in two ways: by helping their depressed partner put into practice the six core elements of Therapeutic Lifestyle Change (TLC), and by serving as an unwavering source of social support.

Helping with TLC

Again, because of the reduced activity in the depressed patient's frontal cortex—the part of the brain that helps translate intentions into actions—most depressed individuals have great difficulty initiating activity. Even things they desperately want to do may go undone. And that includes putting into practice the various elements of the TLC protocol. One of my patients recently put it like this: "I just sit there thinking 'I need to get up and go for a walk while it's still sunny out' or 'I should really call my friend right now,' but then I just keep sitting there on the couch, and nothing happens."

That's where a spouse can come in: they can, in effect, serve as a proxy for their partner's frontal cortex, providing—when necessary—a nudge of initiative that the depressed brain often fails to give. I mentioned this idea a few months ago at a presentation for fellow clinicians, and one of them told me afterward that a little lightbulb went off in her head. As it turned out, her husband had been struggling with depression for some time, and he found it difficult to make himself do many of the things (exercise and light exposure and omega-3 supplementation and social activity) that he knew could help. So she went home that night and talked with him about the whole "frontal cortex angle," asking how he would feel if she were to provide gentle nudges to help him initiate the lifestyle changes he'd been unable to put into practice. To her considerable surprise, he thought it was a fantastic idea.

Of course, it takes great care to make sure this brain-inspired nudging doesn't start to feel like outright nagging—which could lead to resentment and ill will. The best safeguard is simply for the couple to have an open, honest conversation about the issue, and to decide together up front on some basic ground rules: when it's okay to nudge and when it's not, which activities (if any) are off-limits for nudging and which ones need to stay on the front burner. With such clear lines of communication in place, it's possible for a spouse to serve as a superb catalyst for antidepressant lifestyle changes.

Providing Social Support

As we've seen, extended social isolation is unhealthy for anyone, especially for those fighting depression. And yet virtually every depressed patient I've treated has spent far too little time in the company of others, and missed out on the benefits of positive emotional contagion.

Spouses are in a unique position to help on this front, but it doesn't always work out that way. All too often, depressed patients pull away from their marital partners just as they withdraw from everyone else, becoming isolated—physically and emotionally—even within the confines of their homes. Although it can be tempting for spouses in this situation to allow the distance in the marriage to grow (after all, it's hard to maintain closeness with a partner who keeps pulling away), it's a temptation to be avoided.

Simply having a spouse provide their physical presence—even if it's just a matter of spending time together in silence—is of some benefit to depressed individuals, since the mere company of another person can help put the brakes on the brain's depressive stress response. A more potent benefit is provided by caring physical contact—hugging, holding hands, sitting next to each other on the sofa, and so on—which sends a strong anti-stress signal to the depressed brain. It's also helpful for spouses to plan engaging activities together, and to steer conversations away from negative topics that might lead to rumination. (Again, this is not to say that upsetting events shouldn't be discussed, but simply that such conversations should be limited and infrequent.)

Finally, it's important to note that no spouse can serve as an effective resource for their depressed partner unless they're also taking exceptionally good care of their own emotional well-being. Remember, emotional contagion runs in both directions. So, the more the spouse attends to their own needs (making time for friends, regular exercise, restorative sleep, and so forth), the more "immunity" they'll have from their depressed partner's gloom, and the more they'll be able to serve as a source of support and inspiration.

THE IMPORTANCE OF GIVING

It's more blessed to give than to receive. This proverb may sound paradoxical, but psychologists now have the data to back it up. For example, when research subjects were given large sums of money and told either to keep the cash or to spend it on someone else, they consistently reported greater happiness when they gave their bounty away. (This experiment has been replicated in several different variations.) Todd Kashdan, a psychologist at George Mason University, recently found a similar result with the students in his Science of Well-Being course, who were assigned to compare the psychological effects of two activities: 1) something they found innately pleasurable (scuba diving was one option), and 2) a selfless act of kindness for someone else (for example, collecting clothes for a battered women's shelter). Remarkably, students found the latter activity consistently brought them a greater sense of happiness and well-being.

The same general principle holds true for those fighting depression: One of the surest paths to boosting mood is giving to someone else in need. Such giving can take many forms.

In our TLC groups, I've had the joy of watching patients put the principle into practice each week by providing one another with heartfelt support and encouragement—listening to each other's stories, cheering each success, and offering words of comfort with every setback (along with a shoulder to cry on). Many patients have told me this opportunity to give back to others was the single most meaningful thing they experienced during the entire course of treatment.

Likewise, many have grown deeply connected to others through volunteer activities: building houses with Habitat for Humanity, "adopting" a lonely child though Big Brothers Big Sisters, serving as a tour guide with a local museum, knocking on doors for a political campaign, serving meals at a soup kitchen, and working with abandoned animals at the local shelter. The number of volunteer possibilities is nearly infinite, and there now exist some extraordinary online resources to help match people with placements that fit their interests. One of my favorites is www.volunteermatch.org, which has over fifty thousand volunteer organizations in its vast nationwide database.

CARING FOR ANIMALS

We touched briefly in the last section on the possibility of caring for animals, but the topic is so important it deserves a bit more elaboration. As many pet owners know from experience, the bonds we form with animals can be just as emotionally powerful as those we share with other human beings. And caring for animals can be a profoundly therapeutic experience. I've seen patients with symptoms so debilitating they could barely find the energy to eat or get dressed miraculously spring back to life when faced with a helpless puppy or kitten in need of care.

Pets have an almost magical ability to increase our sense of well-being through their affectionate physical contact, which lowers stress hormones and boosts the activity of feel-good brain chemicals like dopamine and serotonin. Pets also provide us with a faithful source of social companionship, and a deep feeling that we truly *matter*: They literally depend on us for their very lives. As we'll see in the next section, this sense of mattering to others is something we're all designed to have, and something we all need.

FINDING COMMUNITY

Twelve thousand years ago, before the invention of agriculture, everyone belonged to a community. Within each intimate hunter-gatherer band, people lived and worked together with a common purpose and a powerful sense of belonging. In a world filled with predators and hostile neighbors, the members of each band were profoundly linked together by their shared fate: Without the group, each individual would die. And, because every person contributed to the well-being of the entire clan (through hunting, foraging, collecting water, child-rearing, scouting, and so on), no one ever had to worry about whether they were valued by others. Simply by being a member of the community, each person was intrinsically important.

For hundreds of thousands of years, this deep sense of belonging was simply part of what it meant to be a human being. It's an experience we all still crave; the longing seems to be embedded in our very souls. Those lucky enough to find authentic community today are much happier (on average) than those who live in its absence.

But it's become increasingly difficult to experience community in the modern world, especially in the United States. The small, intimate societies of our ancestors all have long since been replaced by towns and cities with populations that number well into the millions. And lifelong bonds of commitment—forged between people who rely on one another, moment to moment, for their survival—have been usurped by fleeting ties that often signal nothing more than a desire to pursue leisure activities together (when it's convenient). So, where can we Americans still find authentic community, and the profound sense of belonging it confers?

Church. The most likely place, according to sociologists, is the local church or synagogue.* That's not to say that every house of worship is a gateway to such intimate, meaningful connections. But at least *some* are, and they tend to share a common set of features:

- Size: According to an interesting line of research, people are most likely to flourish in a church that's about the size of a typical hunter-gatherer band. Once the congregation gets much bigger, exceeding two hundred or so members, people often start to feel more anonymous and unimportant. However, some larger churches (even so-called *megachurches*) have effectively addressed this problem by involving members in smaller groups—often known as *home groups*—where they can still find intimate community.

* For the remainder of this section, I'll use the term *church* in the generic sense to refer to any house of worship, of any faith—Christian, Jewish, Muslim, Hindu, Buddhist, and so on.

- Purpose: Nothing binds people together more effectively than a shared purpose and a set of common goals. Churches that provide their members with a clear sense of mission—whether it be caring for the poor and disenfranchised, reaching out to the "unchurched," or trying to change society for the better—tend to foster a greater sense of community than those that don't.
- Investment: Not surprisingly, people who invest heavily of themselves in a church—their time, energy, and resources—are those most likely to find a genuine experience of community there. It's only by spending time with a group of other people on a regular basis—sharing our lives together as we work toward common goals—that any of us can hope to form the deep, intimate connections that make community possible.

Church is not for everyone, of course. Fortunately, other options are available for those who find involvement in a religious community an unattractive prospect. But the same factors that foster community in churches still apply to nonreligious groups: small group size, a strong sense of shared purpose, and a high level of investment among group members.

Volunteer organizations. Many volunteer groups excel at bringing together people who share a specific passion: saving the environment, ending homelessness, protecting battered women, feeding the hungry, promoting a political party, sheltering abandoned animals, and so on. If this prospect sounds appealing, you might reflect on the one or two causes or goals that matter to you the most, and try identifying a group of like-minded souls joined in pursuit of that purpose.

Social organizations. Most towns and cities are host to numerous social organizations and clubs that provide their members with a sense of community. These range from civic groups (like the Jaycees and Rotary and Lion's Clubs) to special interest organizations (like the American Business Women's Association and Veterans of Foreign Wars) to adult sororities and fraternities.

Self-help groups. Organizations such as AA (Alcoholics Anonymous), DBSA (Depression and Bipolar Support Alliance), and NAMI (National Alliance on Mental Illness) bring together individuals dedicated to overcoming various forms of mental illness. In speaking to such groups, I've observed firsthand the tight social bonds that often form among their members.

Interest groups. Myriad groups help bring together people with shared recreational interests: reading, hiking, crafting, cycling, running, writing, rafting, photography, film, visual arts, drama, history, and so on.

Sports leagues. I've also witnessed genuine community spring up among team members in any number of different sports leagues, including softball, basketball, soccer, golf, volleyball, ultimate Frisbee, bowling, and touch football.

The workplace. Increasingly, Americans invest so much of their time and energy at the workplace that it actually becomes their primary vehicle for the experience of community. This is a development I view with some ambivalence, since it would be healthier for most people to invest less of themselves at work—to spend more time cultivating relationships elsewhere. But given the ongoing reality of American workaholism, it's certainly much better for people to experience community at work than never to find it at all.

Developing close bonds with coworkers usually involves carving out ample time to spend with them in a nonwork setting. It also takes a commitment to sharing life's triumphs and failures. But some employment cultures discourage this level of coworker intimacy, so it won't always be attainable, even for those who seek it. In fact, given the loss of balance that easily comes from wrapping up the bulk of one's time and energy in the workplace, I generally advise people to look for their primary experience of community elsewhere.

CONCLUDING THOUGHT

All of us are born to connect, hardwired to live in the company of those who know and love us. When we draw from deep wells of social support—the care and concern of close friends, family, and community—we're more resilient to the slings and arrows of fortune, and we're considerably less vulnerable to depression. Social connection helps push the brain in an antidepressant direction, turning down activity in stress circuitry, and boosting the activity of feel-good brain chemicals like dopamine and serotonin. That's why it makes sense to swim hard against the tide of our "culture of isolation" and to place our relationships at the very top of the priority list. Truly, nothing in life matters more.

9
Habits of Healthy Sleep

Sleep that knits up the ravell'd sleeve of care,
The death of each day's life, sore labor's bath,
Balm of hurt minds, great nature's second course,
Chief nourisher in life's feast.

—**William Shakespeare, *Macbeth***

Why do we sleep? What is sleep *for*? For centuries, scientists had no satisfying answers. As recently as fifty years ago, many thought sleep was useless—a mere period of biological downtime.

That view has now changed. Recent advances in the neurosciences have brought the discovery that adequate sleep is indispensable for both physical and mental well-being—just as Shakespeare intuited four hundred years ago. In fact, it is only during sleep that the body and brain have a chance to do their major repair work—to undo the subtle damage suffered by millions of cells over the course of each day—and to perform a daily tune-up so things continue running smoothly. Sleep is what keeps us firing on all cylinders.

Because sleep is so essential to our well-being, it takes only a few nights of deprivation before adverse effects start piling up: memory and concentration wane; mood turns irritable; judgment grows poor;

reaction times slow; coordination deteriorates; energy dims; and immune function declines.

Even more dire consequences follow prolonged sleep loss. The body starts shutting down, and we begin to experience the sleep deficit as physically painful. That's why intentionally depriving someone of sleep is now regarded as a form of torture,* and rightfully so.

Sadly, sleep disturbance and depression go hand in hand. Not only is disordered sleep one of the telltale symptoms of depression, but it also plays a major role in triggering the illness. As we saw in Chapter 2, the loss of slow-wave sleep—the most restorative phase of slumber—can directly account for many of depression's most debilitating features. Not surprisingly, before the onset of depression, four out of five people suffer from some form of sleep disturbance.

The implications are clear: Anything we can do to improve our sleep can help combat depression and render the disorder less likely to occur in the future.

Fortunately, several elements of the Therapeutic Lifestyle Change (TLC) program carry the potential to enhance sleep. For example, physical exercise profoundly improves sleep quality. It leads to more restorative slow-wave sleep throughout the night, and also helps cut down on the number of nighttime awakenings. Similarly, bright light exposure strengthens the brain's internal body clock, which in turn makes it easier both to fall asleep and to stay asleep throughout the night; it also spurs a desirable increase in slow-wave sleep. And strategies like omega-3 supplementation and anti-ruminative activity and enhanced social connection—by helping slam the brakes on the brain's stress response circuits—can improve both the quality and quantity of sleep.

---

* It's viewed that way by, for example, the *U.S. Army Field Manual*.

For some, putting such lifestyle changes into practice is all it takes to restore healthy sleep each night. But that's not always the case. Many people need additional help on the sleep front. That's why the TLC program has a sixth (and final) element: an array of sleep-enhancement strategies drawn from an effective treatment program for insomnia* that's proven superior to popular sleep medications in long-term clinical trials.

DETERMINING HOW MUCH SLEEP YOU NEED

According to the best research, most adults need about eight hours of sleep each night for optimal physical and emotional well-being. Unfortunately, the average American gets only 6.7 hours. Most of us, therefore, are chronically sleep-deprived. That's why over 90% of Americans ingest caffeine or other stimulants on a daily basis: It helps mask a staggering national sleep deficit, easing drowsiness so we can make it through the day. But caffeine does nothing to reduce the heightened risk of depression brought on by our collective lack of slumber.

Interestingly, people do vary somewhat in their sleep needs. A few lucky souls get by perfectly well on six or seven hours a night, while others require as much as nine and a half hours. Although it's possible that you need much less sleep than average, it's not likely. (Most people greatly underestimate how much sleep they require.)

In my clinical work, I've found it best to have each patient start with a goal of eight hours of sleep each night. And, unless you're

* This treatment approach integrates an array of effective behavioral and cognitive insomnia interventions. One of the best summaries is found in *Cognitive Behavioral Treatment of Insomnia: A Session-by-Session Guide* by Perlis, Jungquist, Smith, and Posner (2005).

certain you need less sleep than that, based on careful attention to your experience over a long period of time, I'm going to ask you to adopt an initial target of eight hours per night, as well. (After a few weeks you can always adjust your nightly sleep goal up or down based on how you respond—a point we'll address later in the chapter.)

Of course, when asked to carve that much time out of their lives for sleep, many people object, at least at first. The most common protest: *I can't afford to spend so much time in bed*. Stacy, a successful executive with a local nonprofit organization, was typical in that respect.

"I'm just not sure eight hours is a realistic goal for me," she said during an early treatment session. "I've got *way* too much to get done. And it seems like things take me longer than they used to. If I let myself sleep more than six hours, I don't think I'll ever be able to keep my head above water."

I reminded Stacy that her depression was going to be hard to clear up until she started getting more sleep, but she still insisted it simply wasn't possible. We were at an impasse, so I came at it from a different angle.

"What happens to your ability to get things done," I asked, "when you get a really good night's sleep? Does it make any difference if, say, you let yourself get a full eight hours?"

She shot back grudgingly, "I suppose I can get more done when I've had a good night's sleep, but I doubt if it's enough to make up for all that time wasted in bed. I don't know, I guess it's possible."

Encouraged by her concession, I asked Stacy if she would be willing to try an experiment—to adopt a goal of eight hours of sleep each night for a full two weeks, after which we could evaluate whether or not it was a good investment of her time. If she concluded that the added sleep truly wasn't worth it, I told her I would drop the subject. To my surprise, she agreed to give it a try.

Since Stacy had already done a good job of implementing some of the other lifestyle changes in the TLC program—and was also willing to put into practice some of the habits of healthy sleep outlined later in this chapter—she encountered little difficulty sleeping for a full eight hours once she set aside the time in her schedule. When I asked her at our next session about the preliminary results of the experiment—only a week into her trial run—she rolled her eyes.

"Okay, fine, you were right—the extra sleep is helping. It's hard to explain it—it's like my head is just clearer. And I've definitely had more energy this week. My husband even said I haven't been as cranky. It's funny: I'm not really any better at getting things done, but that part doesn't even seem to matter. Somehow, I've been finding a way to fit everything in anyway, because the sleep is a priority now."

When it comes right down to it, we usually find the time for things that truly matter to us. As Stacy discovered, when sleep is a priority, we'll make room for it in our busy lives. And, as the research shows quite clearly: In the battle against depression, sleep belongs high up on the priority list.

THE HABITS OF HEALTHY SLEEP

Unlike Stacy, many people set aside adequate time for sleep, only to discover that their bodies still won't cooperate after they've crawled into bed. They're among the sixty million Americans who suffer from insomnia.

This ubiquitous sleep disturbance comes in three varieties. The most common form in depression is known as *terminal insomnia**: waking up too early—usually an hour or two before intended—and being unable to fall back to sleep. *Middle insomnia*, marked by frequent awakenings throughout the night, is also fairly widespread. The final variety—*onset insomnia*—is a hallmark of seasonal affective disorder and many forms of anxiety; it refers to an initial inability to fall asleep at night.

Believe it or not, much of the problem of insomnia stems from unhealthy sleep habits people develop. In this section, we'll identify the most common culprits and outline ten healthy habits of sleep that can help remedy the problem.

Conditioning Your Body to Sleep

One of my friends has perfectly normal blood pressure at home, only to find that it shoots through the roof when he has it measured at the doctor's office. This phenomenon—*white coat hypertension* (that is, blood pressure that spikes only in the presence of white-clad medical specialists)—is a common problem, and it nicely illustrates how the body can be influenced by our surroundings.

Just like Pavlov's iconic dog—trained to salivate merely upon hearing a nightly dinner bell—each of us can be conditioned to respond reflexively to the sights and sounds and tastes and smells of our environment. For example, having endured some unpleasant visits to the dentist's office as a child, I still find my pulse racing every time I

* Technically, terminal insomnia simply means that the awakening comes at the *end* (or termination) of the sleep period.

hear the shrill hiss of a dental drill—even if the sound is just coming from a nearby TV set. Likewise, when I smell fresh-baked apple pie, fond memories of my grandmother's cozy kitchen percolate, unbidden, to the surface of my mind, where they induce an involuntary wave of relaxation.

Our ability to sleep can also be influenced by our surroundings, although most of us are oblivious to the process. Specifically, our brains can be programmed to fall asleep—trained to enter a state of slumber reflexively and automatically—in the presence of certain cues from the world around us. (Conversely, we can also be conditioned to stay awake under certain circumstances.)

When someone consistently enjoys healthy sleep, the sights and sounds and sensations of the bedroom—and the bed, in particular—become strongly associated with the act of sleeping. Night after night, the brain is conditioned to follow a pretty iron-clad rule: When you're in bed, you sleep; when you're not, you don't. And scientists have proven that people benefit from this conditioning, reflexively growing drowsier from the mere act of entering the bedroom, turning out the lights, and crawling into bed.

When a person battles insomnia, a different sort of conditioning takes place. Instead of associating the bed with sleep, they link it with the experience of lying wide awake, tossing and turning in frustration. They often inadvertently weaken their sleep programming even further by pairing the bed with all sorts of non-sleep activities like watching TV, reading, eating, and chatting on the phone.

Unfortunately, the more they lose the benefit of a conditioned sleep-bed association, the more their struggle with insomnia grows. But it's possible at any point to reprogram the body on this front. It simply requires adhering to a basic principle, the first of our habits of healthy sleep.

Habit #1: Use the Bed Only for Sleeping

You can condition your body to fall asleep in bed—and to stay asleep—only if the overwhelming majority of your time in bed is actually spent sleeping. The following guidelines will help make sure this is the case:

- *Anytime you've been lying awake for fifteen minutes, get up, leave the bedroom, and do something relaxing until you feel drowsy enough to return to bed.* This rule is essential because it prevents the bed (and the bedroom) from becoming associated with a state of wakefulness—which would undermine the sleep-bed conditioning process. Although getting out of bed when you've had trouble sleeping may feel like a hassle, it can be made more enjoyable by, say, setting aside a good book or DVD to be brought out only on such sleepless occasions.*
- *Avoid getting into bed anytime you aren't already drowsy.* If you're only allowing yourself a fifteen-minute window for falling asleep, you need to make sure you're already sleepy before climbing into bed; otherwise you'll quickly find yourself hopping right back out again. So, you'll want to avoid any arousing activities—for example, exercising, watching a scary movie, working, or surfing the Internet—right before bedtime.
- *Anything you do to increase your drowsiness should be done somewhere other than the bedroom.* This may seem a little counterintuitive. After all, if you're in another room reading or watching a

---

* Obviously, reading a book or watching a movie to get drowsy—instead of simply staying in bed and resting—might lead to a decrease in your total sleep time, but it's a key part of a process, and it yields greatly improved sleep in the long run. As sleep researchers have discovered, the trade-off is well worth it.

movie to become groggy, won't the walk back to the bedroom unweave the somnolent spell? Wouldn't it make more sense just to read in bed, where you could simply reach over to turn off the light and fall asleep the instant you're ready? Actually, when you're truly drowsy, there's little chance of getting too stimulated merely by walking to your bedroom (assuming you don't decide to do some calisthenics along the way). And, because our goal is to strengthen the association between sleep and bed, anything you do in bed other than sleep—even something relaxing like reading or watching TV—will interfere with the conditioning process.

- *You can make an exception in the case of sex.* For reasons that are still mysterious scientifically, sleep specialists have found that pairing the bed with sex does nothing to weaken the sleep-bed conditioning process. (One theory: Sex helps train the body to associate the bed with positive feelings, which counters the strong feelings of dread many insomniacs have upon getting into bed.) This is the only exception, though.
- *Avoid sleeping anywhere other than your own bed.* Pairing sleep with any other setting—the sofa, the recliner, or a guest room—interferes with the process of programming the sleep reflex to occur in your bed.

Habit #2: Get Up at the Same Time Every Day

Did you know your brain comes with a built-in sleep meter? A cluster of neurons deep in the brain tracks how much shut-eye you've been getting, and it estimates how much more you need at any given time. Based on its calculations, it sets your *sleep drive*, which you can usually feel on a moment-to-moment basis as a sense of drowsiness (or, if sleep drive is low, a sense of wakefulness). When sleep drive is appropriately high at bedtime, problems with insomnia tend to be minimal. And there are some pivotal things you can do to enhance this drive.

When your body clock is working properly, it provides a huge boost to your sleep drive at bedtime each night and sustains it until the next morning. This makes it much easier to get a good night's sleep. But if your internal timepiece starts to malfunction—thinking it's time to wake up when it's only, say, 3:00 in the morning—insomnia is one of the many unfortunate consequences.

One of the best ways to keep the body clock running on time—and, thus, to ensure healthy sleep—is to get up at the same time every morning. I know from my own experience that this isn't always convenient, but it's an essential weapon in the battle against disordered sleep.

Many people are tempted to sleep in on weekends—and pretty much any other time they get the chance (especially if they've been sleep-deprived). But this natural impulse to catch up on sleep turns out to be counterproductive in the long run: It ultimately serves to weaken sleep drive. So, I encourage you to resist the urge to sleep in, even if it means missing out on a golden opportunity for some extra rest. The temporary sacrifice will prove well worth it in the long run, as you find both the quality and quantity of your sleep improving.*

* We can also make an important exception to the "no-sleeping-in rule": After you've established a consistent pattern of healthy sleep, sleeping in for an extra hour or two on occasion will likely do little to throw off your body clock, provided you don't make it a habit.

Habit #3: Avoid Napping

Simply put, anytime you nap, it strongly reduces the brain's sleep drive, which then sets you up for potential insomnia later that night. There's also evidence that napping can cause a reduction in restorative slow-wave sleep. So taking a nap is a bad idea for anyone with sleep difficulties (and anyone who's depressed), even though it might feel like the most natural way in the world to spend a sleepy afternoon.

But for those who have no sleep problems, the occasional nap is unlikely to pose any risk. Some people find they can nap every day and still maintain healthy sleep. (The key point is that if you have disordered sleep, napping will almost always make things worse; but taking a siesta won't pose a problem if your sleep is already healthy.)

Habit #4: Avoid Bright Light at Night

Even though indoor lighting is dim in comparison with direct sunlight, a well-lit room is still about as bright as the clear sky at sunset. As we saw in Chapter 7, indoor light can trick the brain into thinking it's still not nighttime yet, even if it's been pitch dark outside for hours. Such trickery can interfere with sleep, because the brain won't allow your sleep drive to kick into high gear until it thinks the sun has been down for at least an hour or so.

Many people who have onset insomnia—trouble falling asleep at night—are unwitting victims of this phenomenon. They keep all the lights on until the moment just before their head hits the pillow, and then they wind up having to lie awake in the dark for an hour before their brain finally gets the message that it's time for sleep.

Fortunately, there's a simple solution: Turn off all the lights about an hour before bedtime, and use only candlelight or very dim lamp light from that point on. You'll need to turn off your computer late at night as well, because its monitor (at close range) is bright enough to simulate twilight. (A TV screen is usually okay, provided you sit across the room with all the other lights out).

Light exposure in bed. Once you're in bed, it's best to keep your bedroom pitch dark. One of my patients discovered this the hard way last year. After having a few nightmares, her five-year-old son begged her to start leaving the hallway light on overnight so he could spot any monsters trying to sneak into his room. She agreed, and since her bedroom was on the same hallway (and she kept her door ajar so the cat could come and go), a fair amount light came streaming into her room each night. Although she didn't mind—she said she hardly even noticed the increased light—her sleep quickly started to deteriorate, with frequent awakenings throughout the night.

It takes very little light—even when it's filtered through our eyelids—to convince the brain that it's daytime and (therefore) time to be fully awake. So I advise you to turn out all nightlights, bathroom lights, and any other light sources (TVs, for example) before you climb into bed. Likewise, if there are certain times of year when the sun rises before your usual wakeup time, you'll likely benefit from installing blackout curtains in your bedroom. (A much cheaper alternative is to start wearing a sleep mask; they do a great job of blocking out ambient light.)

Late sunlight exposure. Sunlight exposure in the early evening can suppress sleep drive for hours. And when such exposure occurs several nights in a row, it can even throw off the body clock, making you want to go to bed and wake up much later than usual. Therefore, unless you actually need to recalibrate your body clock like this*—a process described in detail in Chapter 7—it's wise to avoid getting regular sunlight after about 7:00 in the evening. (You can always wear sunglasses, however, if you still want to enjoy being outside past that hour in the summer.)

Habit #5: Avoid Caffeine and Other Stimulants

As you might expect, stimulants like caffeine and nicotine strongly suppress sleep drive. Caffeine has a typical half-life in the body of about four hours. (This means that every four hours, your blood level drops by 50%.) So, let's say you have a strong cup of coffee—with 200 milligrams (mg) of caffeine—at noon. By 4:00 in the afternoon, you still have 100 mg of caffeine in your body, and at 8:00 pm, there's still 50 mg in your system. Even at midnight, you're left with 25 mg of caffeine coursing through your veins; that's about the equivalent of a cup of green tea, and it's enough to disrupt your sleep.

You probably won't have any problem with a single cup of coffee or tea (or a caffeinated soda) first thing in the morning, because your body still has a full sixteen hours or so to clear it from your system before bedtime. But it's a good idea to avoid caffeine after you've been awake for more than a few hours. (Also, please note: Oral contraceptives can extend the half-life of caffeine by several hours, so even greater caution with caffeine intake is required.)

---

* If you tend to wake up far too early, such recalibration could be helpful.

Habit #6: Avoid Alcohol at Night

Many people with onset insomnia use alcohol in an effort to increase drowsiness before heading off to bed. This strategy sometimes works, but it also causes a horrible rebound effect—with frequent awakenings and poor-quality sleep throughout the night. For this reason, it's a good idea to avoid any alcohol within a few hours of bedtime.

Habit #7: If Possible, Keep the Same Bedtime Every Night

By going to bed at the same time each night, you program your body to give a massive boost to sleep drive—usually starting about thirty to forty-five minutes before bedtime. The ensuing drowsiness makes it much easier to fall asleep.

However, you may still face the occasional night when you're simply too wound up at bedtime to drift off to sleep. On such nights, it's best to delay going to bed for a while, and to engage instead in some form of relaxing activity until you're drowsy enough to climb into bed and fall asleep fairly quickly (that is, within about fifteen minutes).

Habit #8: Turn Down Your Thermostat at Night

There's evidence that a mild drop in temperature at night helps increase sleep drive. This may seem a little puzzling until you consider that our remote ancestors always slept outside (or in open huts), where it got noticeably colder right around bedtime. And, since our bodies are still largely designed for life in the Pleistocene, a nighttime dip in temperature actually sends us a primal signal that it's time to sleep. Accordingly, you may want to try lowering your thermostat by about five degrees an hour before bedtime.

Habit #9: Avoid Taking Your Problems to Bed with You

Nancy Hamilton, a noted sleep researcher, recently passed along a memorable formula for falling asleep: "All it takes is a tired body and a quiet mind." We've now addressed the *tired body* part of the formula in our review of the many ways to enhance sleep drive, so we'll turn our attention to strategies for cultivating a quiet mind.

For many people, the prime time for dwelling on negative thoughts is when they're lying in bed, trying to fall asleep. Such rumination revs up the brain's stress response circuits, and this, in turn, makes it virtually impossible to fall asleep. So it's crucial to make sure you don't succumb to any bouts of bedtime brooding.

As we saw in Chapter 5, the best way to put an end to rumination is by redirecting your attention to some type of engaging activity. But this particular strategy seems tricky to put into practice while you're lying in bed, waiting to fall asleep. What sort of activity could you possibly engage in, anyway?

There's really only one option: *mental activity*. The challenge is to find some sort of mental task that's engrossing, and yet simultaneously relaxing enough to allow you to fall asleep. Apparently, some people find counting imaginary sheep helpful—if the old cliché is to be believed. I have to admit, though, I've never met a person for whom this worked. But I have had patients tell me they've successfully directed their thoughts away from rumination with one or more of the following mental exercises:

- *Replay scenes from a favorite movie in your head.* On nights when the tendency to ruminate is particularly acute, you can even try watching a relaxing film right before you turn in for bed: This will keep all the movie's details fresh in your mind as you attempt to replay them.
- *Visualize a relaxing scene.* Many people find it easiest to choose a favorite vacation spot or some other pleasant venue. Some, for example, like to imagine themselves walking along a scenic beach or a majestic mountain pass; for others, it's sitting in a childhood tree house or strolling through a verdant forest. It simply has to be some place you know well and can bring to mind with great clarity.
- *Play a round of golf in your mind's eye.* Visualize in detail the look of every fairway and bunker and green, the smell of the cut grass, the feel of the wind, the sound of birds and crickets, and so forth. (I also find it helpful to imagine myself playing at the skill level of a Tiger Woods; otherwise the mounting frustration over my erratic swing can quickly undo any relaxation I might otherwise achieve.)
- *Use progressive muscle relaxation.* This highly effective relaxation technique simply involves momentarily tightening and then relaxing each major muscle group in the body. It's easy to learn, and high-quality tapes and CDs are available to guide you through the process. Because this technique takes a bit of concentration, it's an effective antidote to rumination, and a particularly useful activity on nights when you need to get your thoughts off something that's troubling you.
- *Use another proven relaxation technique. Diaphragmatic breathing* involves learning how to inhale and exhale slowly and deeply from the diaphragm (the large muscle that sits right below the

lungs). *Autogenic training* makes use of guided imagery to create a pleasant feeling of warmth in each part of the body. Both are highly effective in focusing attention and preparing you for sleep.

Although each of these strategies can redirect your attention away from upsetting thoughts, in some cases the problem of nighttime rumination can best be addressed by doing something before you turn in for the night. Specifically, if you have troubling thoughts on your mind in the evening, you can try one of these strategies to make rumination in bed less likely:

- *Talk things through with a trusted confidant.* This allows you to get any distressing thoughts off your chest, which usually weakens the desire to keep mulling them over later.
- *Write down your ruminative thoughts.* This process often makes it easier to leave them behind for the night.
- *Fill your mind, right before you go to bed, with explicitly positive thoughts and images.* Because of the contextual nature of human memory, loading your mind with such positive information will temporarily make it more difficult to recall any upsetting memories, and much harder to get stuck in a ruminative thought process.

Habit #10: Don't Try to Fall Asleep

Sleep is an inherently paradoxical state: The harder you try to attain it, the more elusive it becomes. Sleep can never be stalked and caught—like some sort of wild animal—when you hunt it with intense, focused effort. Instead, it will appear unbidden, sneaking up on you gently after you've fully let go of the struggle.

This means it's always counterproductive to worry about how long it's taking you to fall asleep—a process that quickly turns into outright rumination. That's why sleep specialists generally advise you to turn your clock away from the bed, so you can't see at a glance what time it is.*

Likewise, whenever you lie in bed worrying about the negative consequences of sleep deprivation the next day, it will make it much harder to fall asleep. If you find such worrisome thoughts springing up on occasion, you may find it helpful to remind yourself that a single night of poor sleep is never catastrophic (though it can certainly be frustrating). Also keep in mind that temporary sleep deprivation actually serves to increase sleep drive on the following night. In other words, tonight's sleep loss means tomorrow night's sleep will likely prove much better. And, ironically, once you let go of any worry over lost sleep, there's a good chance you'll soon drift off anyway.

THE PROBLEM OF HYPERSOMNIA

Our review of the habits of healthy sleep has focused so far on insomnia and related sleep disturbances. But about 20% of people with depression suffer from *hypersomnia*—sleeping far too much. What can be done for them?

As it turns out, many cases of depressive hypersomnia result from inefficient sleep: multiple awakenings through the night and a re-

* Then again, we saw earlier that it's important to get up out of bed anytime you've been lying awake for fifteen minutes—a rule that would seem to require you to have access in bed to a visible clock. It's generally best, however, if you simply leave the bedroom when you *estimate* that fifteen minutes have passed; most people quickly get very good at guessing in this fashion, and this allows them to avoid staring at the clock all night.

duced amount of restorative slow-wave sleep. Because people with this problem get such poor quality sleep, they may find themselves in bed for twelve or fourteen hours a night, and yet still feeling tired.

Fortunately, as we've seen, several elements of Therapeutic Lifestyle Change help increase slow-wave sleep—especially exercise and sunlight exposure—and adopting the habits of healthy sleep we've covered in this chapter can also provide an enormous boost to sleep quality. I've consistently observed good outcomes among hypersomnia patients in our TLC groups as they've put these various strategies into practice, and most eventually found their sleep returning to normal.

WHEN ALL ELSE FAILS

In the great majority of cases, employing these ten habits of healthy sleep—in tandem with the other antidepressant elements of Therapeutic Lifestyle Change—will effectively put an end to the common sleep problems that characterize depression. But there are some important exceptions. Most arise from the presence of medication side effects, undiagnosed sleep disorders, or other medical conditions.

Oddly enough, some common antidepressant medications carry the potential to interfere with sleep. Often this involves repeated awakenings due to periodic limb movements. (Stimulants such as caffeine and amphetamines can have a similar effect.) In a similar vein, the frequent use of some sleep medications can lead to rebound insomnia on any night when the drugs are not used.

Sleep disorders constitute another important cause of poor quality sleep. For example, some people suffer from a serious, potentially life-threatening condition known as *sleep apnea*. It involves dozens (often hundreds) of mini-awakenings throughout the night as breathing stops temporarily—usually due to an airway obstruction in the throat. Others suffer from *periodic limb movement disorder,* in which the legs or arms twitch repeatedly throughout the night, greatly reducing sleep quality. With such sleep disorders, the patient usually has no idea anything is wrong, other than a relentless sense of sleepiness and fatigue that stems from chronically poor sleep.

Numerous other medical conditions can also interfere with sleep. Chronic pain is the biggest culprit: It's virtually impossible to sleep soundly when intense physical discomfort keeps intruding into your consciousness. Allergies, colds, and other respiratory conditions also carry the potential to disrupt sleep all night long, as do diseases like *hyperthyroidism* and *pheochromocytoma* (adrenal tumor), which are capable of keeping the body continuously revved up. The list of medical causes of sleep disturbance is a lengthy one—and the topic is so complex that it warrants a book in its own right.

Therefore, if you have sleep problems that persist even after putting into practice the strategies we've reviewed in this chapter, I strongly recommend that you see your doctor or other health care professional for help as soon as possible. Remember: Our bodies were designed to sleep rather effortlessly anytime we go to bed with a tired body and a still mind. If you can't do so, it's a sign you need medical attention.

PART THREE

MAKING THE CHANGE

10

Putting It All Together

Although we've already explored several potent strategies for fighting depression (omega-3 supplementation, anti-rumination activity, exercise, sunlight exposure, social connection, and healthy sleep), we haven't yet discussed how to put everything together into a complete package. How, in other words, can you incorporate all six antidepressant strategies into your life at the same time?

It's not a trivial challenge. When I first began describing the Therapeutic Lifestyle Change (TLC) program to my colleagues, back before we'd started recruiting any patients into our first treatment study, some warned me that the program was too ambitious. Quite simply, my colleagues thought people would find it too difficult to make so many changes all at once.

They had a point. In fact, I agreed: TLC *is* an ambitious program, and it does require a great deal of dedication. But I wasn't worried. I knew from years of experience that most depressed individuals are willing to do whatever it takes to escape the illness, to find relief from its relentless, debilitating pain. They simply need some clear, practical direction about how to make the necessary changes, as well as a bit of coaching along the way.

Still, as I put the TLC program together, my top priority was to make sure it was truly doable. That meant breaking things down into small, manageable stages—to be implemented gradually, one at a time, over the span of several weeks. It also meant starting with the easiest changes up front, and then introducing more challenging elements later in treatment, after patients had gained some momentum (and confidence). Fortunately, this week-by-week approach has proven to be highly successful—much more so than I could have predicted.

In the pages that follow, you'll find a weekly step-by-step outline of the Therapeutic Lifestyle Change program. The recommended schedule is based on the assumption that you haven't yet made any of the six core therapeutic lifestyle changes. However, if you've already made progress with some of these steps (for example, if you're currently exercising on a regular basis), you'll be able to skip past those corresponding parts of the schedule.*

BEFORE YOU BEGIN: SEE YOUR DOCTOR

Depression can be triggered by several medical conditions, including diabetes, heart disease, sleep apnea, thyroid problems, mononucleosis, and hormonal imbalance. Likewise, numerous drugs, including some psychiatric meds, can induce depressive symptoms as a side effect.† For this reason, I believe it's crucial for every person suffering from depression to see their doctor for a complete physical exam, just to make sure the disorder isn't the direct result of another serious ill-

* The protocol is also based on the assumption that you're currently battling symptoms of depression. But you can still benefit from implementing the protocol even if you're not depressed: It will help dramatically reduce your risk of future depression.

† Both medical and drug-related causes of depression are discussed in some detail in Chapter 11.

ness or an adverse drug reaction (either of which could require immediate medical attention.)

In fact, I advise you to schedule an appointment with a physician*—if you haven't already done so in the recent past—as the first step toward putting the principles of Therapeutic Lifestyle Change into practice. During your appointment, you can also get your doctor's clearance to begin an aerobic exercise routine, use a light box, and take the various nutritional supplements included in the TLC protocol. And, if you don't know how to take your pulse already, your doctor can teach you during the appointment.

MEASURING YOUR PROGRESS

How can you tell, as you proceed through the protocol, if you're making any real progress—getting any better—from one week to the next?

Although you could always try to guesstimate your depression level each week, such ballpark guesses tend to be wildly inaccurate. It's much more useful to have a precise measurement. That's why you'll find a superb depression scale in Appendix A that you can use to track your symptoms each week as you adopt each change in your lifestyle. It usually takes only a few minutes to fill out and score this brief questionnaire, and then plot your score on the graph provided in Appendix B.

So, before you begin putting the TLC program into practice, take a moment to complete this scale. It will give you a nice baseline measurement of your depressive symptoms; this in turn will allow you to tell, during the weeks ahead, whether or not the recommended lifestyle changes are helping as they should.

* You could, alternatively, see a licensed nurse practitioner or physician's assistant.

THE TLC PROTOCOL

Week 1

Supplements. During your first week, I suggest starting with a simple change that takes only a minute of your day, but that still has a surprisingly potent effect on the brain: nutritional supplementation. There are five products you'll need to buy. (All can be found at a local health food store or drug store, but they're usually less expensive when purchased online.)

- Omega-3: This is best obtained in the form of high-quality fish oil capsules (or liquid). Try starting at a total omega-3 dosage of 1000 mg of EPA and 500 mg of DHA* each day.
- Vitamin D: If, like most Americans, you're not synthesizing enough vitamin D in your skin—through regular brief exposure to the sun's UV rays—it is important to take a supplement. I recommend a dose of 50 mcg each day, in the form of vitamin D_3.
- Multivitamin: Because omega-3s are fragile molecules, they need some help in the body to do their job. Specifically, they require the protection provided by antioxidants, found in reasonably high quantities in any good daily multivitamin.
- Vitamin C: For added antioxidant protection, I also suggest taking a 500 mg supplement of vitamin C each day.
- Evening primrose oil: Evening primrose oil provides your brain with an essential fat called GLA, which can get depleted when

* Many supplements contain a 2:1 ratio of EPA to DHA, which allows you to get an exact ratio of 1000 mg of EPA and 500 mg of DHA. But some have a higher concentration of DHA, so they provide more than 500 mg of DHA for every 1000 mg of EPA. That's perfectly fine, as well. The important thing is to get 1000 mg of EPA and *at least* 500 mg of DHA.

you take high doses of omega-3s. You need only a little of this oil, though—just one 500 mg capsule each week.* It's important not to exceed this dose, because taking too much can cause unwanted inflammation.

Rumination. In addition to starting nutritional supplementation this week, you can take an important first step toward ending rumination. Specifically, I suggest that you try noticing throughout the day each time you find yourself brooding over negative thoughts. As described earlier, it's impossible to stop rumination without learning first how to detect the process when it's happening. (Most depressed individuals spend a great deal of time brooding without any real awareness that they're doing so.) Several strategies for learning how to notice rumination are discussed on pages 94–100.

Depression Scale. At the end of each week, complete the depression scale and compare the result with your baseline score to see if any changes have occurred.

Week 2

Supplements. Continue as in Week 1.

Rumination. Now that you've become more skilled at noticing your ruminative thoughts (after a week's worth of practice), begin interrupting these thoughts by redirecting your attention each time they occur. You can do this by applying the many techniques described in Chapter 5, including making a list of engaging activities to try this week; identifying and avoiding the specific situations that commonly

* This provides 40 to 50 mg of GLA—a full week's supply.

lead you to ruminate; and scheduling at least one activity each day to take the place of those high-risk situations.

Exercise. You won't start the exercise part of the program until Week 3, but you'll need to make sure you have a few things in place by then. First, pick up a heart rate monitor, or if you can't afford one right now, make sure you can reliably take your pulse. Second, choose the form of exercise you'll be starting with, and make sure you have access to any necessary equipment. (For some people, this will mean lining up a gym membership.) Finally, unless you've already been working out on a regular basis, you may want to consider hiring a personal trainer for at least the first six weeks to help you get started. (You can contact any local gym or health club for referrals.)

Depression Scale. Complete the depression scale and record your score.

Week 3

Supplements. Continue as before.

Rumination. Keep working to improve your ability to notice rumination, and try to get to the point where you can catch yourself the moment it begins. Likewise, keep experimenting with different activities to interrupt it. Every time you find something that works, try other activities that seem similar. For example, if you find that playing Scrabble™ online is helpful, you might experiment with some other online games. Finally, continue avoiding high-risk situations and substituting more engaging activities in their place. Schedule at least one such activity each day.

Exercise. Mark off in your schedule three hour-long blocks of time for exercise this week. (Even though you won't be exercising for the full hour, this will leave enough time for you to cool down and clean up afterwards.) Each time you work out, the goal is to exercise intensely enough to get your heart rate in the target aerobic range (refer to Chapter 6, Table 6-1) and keep it there for thirty minutes. If you haven't been active in some time (or even if you have), I strongly recommend that you begin with brisk walking, because it is by far the easiest, most natural aerobic activity for most people to pick up.

Light. If you're going to be using a light box for your bright light exposure, order it this week so it will be on hand for Week 4.

Depression Scale. Complete the depression scale and record your score.

Week 4

Supplements. Continue as before.

Rumination. Continue as before.

Exercise. Continue as before. If you weren't successful last week in exercising aerobically three times, that's a good indication that hiring a personal trainer may be necessary to help you get started.

Light. Begin scheduling thirty minutes of bright light exposure each morning, as outlined in Chapter 7. (Or, if you're consistently waking up too early in the morning, begin scheduling thirty minutes of exposure roughly five hours before your planned bedtime.) Also look for other opportunities to get the benefit of natural sunlight exposure during the day (especially from 11:00 am to 3:00 pm, when vitamin D synthesis is possible).

Depression scale. Complete the depression scale and record your score.

Week 5

Supplements. Continue as before.

Rumination. Continue as before.

Exercise. Continue as before. If you aren't satisfied at this point with your chosen form of exercise, try experimenting with another one from your list (pages 123–124) instead.

Light. Continue as before.

Social support. Schedule at least three social activities for the week ahead, writing them in your calendar. It's best to spend time with friends or loved ones whom you can see in person. When that's not possible, substitute phone calls (or video chats) with out-of-town friends and relatives. Another alternative is time spent on supportive online forums for depression (see pages 176–177).

Depression scale. Complete the depression scale and record your score.

Week 6

Supplements. Continue as before.

Rumination. Continue as before.

Exercise. Continue as before. If you've still not been successful in exercising aerobically at least three times each week, you will almost certainly need to hire a personal trainer to help you with this part of the program.

Light. Continue as before.

Social support. Schedule at least four social activities for the week ahead, writing them in your calendar. In addition, evaluate whether or not you have any truly toxic relationships in your life;

if you do, try working to improve the relationships that are open to improvement (see pages 177–178) and limiting your contact with any irredeemably toxic individuals by at least 50% in the week ahead.

Sleep. Adopt the goal of getting adequate sleep each night: seven to nine hours, depending on your body's needs (see pages 195–197). Put into practice the first two habits of healthy sleep: use your bed only for sleeping and wake up at the same time every morning.

Depression scale. Complete the depression scale and record your score.

Week 7

Evaluation. You've now been putting the principles of Therapeutic Lifestyle Change into practice for six weeks. Most people will see at least some benefit by this point. Please take a moment to look at your weekly depression scores, going all the way back to the first score before you started the TLC program. Do you see a clear trend toward improvement, with your current level of symptoms at least 25% lower than when you began? If not, it will be important to skip ahead now to Chapter 11, which focuses on troubleshooting, and also to consider immediately contacting a licensed therapist for assistance (including help with putting the TLC program into practice), if you haven't done so already.

Supplements. Continue as before. However, if you haven't seen at least a 50% reduction in your symptoms from baseline (when you began the TLC program), consider increasing your omega-3 dose to 2000 mg each day of EPA (with at least 1000 mg of DHA).

Rumination. Continue as before.

Exercise. Continue as before. If you haven't seen at least a 50% decrease in your baseline depressive symptoms, consider bumping up your exercise regimen to at least five thirty-minute workouts each week.

Light. If your depression scale score is now below 10, you can decrease bright light exposure to fifteen minutes each day.

Social support. Schedule at least five social activities for the week ahead. Also, try limiting your contact with any irredeemably toxic individuals by an additional 50% in the week ahead.

Sleep. Continue as before. Also, work to incorporate the remaining habits of healthy sleep (habits 3 through 10, outlined in Chapter 9, pages 203–210).

Depression scale. Complete the depression scale and record your score.

Week 8

Supplements. Continue as before.

Rumination. Continue as before.

Exercise. Continue as before.

Light. If your depression scale score is now below 10, you can decrease morning/evening bright light exposure to fifteen minutes each day.

Social support. Schedule at least one social activity each day. In addition, target at least one form of community involvement to participate in during the upcoming week. Finally, try eliminating your contact with any irredeemably toxic individuals.

Sleep. Continue as before.

Depression scale. Complete the depression scale and record your score.

Weeks 9 through 12

Supplements. Continue as before.

Rumination. Continue as before.

Exercise. Continue as before.

Light. When your depression scale score drops below 10, you can decrease bright light exposure to fifteen minutes each day. Continue adding another fifteen to thirty minutes' worth of sunlight exposure (when it's available) during the day.

Social support. Continue as before, and increase your community involvement to at least two forms of activity each week.

Sleep. Continue as before.

Depression scale. Complete the depression scale and record your score.

Evaluation. By the end of twelve weeks (roughly three months), the great majority of our TLC patients at the University of Kansas have experienced significant improvement in depressive symptoms. At a minimum, we expect to observe at least a 50% decrease in severity from pretreatment, at which point most people no longer meet the full diagnostic criteria for major depression, and the overall trajectory points toward complete recovery. If you don't see such improvement* when looking at your own depression scores, please turn to Chapter

* In other words, you should see at least a 50% reduction in your initial depression score (the one obtained before you began putting these lifestyle changes into practice).

11, which focuses on troubleshooting, and consider contacting a licensed therapist for assistance.

OVERCOMING DEPRESSION FOR LIFE

If you've successfully applied the six major elements of Therapeutic Lifestyle Change as outlined in the preceding section, you've taken an important step toward the goal of long-term freedom from depression. However, even after you've experienced relief from the acute agony of depressive illness, there's never room for complacency when battling such a relentless foe. As we've seen, the rate of relapse in depression is very high: Over half of those who recover from depression will face the disorder again at some point.

Fortunately, you can reduce this risk dramatically. There's abundant evidence that each of the major lifestyle changes we've outlined can protect against the return of depression. The key is to make sure you stay at it—that you continue living the depression cure every day in the months and years ahead.

The best analogy might be that of adult-onset (Type II) diabetes, a serious illness that can often be controlled through a strict regimen of diet and exercise. If a diabetic fails to follow the appropriate lifestyle regimen, however, blood sugar skyrockets, and damage to the body's major organs (heart, kidneys, brain, eyes) usually follows. That's why doctors tell those afflicted by the disease, in no uncertain terms, that diabetes is a lifelong illness—they will always have it—but it can be successfully managed; they can remain healthy if they work on it each and every day.

Depression is very much the same. You can eliminate the symptoms, but the disorder's enduring imprint on the brain, with its corresponding risk of relapse, is always there.* Still, you're largely in control of your own fate. You have a superb chance of remaining healthy if you're willing to work at it—to make the antidepressant lifestyle regimen a nonnegotiable priority in your life.

In addition, there are two general principles of relapse prevention that will help ensure your depression remains a thing of the past:

Stress management. Depression can be triggered by the brain's runaway stress response, and the illness often follows closely on the heels of taxing life events. So, even though the regimen we've outlined is effective in putting the brakes on the brain's stress response circuits, it's best—when possible—to eliminate the major sources of stress from your life.

In Chapter 8, for example, we discussed the importance of identifying and limiting so-called *toxic relationships*, which can stand in the way of a full recovery from depression. Likewise, it's crucial to avoid the strain of such unhelpful social ties after the illness has receded. Here's a good rule of thumb to keep in mind: Any relationship that consistently provokes a high level of stress is one that adds to your risk of future depression.

Another particularly disruptive social stressor is the decision to relocate geographically. We've become such a transient society that most people barely think twice about moving halfway across the country, even if it means severing all of their important social bonds in the process. But we're simply not designed to be uprooted like that. It

* That sounds depressing, so let me sound a more hopeful note: With each passing month of recovery, depression's imprint on the brain grows more and more faint.

takes a huge toll on our mental health, kicking the brain's stress circuits into high gear. Not surprisingly, relocation is a common trigger of depression. This is not to say that one should never consider moving away from friends and family, but the anticipated benefits of such a move (such as a good job or educational opportunity) should be carefully weighed against the costs—the increased stress and the temporary lack of social support the move will entail.

It's also important to limit stress in the workplace. For example, a few years ago one of my patients found herself in a hostile, unsupportive work environment. Her boss was prone to harsh, critical outbursts (even though he greatly valued her as an employee), and her coworkers treated her as an outcast because of her political views. (She was an outspoken liberal in an office filled with conservatives.) Rather than quit her job, which would have brought its own set of stresses, she began exploring ways to improve things at work. A frank, open conversation with her boss led him to apologize for his occasional outbursts: He also pledged to treat her with greater consideration in the future. And she was successful in connecting with two coworkers around common interests that had nothing to do with politics. (At my suggestion, she also found noise-cancelling headphones a great benefit when conservative talk shows were blaring on the office radio.)

Vigilance. When it comes to staying healthy and depression-free, it's crucial to stay ever attuned to the possible emergence of new symptoms, and to do whatever it takes to nip them in the bud. Preventing the onset of depression is a lot like stopping a snowball that's rolling down a hill. If you catch it quickly, before it has a chance to build up much size or momentum, it's easy to halt it in its tracks. But if you wait too long, it becomes an unstoppable juggernaut that crushes everything in its path.

Some situations are particularly likely to trigger the return of some depressive symptoms, and you'll need to be especially attentive when you face them. Common high-risk situations to watch out for include the death of a loved one, the experience of divorce (or other romantic breakup), bouts of physical illness, caring for a sick relative, geographic relocation (or the loss of a close friend due to relocation), the loss of employment, an unexpected financial setback, and even extended periods of gloomy weather (and corresponding low sunlight exposure).

As soon as you begin to notice the return of any depressive symptoms, even if they're relatively mild, it's important to address them immediately. The following three principles can be helpful in that respect:

- First, it's often possible to render obvious triggering events less stressful. For example, when overwhelmed by the task of caring for her elderly mother, one of my patients was able to reduce her stress load by hiring a home-health nurse. I've observed, though, that people often resist opportunities to lighten their burdens like this. Many times it's because they feel they don't deserve the help, and sometimes they're simply unwilling to ask for it. But such help can make an enormous difference in keeping stress at a manageable level.
- It's also important to evaluate, with complete honesty, how effectively you've been putting the six principles of Therapeutic Lifestyle Change (TLC) into practice every day. Have you slacked off in any areas? If so, it will be helpful to renew your commitment to implementing each one—to make certain

you're getting the full antidepressant benefit of the TLC protocol each day.

- If, on the other hand, you've experienced some breakthrough symptoms of depression despite sticking to the entire TLC regimen, it's usually a good idea to check in with your doctor if the symptoms last more than a few days. (I'd advise you to check in *immediately*, however, if you're having suicidal thoughts.) In addition, you can try turning things up a notch on the therapeutic lifestyle front for a few weeks—taking advantage of the potent ability of these simple strategies to clamp down on the brain's runaway stress response (and corresponding depressive symptoms). For example, you might consider immersing yourself in your social support network, spending as much face time as possible with those who can love and nurture you through your time of distress.

A complete set of strategies for enhancing the antidepressant effect of the TLC regimen is outlined in the following chapter, along with a detailed troubleshooting guide.

11

When Roadblocks Emerge: A Troubleshooting Guide

The Depression Cure. Admittedly, this is a bold title—inspired by the promise of reclaiming the protective legacy of an antidepressant way of life. But not everyone who picks up this book will find the cure they've been looking for, at least not right away. Some will still find themselves battling depressive symptoms, even after attempting to make all the recommended changes. What if you happen to be one of them? What should you do then?

The answer hinges on how successful you've been in putting the full Therapeutic Lifestyle Change (TLC) protocol into practice. In most cases, when I've seen someone continue to struggle with depression after trying the TLC program, it's because they've run into some important roadblocks that kept them from making the necessary changes. Fortunately, several troubleshooting strategies can help address these obstacles to recovery.

Every once in a while, however, someone does a pretty good job of making the recommended lifestyle changes, and yet they still face lingering symptoms of depression.* In such cases, several additional

* However, I've never seen someone utilize the entire TLC protocol without significant improvement in their depressive symptoms.

treatment recommendations* may prove helpful. We'll cover them in some detail in the concluding section of this chapter.

THE BEST OF INTENTIONS

We are all creatures of habit. The brain's reward pathways light up with pleasure every time we indulge in one of our habitual behaviors, no matter what it happens to be—reading the paper, flossing teeth, walking the dog, making the bed, and so on. That's why we find it so hard to change our typical way of doing things. Keeping our usual m.o. is usually much more rewarding than adopting a new one. (It takes a few weeks of real effort before any new behavior turns into a full-fledged habit—after which it finally becomes rewarding and, thus, self-sustaining.)

The bottom line: Lifestyle change is much easier said than done. Think about the millions of people who resolve each year to start working out, to eat healthily, to stop smoking, to watch less TV, or to get more sleep—and how few succeed. If lifestyle change were simple, we wouldn't be facing an epidemic of obesity, with two-thirds of American adults now overweight.

Compound this difficulty with the fact that depression makes it particularly hard for someone to initiate new activity. As we've seen, the disorder shuts down circuits in the left frontal cortex, the part of the brain that allows us to put our intentions into action.

By all rights, then, Therapeutic Lifestyle Change might look like some sort of cruel pipe dream—something that sounds great on paper but that proves impossible to put into practice in the real world. And yet I've watched countless depressed individuals find a lasting cure

* Some other diagnostic possibilities may also need to be considered.

by making the TLC program a central part of their lives. How did they succeed?

In most cases, they had help. They needed help. While I've known a few dozen people over the years who've been able—completely on their own—to put the TLC protocol into practice after simply hearing about it (in a newspaper or magazine article or a talk I'd given), such individuals are the exception, not the rule. Typically, their depressive symptoms were on the milder end of the continuum, so they still had enough energy and initiative to make the necessary changes.

So, if you've failed on your own to make some of the therapeutic lifestyle changes described in *The Depression Cure*, please know that you're not alone. Among the clinically depressed, such difficulties are par for the course. But with the help of some good coaching, you're still likely to benefit from everything in the TLC protocol—omega-3 supplementation, anti-ruminative activity, aerobic exercise, sunlight exposure, increased social support, and healthy sleep.

You simply need to find someone who can help you translate your intentions into action. By gently encouraging you each step along the way as you put the protocol into practice, a TLC coach can, in effect, play the role of your left frontal cortex—shoring up your ability to initiate the changes you've already committed to making.

Finding a TLC Coach

Where can you find such coaching? There are two different options worth exploring: You can use either a professional therapist or an amateur coach. We discuss both options in this section.

A professional therapist. In my experience, most depressed individuals, especially those struggling with the TLC protocol, can benefit from the expert guidance of a trained therapist. But there's a bewildering array of licensed mental health practitioners to choose from: psychiatrists, clinical psychologists, counseling psychologists, social workers, nurse practitioners, and other assorted counselors and therapists. Generally speaking, those with the best, most advanced training in helping people change the way they live—the crux of the TLC protocol—are clinical psychologists. (Please keep in mind, however, that highly trained psychiatrists, nurse practitioners, and clinical social workers can be effective in this coaching role, as well.)

Over the past few years, I've been contacted by depressed individuals all over the country looking for a professional in their area to help them put the principles of TLC into practice, and I direct them to a highly skilled therapist whenever I can. But it has to be someone who is willing to work with them on implementing the antidepressant lifestyle changes outlined in *The Depression Cure* (as opposed to other traditional psychotherapy activities, such as exploring the details of childhood). In addition, I always look for a therapist who's been trained in *behavior therapy*—the type of treatment that focuses on changing what we *do*.

A superb resource for finding such therapists in your area is the *European Association of Behavioural and Cognitive Therapies* (EABCT). Another option is to ask for a referral for a skilled behavior therapist from your doctor or other trusted professionals in your community.

When you contact a psychologist or other mental health professional to serve as your TLC coach, please bear in mind that all therapists are not created equal (even among those who are highly

---

* You can find the EABCT directory at http://eabct.glimworm.com/index.jsp

trained). There are some that you'll "click" with right away and some that you won't. According to the best research, you'll likely have a good intuitive sense of how well you're going to hit it off with a therapist within the first session or two. So, if it doesn't feel like a reasonably good fit early on, it's probably best to consider moving on to the next name on your referral list.

An amateur coach. A completely different approach to coaching, however, can sometimes be a viable option: the amateur coach. Some people are in the fortunate position of having a loved one—a spouse, parent, sibling, child, or close friend—who is both willing and able to serve as their TLC coach. Although this approach has some potential pitfalls, I've also seen it work very well, as long as the following conditions are met:

- Rapport: There has to be a strong, trusting relationship in place—with rock-solid rapport—between the coach and the person he or she is helping. This is crucial, because TLC coaches sometimes need to push their depressed charges out of their comfort zones. Even when they do this with great tact and gentleness, it will come across as nagging—and damage the underlying relationship—if the level of rapport is not high at the outset.
- Knowledge: The coach also needs to become knowledgeable about the ins and outs of the entire TLC protocol. This is not a difficult task, but it does require a significant time commitment.
- Dedication: Clearly, coaching someone through the TLC program takes a high level of dedication. It requires checking in with them on a regular basis, providing timely prompts for each major area of lifestyle change. Early in the process, this can even mean

arranging for several different prompts each day—depending on how much difficulty the depressed individual has with initiating activity. (As the weeks pass and symptoms improve, much less prompting will usually be necessary.)

Troubleshooting Tips

Whether or not you choose to take advantage of a TLC coach, you can overcome some of the most common obstacles to implementing the program by attending to a set of basic troubleshooting tips. Although these are described, one lifestyle element at a time, at various places throughout the book, Table 11-1 provides a handy summary of the best strategies for addressing major TLC trouble spots.

WHEN TLC ISN'T ENOUGH

Occasionally, someone will do a good job of adopting all the major lifestyle changes recommended in the TLC program, but will still suffer from serious depressive symptoms. Such a dilemma has several potential causes—mostly due to various medical conditions or other co-occurring forms of mental illness—and these need to be addressed with the help of a trained clinical professional.

Medical Complications

Because depression is literally a form of physical illness, it makes sense that the disorder can sometimes be caused by another serious medical

TABLE 11-1. *TLC Trouble Spots and Solutions*

TLC Element	*Problem*	*Potential Solution*
Omega-3 Supplement	*Trouble remembering to take supplements every day*	Give yourself an unavoidable visual reminder. For example, store the bottle on your nightstand, on your pillow, or next to your toothbrush.
	Burping up fishy taste, or indigestion or discomfort	Switch to a pharmaceutical grade fish oil supplement, one that's been molecularly distilled.
	Can't take fish oil (vegetarian or seafood allergy)	Use both flaxseed oil and an algae-based omega-3 supplement to get necessary EPA and DHA.
Anti-ruminative Activity	*Trouble catching rumination when it's happening (in "real time")*	Several times each day, stop whatever you're doing to monitor and observe your thoughts. If needed, use prompts, such as programmable alarms on your cellphone, PDA, or pager; calls from your TLC coach; or regular breaks in your schedule (such as a trip to the bathroom).
	Low motivation to stop rumination (it feels beneficial or useful)	Give yourself permission to ruminate on a specific problem, but with a strict time limit of no more than ten minutes a day. (After that, you've hit the point of diminishing returns, and no additional insights are likely to emerge.)
	Difficulty stopping rumination	Make a list of your most engaging activities (both social and solo) and experiment with each during bouts of rumination to determine which are the most effective at stopping rumination. Also, try writing down ruminative thoughts, and then walking away from them.

Aerobic Exercise	*Can't get started, or can't stick to an exercise regimen*	Hire a personal trainer or find an exercise buddy who will hold you accountable and provide appropriate prompts.
	Ruminating during exercise	Exercise to engaging music or books-on-tape or switch to a more engaging, social form of exercise.
	Not enjoying exercise	Find an exercise partner (or trainer); experiment with more game-like physical activities; try taking brisk walks immersed in the beauty of nature.
Bright Light Exposure	*No reliable natural sunlight available right now (too cloudy or cold, days too short, and so on)*	Buy a 10,000-lux light box.
	Eyes can't tolerate the light box, or feeling jittery or nauseated	Try doubling the distance from the light box for a week, and then gradually moving closer.
	Can't make time in my morning routine for light exposure	Try sitting in front of the light box (or outside on sunny mornings) during breakfast; place the light box safely on the bathroom counter while grooming; use the light box during the first fifteen to thirty minutes at work.
Social Connection	*Low motivation to socialize; feel like withdrawing*	Remind yourself that this is completely normal in depression: Your brain thinks you're physically ill and need to withdraw. But social activity helps fight depression. If needed, use a TLC coach for prompting and encouragement.

	It feels like existing relationships have been damaged by depressive withdrawal	Confide about depression to friends and loved ones, explain how it causes withdrawal, and ask for help reestablishing each relationship.
	Spending time with some friends and loved ones makes me feel worse, not better	Avoid joint rumination, focusing instead on joint activities. Also, identify any toxic relationships, and begin to limit time spent with such individuals.
	Few friends or loved ones to spend time with	Try reconnecting via phone or video chat (Skype) with friends or loved ones that live elsewhere; join an online depression forum to receive support from others struggling with the illness; become involved in a community organization.
Sleep	*No time in busy schedule for eight hours of sleep each night*	Make sleep your top priority, realizing that healthy sleep leads to greater efficiency in everything else, more than making up for any lost time spent in bed.
	Trouble falling asleep	Avoid stimulating activity and use only dim light an hour before bedtime; avoid caffeine except in the morning; turn down the thermostat at bedtime; increase morning bright light exposure and avoid late sunlight exposure; follow all the principles of healthy sleep outlined in Chapter 9.
	Trouble staying asleep	Avoid early morning bright light exposure and substitute exposure in late afternoon or early evening; use blackout curtains in the bedroom; increase exercise; follow all the principles of healthy sleep outlined in Chapter 9.

condition. Many different types of medical illness can, under some circumstances, trigger the onset of clinical depression; they can also make the disorder very difficult (sometimes impossible) to treat effectively until the underlying medical issue is addressed.

Therefore, if you've found the TLC protocol ineffective in clearing up your depression, it's absolutely essential that you see a physician right away for a complete medical evaluation—to rule out any number of illnesses that might be keeping you depressed. Some of the more common medical culprits are

- Diabetes
- Hypothyroidism (low thyroid function)
- Sleep apnea
- Mononucleosis
- Persistent infection
- Hormonal imbalance
- Malnutrition
- Heart disease
- Cancer
- Stroke
- Brain injury
- Parkinson's disease
- Alzheimer's disease

In addition, many medications—even some of the drugs commonly used in treating mental illness—carry the potential to trigger depression, and they can also maintain the disorder once it's begun. Your physician can help you evaluate this possibility, as well. It will be especially important to bring it to your doctor's attention if you're taking any of the following types of medication:

- Benzodiazepines (Rivotril, Ativan, Valium)
- Tranquilizers/sedatives
- Beta blockers
- Antihistamines
- Birth control pills
- Steroids
- Non-steroidal anti-inflammatory drugs (NSAIDs)
- Antipsychotics
- Antihypertensives (blood pressure medications)

Psychiatric Complications

There is strong research evidence that the various elements of Therapeutic Lifestyle Change are effective not just in the treatment of depression, but also in the reduction of symptoms across a number of other psychological domains. TLC can reduce anxiety, soothe irritability, put the brakes on impulsive behavior, weaken addictive cravings, and tighten erratic thinking.

Nevertheless, some forms of mental illness may make it difficult to fully recover from depression until they're directly addressed in treatment by a skilled clinician. The more common such co-occurring conditions are described in this section.

Post-Traumatic Stress Disorder (PTSD). Following severe trauma, many people suffer PTSD—a painful syndrome that involves intrusive traumatic memories and nightmares, emotional numbing, relentless tension, extreme vigilance, exaggerated startle reflex, and avoidance of people and situations associated with the trauma. Because PTSD keeps the brain's stress response circuits in overdrive, it can powerfully interfere with recovery from depression.

Fortunately, the disorder has a high rate of treatment response to skilled psychotherapy.

Other anxiety disorders. Despite TLC's ability to reduce overall anxiety, several specific anxiety disorders usually require a more focused intervention to bring about full recovery. These include obsessive-compulsive disorder, panic disorder, agoraphobia, social anxiety disorder, and specific phobias. All can be successfully treated in the majority of cases by behavior therapy.*

Substance abuse and dependence. Alcohol and other drugs of addiction have an array of harmful effects on brain function, and they typically also bring about high levels of depressive life stress. They also wreak havoc on the user's social support networks. In brief: Substance use disorders can make it impossible to recover from an episode of depression until effectively addressed in treatment.

Bipolar disorder. Individuals with bipolar disorder (formerly known as manic-depression) suffer not only bouts of depression, but also episodes of *mania*—several days or more of elevated (or irritable) mood, increased energy, reduced need for sleep, rapid speech, heightened self-esteem, frenzied activity, and recklessly impulsive behavior. (Some bipolar patients experience similar, less debilitating, episodes known as *hypomania*.) Although there is some evidence that Therapeutic Lifestyle Change elements can reduce symptoms of depression in bipolar disorder, it's also clear that optimal treatment of the illness often involves the use of mood-stabilizing medications such as Lamictal, lithium, Depakote, or Trileptal.

Psychotic disorders. Illnesses such as schizophrenia, delusional disorder, and schizoaffective disorder are distinguished by thoughts or perceptions that don't correspond with reality—for example, hearing

* A related form of treatment, CBT, is also effective for most anxiety disorders.

voices or succumbing to unfounded, paranoid fantasies of persecution by others. Such symptoms can interfere with functioning on multiple levels, and can easily cause or maintain an episode of depression. Psychotic disorders are often at least partially responsive to antipsychotic medications.

Eating disorders. The two most serious eating disorders, bulimia nervosa and anorexia nervosa, involve such compromised nutrition that brain function is adversely affected. Both conditions can cause a host of serious physical complications—anorexia can even be fatal when left untreated—and they require *immediate* attention from trained medical, psychological, and nutritional specialists.

Personality disorders. To a psychologist, your personality is simply *the way you normally think, feel, and behave.* As such, personality is usually pretty stable over time and across different situations. Even though we all have our little foibles and peccadilloes, some people have personality traits that cause quite a bit of distress, even to the point of interfering with their ability to function. There are individuals, for example, who have great trouble forming healthy relationships due to their profound insecurity. Others suffer from such extreme perfectionism that they are continually stressed out from an inability to live up to their own high standards. Still others have a penchant for generating drama and chaos, with a knack for setting off the kind of painful life events known to trigger (and maintain) depression.

The field's diagnostic Bible, the *DSM-IV,* refers to these various dysfunctional patterns by the term *personality disorders.* And, until such disorders are addressed in treatment, they can make it difficult to benefit fully from the TLC protocol.

Although there is a paucity of solid research evidence on the various forms of psychotherapy available for personality disorders, the one notable exception is *dialectical behavior therapy* (DBT). It's tremendously helpful in treating borderline personality—a condition characterized by intense, out-of-control emotions, impulsive behaviors, desperate attachments, and an unstable sense of self. But DBT appears promising for several other forms of personality dysfunction, as well.

Another treatment approach with some research support—and one that I've found particularly useful in my clinical practice with personality disordered patients—is *schema therapy*, developed by Dr. Jeffrey Young of the New York Center for Cognitive Therapy. It involves identifying and changing the harmful core beliefs, or *schemas,* about oneself and others; such schemas cause extraordinary suffering, and they can make it impossible to form satisfying relationships.

TAKING ANTIDEPRESSANT LIFESTYLE TO THE NEXT LEVEL

As we've seen, our remote hunter-gatherer ancestors were extraordinarily resilient in the face of difficult life circumstances, and largely free from the scourge of depressive illness. They were protected by a set of habits that benefit the brain more powerfully than any known antidepressant medication. The Therapeutic Lifestyle Change program is designed to help people reclaim this protective legacy from the ancestral past. It's a treatment approach based on the best research findings from clinical labs around the world, an approach that's proven effective for the great majority of depressed patients who put it into practice.

However, the TLC program was designed with an important consideration in mind: I wanted to make sure the treatment was truly doable, that depressed patients would actually be able to make the changes I was asking of them. As a result, I ended up leaving some potentially helpful things out of the basic program—despite good research support for their ability to fight depression—simply because I didn't want to overwhelm patients with too many lifestyle changes to juggle all at once.

So, while the standard TLC regimen is already highly effective for most people, some additional strategies may prove helpful if your depressive symptoms have not fully cleared up after you've made each of the treatment's recommended lifestyle changes. It's possible, in other words, for you to *take antidepressant lifestyle change to the next level*, provided you're willing to put even more time and effort into the process of recovery. In this section I describe the several options worth considering.

Upping the Exercise Dose

Whereas our hunter-gatherer forebears engaged in vigorous physical activity for several hours each day, the TLC protocol calls for a total of only ninety minutes of aerobic exercise each week. Frankly, that's a low dose of exercise, given the robust antidepressant effect of physical activity on the brain. Although this modest amount of exercise is still potently antidepressant, many people would likely experience even greater clinical benefit from a higher level of activity.

According to fitness researchers, the beneficial effects of exercise on the body steadily increase as we ramp up our weekly workout time—yielding more energy, better cardiac and pulmonary function, improved metabolism, and so on. Remarkably, the health dividends of exercise appear to increase up to a dose of at least an hour each day.

A few years ago I decided to experiment with a more ambitious workout regimen myself, mostly so I could see firsthand if it really made any noticeable difference. I went from exercising thirty minutes every other day to working out an hour each day, and the effects were immediate and compelling: My sleep quality, energy level, stamina, calmness, mental clarity, and sense of well-being all significantly improved. The benefits proved well worth the extra time investment, so I've stayed with it. Now, if I skip even a single daily workout, the next day I'll feel relatively sluggish, antsy, and just not as sharp.

Researchers have yet to study the effectiveness of such a "high dose" exercise regimen in combating depression (in part, because it's difficult to get people to volunteer for that much exercise). But I have no doubt the added activity is beneficial for the brain, just as it's already proven to be for the rest of the body. So, if you're already getting ninety minutes of aerobic activity each week (as recommended in the standard TLC protocol), you might want to consider bumping it up—experimenting with gradually higher levels of activity for the next several weeks to see if you notice a difference in your depressive symptoms (and other dimensions of well-being). I recommend adding an extra sixty minutes or so to your routine each week, until you're up to an hour of exercise each day (roughly four hundred minutes a week).

Increase Omega-3

The starting omega-3 dosage recommended in the TLC protocol—1000 mg of EPA and 500 mg of DHA per day—is adequate for most people, but it's not high enough to get everyone's blood levels of omega-6 and omega-3 fats in balance. Even some who try doubling this standard dosage still won't achieve the proper fatty acid ratio for optimal brain function. As we saw in Chapter 4, the only way to ensure this ideal balance is with a blood test, which will allow your doctor to evaluate the ratio of omega-6 and omega-3 fats in your blood plasma. (Remember, the target ratio is 2 to 1.) Although having your blood drawn is inconvenient, it can help ensure that your brain is getting all the omega-3 fats it needs.

Decrease Dietary Sugar

As we've seen, chronic inflammation—the body's immune response running amok—is a major culprit in depressive illness. It's an insidious process that, over time, ravages both body and brain. And even though we can help get the body's inflammation response under control by increasing our intake of omega-3 fats, a dangerous pro-inflammatory villain is lurking at the heart of the modern Western diet: sugar.

The typical American now consumes a staggering eighty pounds of processed sugars* each year. That's twenty-five teaspoons of sugar—the equivalent of four hundred calories—every day. This ubiquitous sweetener now makes up an unfathomable 20% of our diets. And each little white grain carries the potential to nudge the brain a little further away from the state of healthful balance needed to break the grip of depressive illness. (Please note that the natural sugars found in fruits and vegetables pose no such hazards to the brain.)

Unfortunately, neuroscientists have recently discovered that sugar is potently addictive. It can light up the brain's pleasure centers

* This figure includes related sugary sweeteners like high-fructose corn syrup.

just like cocaine or heroin. This makes the "sugar habit" incredibly difficult to break. Most of us have been hooked on the stuff since childhood.

But it *is* possible to cut way back on sugar intake—enough to reduce the sweetener's potential depressive impact—with just a bit of effort. It's simply a matter of finding reasonable, satisfying substitutes for the major sources of sugar in your diet: the soft drinks, candy, ice cream, juices, snack bars, breakfast cereals, and other assorted sweets.

Although simply switching to soft drinks and snacks laced with artificial sweeteners might seem like an obvious strategy, I'm hesitant to recommend this approach. Instead, I recommend substituting natural, healthy alternatives to the sugars in your diet. For example, honey is *anti*-inflammatory, and it has an array of other health benefits. (It's antibiotic, antiviral, and even seems to help protect against adult-onset diabetes.) And while it's probably not a good idea to eat honey by the bucketful—"everything in moderation" is a great nutritional rule of thumb—using it to sweeten your drinks, and the occasional snack, will certainly help take the sting out of eating less sugar. Other natural sweeteners to keep in mind include *stevia* (also known as *sweetleaf*), a South American herb that's actually a little sweeter than sugar, and *Xylitol*, a plant derivative now recommended by dentists to help fight cavities.

The healthiest sugar substitute of all is *fructose*, the natural sweetener found in all fruits. Although not as sweet as processed sugar itself, fructose is much better for the body and brain. And fortunately, as you work to eliminate the major sources of dietary sugar from your life, you'll notice that fruit will begin to taste much sweeter. (In essence, your taste buds will quickly recalibrate, so that fruit starts to taste about as sweet as candy bars and cakes used to.) This happy development, in turn, will make it much easier to continue keeping sugar intake to a minimum.

Eat More Tryptophan

The brain makes its entire supply of serotonin, a feel-good neurotransmitter, out of a protein called *tryptophan*. Most of us get plenty of tryptophan in our diets; it's found in abundance in meats like turkey, chicken, beef, pork, and fish, as well as cheese, eggs, milk, beans, and soy products. But when we're severely strained, stress hormones can limit the amount of tryptophan available to the brain, which in turn causes serotonin activity in the brain to plummet. This can, in turn, trigger a vicious feedback loop: Depression causes elevated stress hormones, which suppress tryptophan levels in the bloodstream, which reduce serotonin activity in the brain, which deepens the depression, and so on.

One way to help break this cycle is to increase dietary tryptophan intake—to eat several servings of meat, eggs, dairy, and soy products each day. Another alternative is to take a tryptophan supplement, a strategy with some research support in fighting depression. (A typical dose in published studies is 1 to 3 grams daily.) However, because there have been alarming reports of life-threatening impurities found in over-the-counter tryptophan supplements, I strongly advise against going that route. A more reliable form of the protein is available in prescription form (it's sold in the US as *Tryptan*), but you can safely get an equivalent dose of tryptophan by simply adding about four small (3-ounce) servings of meat or other tryptophan-rich foods to your diet each day.

(Although you may worry that adding so much extra protein to your diet will result in weight gain, there's pretty solid research evidence that tryptophan suppresses appetite, which can result in a net calorie decrease despite the added protein intake.)

Increase Vitamin D

I've suggested a daily Vitamin D_3 dose of 50 mcg per day, based on so-called "tolerable upper intake levels" published by the Institute of Medicine. However, this guideline is now over ten years old, and research has been published in the meantime to support the safety of higher doses. One recent study, for example, found that some people (about 25% of those in the study) needed 100 mcg of Vitamin D_3 each day to get maximal benefit; tellingly, no one experienced any adverse side effects at that higher dose. If you're still battling depressive symptoms after supplementing at 50 mcg per day, you may want to consult with your doctor about bumping the dosage up to 100 mcg. (Since that's above the recommended upper intake level, it would be inadvisable for anyone to take such a high dose without medical supervision.)

Get More Sunlight Exposure

When we're exposed to sunlight, it stimulates activity in brain circuits that use serotonin, with a resultant antidepressant effect.* Although the TLC protocol recommends bright light exposure—either through

---

* In addition, sunlight exposure helps regulate the internal body clock, improves sleep quality, and (under some circumstances) stimulates synthesis of vitamin D—all of which provide an antidepressant benefit.

direct sunlight or its light box equivalent—of about thirty minutes each day, some people will find additional benefit from extending this daily exposure out to sixty minutes or more. Individual results will vary quite a bit, however, so the wisest approach is simply to experiment with several different daily "doses" of light exposure, observing and monitoring the effect of each dosage level, and remaining vigilant for possible unwelcome side effects of extended exposure (jitteriness or nausea, for example).

STRESS REDUCTION

If you've put the entire TLC protocol into practice and still find yourself battling depressive symptoms, it may prove useful to take an inventory of the major stressful circumstances in your life. I encourage you to write them down, and to rate each one (on a 10-point scale) in terms of how much strain it causes on a day-to-day basis.

Two distinct strategies can be used to limit the effect of each major stressor: We can work to improve the stressful situation itself, or we can enhance our ability to *cope* with the situation, even when it can't be "fixed" in any meaningful way.

Improve the situation. Fortunately, in many cases, there are at least some steps you can take to render things less stressful. We've discussed many such strategies in Chapter 8, such as enlisting the help of someone to ease your most stressful burdens or finding a confidant who can serve as a sounding board. (In many cases, simply talking over a stressor with a loved one will serve as a catalyst for fresh insights about how to improve the situation.)

Improve your ability to cope. Life tosses out its share of heartaches to everyone. Death, illness, failure, and loss are simply part of the human condition—painful circumstances that can't be improved, no matter how masterful our problem-solving abilities may be. And whenever we're faced with such agonizing stressors, our ability to cope with them successfully will determine whether or not we keep depression at bay.

The most effective coping strategy—by far—involves turning to loved ones, friends, and extended community for intensive social support. As we've seen, the physical and emotional presence of others provides a powerful safety cue for the brain, coaxing it to put the brakes on its stress response circuits even in the face of painful life circumstances. As a result, social support is a potent buffer against the experience of depression.

Then again, not everyone is lucky enough to have such a protective network in place. But it turns out that even *one* caring, committed individual can make all the difference—even if that person is a clinician you see for only one or two sessions a week.

In many cases, our ability to cope with difficult events also hinges on the way we interpret them. Sometimes things are not as catastrophic as we think they are. Good psychotherapists are highly trained to help their depressed patients see such stressful situations in a less dire light. But a good friend or loved one can sometimes play a similar role—pointing out the subtle and not-so-subtle ways that depression might cause a situation to look bleaker than it truly is.

I've also seen many individuals find enormous comfort and strength through participation in a faith community. And the benefit often goes far beyond the wonderful social support such communities can provide. It also comes from adopting an interpretive point of view that says, in effect, "As agonizing as this situation seems right now, there's a mysterious way in which it's not as bad as I think it is." I've also witnessed several of my nonspiritual patients find a similarly helpful reinterpretation of stressful circumstances through the practice of mindfulness meditation,* which helps promote a deep, radical acceptance of each moment life presents us with.

The principles of Therapeutic Lifestyle Change have proven to be extraordinarily effective in treating depression in patients of all ages. Equally important, however, is their ability to protect against the future onset of illness.

Remember, we were never designed for the sedentary, socially isolated, sleep-deprived, poorly nourished, indoor, frenetic pace of modern American life. Our brains, our bodies, our minds, our hearts, and our souls were all built for something different—for a life filled with abundant physical activity, social connection, healthful sleep, balanced nutrition, natural sunlight, and the sort of meaningful, engaging activities that leave little time for depressive rumination. By living the lives we were meant to lead, reclaiming the protective features of the past and integrating them into the present, we can overcome depression for the long haul. We can vanquish that treacherous foe once and for all. We can live the depression cure.

* An increasingly popular technique now taught in most large and medium-sized metropolitan areas throughout the country. There are also several superb instructional books on mindfulness meditation, including classics such as Jon Kabat-Zinn's *Full Catastrophe Living* and *Wherever You Go, There You Are*, and Thich Nhat Hahn's *The Miracle of Mindfulness*.

Appendix A: Depression Scale

Following is a list of some ways you may have felt or behaved. Please make a copy and indicate how often you experienced these things *during the past week* (circle one number on each line):

During the past week . . .	Rarely or none of the time (< 1 day)	Some (a little of the time) (1–2 days)	At least half the time (3–4 days)	Just about all the time (5–7 days)
1. I was bothered by things that usually don't bother me.	0	1	2	3
2. I did not feel like eating; my appetite was poor.	0	1	2	3
3. I could not shake off the blues, even with others' help.	0	1	2	3
4. I felt that I was just as good as other people.	3	2	1	0
5. I had trouble keeping my mind on what I was doing.	0	1	2	3
6. I felt depressed.	0	1	2	3
7. I felt that everything I did was an effort.	0	1	2	3
8. I felt hopeful about the future.	3	2	1	0
9. I thought my life had been a failure.	0	1	2	3

10. I felt fearful.	0	1	2	3
11. My sleep was restless.	0	1	2	3
12. I was happy.	3	2	1	0
13. I talked less than usual.	0	1	2	3
14. I felt lonely.	0	1	2	3
15. People were unfriendly.	0	1	2	3
16. I enjoyed life.	3	2	1	0
17. I had crying spells.	0	1	2	3
18. I felt sad.	0	1	2	3
19. I felt that people disliked me.	0	1	2	3
20. I could not "get going."	0	1	2	3

Scoring: Your score is the sum of all 20 circled numbers.

Center for Epidemiological Studies Depression Scale (CES-D). Radloff, LS (1977). The CES-D scale is a self-report depression scale for research in the general population. *Applied Psychological Measurement, 1,* 385–401.

Appendix B: Tracking Chart for Depression Symptoms

Please make a copy of the following grid, and then record your depression scale score (from Appendix A) on the grid to help track your symptoms through each week of the Therapeutic Lifestyle Change program.

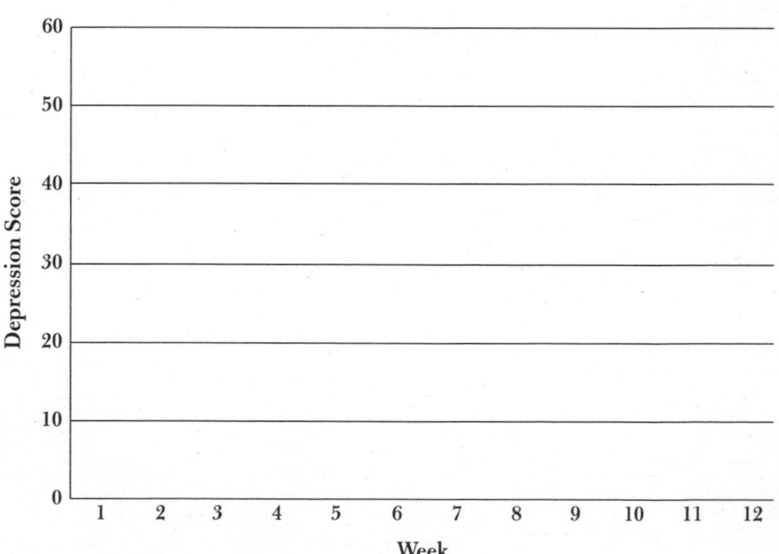

Notes

CHAPTER 1: THE EPIDEMIC AND THE CURE

4 **They work for fewer than half.** Nierenberg et al., 2008.

4 **The United States hasn't declined: It's increased.** Compton et al., 2006.

4 **About one in four Americans.** Kessler et al., 2005.

4 **Roughly ten times higher today.** Seligman, 1990.

5 **Amish communities have a rate of depression.** Egeland and Hostetter, 1983. More recent evidence comes from the work of Miller et al., 2007.

5 **Across the entire industrialized world.** Andrade et al., 2003. Of the many converging lines of evidence, this reference documents one of the most compelling: higher rates of depression among more recent birth cohorts in ten nations.

5 **Fraction of that observed in the West.** Weissman et al., 1996.

5 **Anthropologist Edward Schieffelin.** Schieffelin, 1985.

6 **Until about twelve thousand years ago.** Diamond, 1997.

6 **They've changed very little.** Tooby and Cosmides, 1990.

6 **A staggering 65%.** Ogden et al., 2006.

7 **A mere 4%.** Rampersaud et al., 2008.

9 **Over three times higher.** Karwoski, 2008; Ilardi et al., 2007; Ilardi et al., 2009.

10 **More omega-3 fat than we do.** Simopoulos, 2006.

10 **Countries with the highest levels.** Peet, 2004.

10 **British researchers recently studied.** Peet and Horrobin, 2002

13 **Remarkably good shape.** Cordain et al., 1998.

13 **Compared aerobic exercise and Lustral.** Blumenthal et al., 1999. The finding was later replicated by Blumenthal et al., 2007.

13 **To become depressed again.** Babyak et al., 2000.

16 **Winter daylight is scarce.** Mersch et al., 1999.

17 **The typical village.** Dunbar, 1996.

20 **Lack a supportive social network.** Harris, 2001.

20 **Disrupted sleep is one.** Thase, 2005.

21 **80% of depressed patients.** Armitage, 2000.

21 **About 10 hours a night.** Bower, 1999.

21 **We clock in.** Sleep in America Foundation, 2008.

24 **Our clinical trials.** Ilardi et al., 2007; Karwoski, 2008; Ilardi et al., 2009.

CHAPTER 2: MAKING SENSE OF DEPRESSION

31 **Brain's runaway stress response.** Nemeroff and Vale, 2005.

32 **When the stress response lasts.** Steiger, 2007.

33 **The illness is most often triggered.** Hammen, 2005.

34 **Left frontal hemisphere.** Henriques and Davidson, 1991; Coan & Allen, 2003.

35 **Actually start shrinking.** Frodl et al., 2008.

35 **Rats are experimentally deprived.** Rechtschaffen et al., 2002.

36 **The best studies.** Hamet and Tremblay, 2005, for example.

37 **A recent large-scale study.** Caspi et al., 2003.

38 **Social support networks.** Harris, 2001.

38 **British team of researchers.** Brown and Harris, 1978.

38 **Emotionally abusive spouse.** Harris, 2001.

39 **Prone to depression.** Nolen-Hoeksema et al., 2008.

39 **Researchers have found that estrogen.** MacQueen and Chokka, 2004.

40 **Testosterone has been strongly linked.** Seidman, 2003.

40 **Exercise changes the brain.** Ploughman, 2008.

41 **It rises to well over 50%.** Mueller et al., 1999.

41 **Toxic imprint on the brain.** Post, 1992.

CHAPTER 3: TREATING DEPRESSION

44 **Over one hundred fifty million antidepressant prescriptions.** Stagnitti, 2008.

45 **Only 23% were depression-free.** Corey-Lisle et al., 2004.

45 **Only 28% of study patients.** Trivedi et al., 2006. This was the remission rate observed with a widely used clinician-based rating scale; the rate with a patient self-report scale was similar, but slightly higher.

46 **He found that in 56%.** Kirsch et al., 2002.

47 **Among severely depressed patients.** Khan et al., 2002.

48 **Roughly half of all depressed patients.** Trivedi et al., 2006 (NEJM—augmentation article).

48 **Up to 50%.** Mueller et al., 1999.

49 **Goes off his or her prescribed medications.** Olfson et al., 2006.

50 **Combed through their database.** http://www.fda.gov/cder/drug/antidepressants/SSRIlabelChange.htm.

50 **It may afflict the majority.** Opbroek et al., 2002.

51 **Many people taking SSRIs.** Werneke et al., 2006.

51 **Potential to cause insomnia.** Mayers and Baldwin, 2005.

54 **Cognitive-behavioral therapy is every bit as effective.** Parker et al., 2008.

54 **Leads to complete recovery.** DeRubeis et al., 2005; Keller et al., 2000.

56 **In a recent study.** Dimidjian et al., 2006.

58 **A definitive set of studies.** Svartberg and Stiles, 1991.

59 **As high as 65%.** Husain et al., 2004.

59 **Most ECT patients.** Odeberg et al., 2008.

60 **Permanent brain damage.** Reviewed in Breggin, 1999.

60 **Up to 70%.** Freeman & Kendell, 1986. More recently, Sackeim et al., 2007, observed compelling evidence of enduring memory deficits following ECT in the most rigorous study of the issue to date.

60 **Drop in IQ.** Lipman et al., 1993.

60 **Sales of antidepressant drugs.** IMS MIDAS®, MAT December 2006.

CHAPTER 4: BRAIN FOOD

66 **Insanely high doses.** Page et al., 1999.

66 **Supplementing their diets.** Carzelon et al., 2005.

67 **Our hunter-gatherer ancestors.** Simopoulos, 2006.

67 **A staggering 16 to 1.** Simopoulos, 2002.

68 **"Civilized" early farmers.** Cohen, 1989.

68 **Brains even grew smaller.** Ruff et al., 1997.

69 **Consumption of omega-6 fats.** Pollan, 2008.

70 **Depression tends to be less common.** Peet, 2004.

70 **Lower omega-3 blood levels.** Peet et al., 1998.

70 **The message of serotonin.** Chalon, 2006; McNamara and Carlson, 2006.

70 **Scramble dopamine signals.** McNamara and Carlson, 2006; Chalon, 2006.

71 **Inflammation is also one.** Miller, 2009 (in press).

74 **Published research so far.** Reviewed in Ross et al., 2007.

75 **Help stabilize heart rhythm.** Masuelli et al., 2008.

76 **The best supported daily dosage.** Ross et al., 2007.

80 **Cut back its production of GLA.** Sears, 2007.

82 **Help suppress some allergic reactions.** Miyake et al., 2007.

82 **Ratio on this blood test.** http://www.drsears.com/tabid/399/itemid/68/AAEPA-Blood-Test-Services.aspx

84 **Ratios barely budged.** Young et al., 2005.

85 **Their rates of depression.** Hibbeln, 1989.

CHAPTER 5: DON'T THINK, DO

93 **Amplify negative emotions.** Ciesla and Roberts, 2007.

93 **When we ruminate.** Moulds et al., 2007.

94 **Link between depression and rumination.** Nolen-Hoeksema et al., 2008.

94 **Some surprising quirks.** Marcus, 2008.

95 **Brain uses our mood.** Duncan and Barrett, 2007.

100 **Study of depressed teenagers.** Rose et al., 2007.

CHAPTER 6: ANTIDEPRESSANT EXERCISE

114 **Majority of Americans.** U.S. Department of Health and Human Services, 1999.

115 **Several hours each day.** Cordain et al., 1998.

116 **Long list of health benefits.** Penedo and Dahn, 2005.

116 **Ambitious study of exercise.** Blumenthal et al., 1999.

117 **Stimulates the brain's release.** Vaynman and Gomez-Pinilla, 2006.

120 **Researchers have looked.** Barbour et al., 2007.

126 **Exercising with others.** Blumenthal et al., 2007. Those exercising in a group setting had better outcomes than those working out alone, but the difference between the two groups was not statistically significant.

CHAPTER 7: LET THERE BE LIGHT

136 **Over one hundred times brighter.** Eastman, 1990.

137 **The production of serotonin.** Praschak-Rieder et al., 2008.

137 **The mood-elevating effects.** Goel and Etwaroo, 2006.

137 **More social contact.** Aan Het Rot et al., 2008. This study also observed an effect of bright light in rendering people less quarrelsome and less prone to fighting.

139 **Study of Montreal residents.** Guillemette et al., 1998.

140 **The average American.** Rosen and Rosenthal, 1991.

141 **It's been evaluated.** Golden et al., 2005.
141 **Yields even better results.** Lam et al., 2006.
145 **Blue light turns out.** Wu et al., 2006.
156 **Hundreds of genes.** Marhsall, 2008.
157 **Low blood levels.** *Health News*, 2008.
157 **Recent clinical trial.** Gloth et al., 1999.
158 **Vitamin D deficient.** Holick, 2009.
159 **Canadian medical researchers.** Vieth et al., 2001.
159 **Patients taking 1000 mcg.** Kimball et al., 2007.

CHAPTER 8: GET CONNECTED

163 **They're exquisitely attuned.** Newton, 2008.
164 **"Alone time" is virtually unknown.** For example, Chagnon, 1996.
164 **Nearly 25% of Americans.** McPherson et al., 2006.
166 **Enhances social connectedness.** Harris, 2001.
167 **Compared with our counterparts.** Putnam, 2000.
167 **Recent landmark study.** McPherson et al., 2006.
177 **Psychologists have documented.** Leiberg and Anders, 2006.
177 **Joint rumination is.** Byrd-Craven et al., 2008.
185 **Science of Well-Being.** *New York Times*, January 7, 2007.
188 **Interesting line of research.** Dunbar, 1996.

CHAPTER 9: HABITS OF HEALTHY SLEEP

193 **Adverse effects start.** See, for example, Chee and Chuah, 2008.
194 **Physical exercise profoundly improves.** Dworak et al., 2008.
195 **Most adults need.** Dement, 2000.
195 **The average American.** Sleep in America Foundation, 2008.
195 **Over 90% of Americans.** Lovett, 2005.
201 **A sleep meter.** Dement, 2000.
211 **Some common antidepressant medications.** Mayers and Baldwin, 2005.

CHAPTER 10: PUTTING IT ALL TOGETHER

225 **Our TLC patients.** Ilardi et al., 2007; 2009.
226 **Rate of relapse.** Mueller et al., 1999.

CHAPTER 11: WHEN ROADBLOCKS EMERGE

232 **Left frontal cortex.** Henriques and Davidson, 1991.
240 **Medical illness can.** Gill and Hatcher, 2007.
240 **Drugs commonly used.** Dhondt et al., 1999.
241 **Reduce anxiety.** Knapen et al., in press.
241 **Soothe irritability.** Sagduyu et al., 2005.
241 **Impulsive behavior.** Hallahan et al., 2007.
241 **Addictive cravings.** Hosseini et al., in press.
241 **Erratic thinking.** Wu et al., 2008.
242 **Depression in bipolar disorder.** Stoll et al., 1999.
245 **According to fitness researchers.** Blair et al., 2004.
247 **Sugar is potently addictive.** Lenoir et al., 2007.
249 **Amount of tryptophan.** Russo et al., 2003.
250 **One recent study.** Vieth et al., 2001.

Bibliography

Aan Het Rot, M., D. S. Moskowitz, and S. N Young. "Exposure to bright light is associated with positive social interaction and good mood over short time periods: A naturalistic study in mildly seasonal people." *Journal of Psychiatric Research,* 42 (2008): 311–319.

American Psychiatric Association. *Diagnostic and statistical manual of mental disorders: DSM-IV-TR. 4th ed., text revision.* Washington, DC (2000).

Andrade, L., J. J. Caraveo-Anduaga, P. Berglund, R. V. Bijl, R. De Graaf, W. Vollebergh, E. Dragomirecka, R. Kohn, M. Keller, R. C. Kessler, N. Kawakami, C. Kilic, D. Offord, T. B. Ustun, and H. U. Wittchen. "The epidemiology of major depressive episodes: Results from the International Consortium of Psychiatric Epidemiology (ICPE) Surveys." *International Journal of Methods in Psychiatric Research,* 12 (2003): 3–21.

Armitage, R. *Canadian Journal of Psychiatry,* 45 (2000): 803–809.

Babyak M., J. A. Blumenthal, S. Herman, P. Khatri, M. Doraiswamy, K. Moore, W. E. Craighead, T. T. Baldewicz, and K. R. Krishnan. "Exercise Treatment for Major Depression: Maintenance of Therapeutic Benefit at 10 Months." *Psychosomatic Medicine,* 62 (2000): 633–638.

Barbour K. A., T. M. Edenfield, and J. A. Blumenthal. "Exercise as a Treatment for Depression and Other Psychiatric Disorders: A Review." *Journal of Cardiopulmonary Rehabilitation and Prevention,* 27 (2007): 359–367.

Blair S. N., M. J. LaMonte, and M. Z. Nichaman. "The Evolution of Physical Activity Recommendations: How Much Is Enough?" *American Journal of Clinical Nutrition,* 79 (2004): 913S–920S.

Blumenthal J. A., M. A. Babyak, P. M. Doraiswamy, L. Watkins, B. M. Hoffman, K. A. Barbour, S. Herman, W. E. Craighead, A. L. Brosse, R. Waugh, A. Hinderliter, and A. Sherwood. "Exercise and Pharmacotherapy in the Treatment of Major Depressive Disorder." *Psychosomatic Medicine,* 69 (2007): 587–596.

Blumenthal J. A., M. A. Babyak, K. A. Moore, W. E. Craighead, S. Herman, P. Khatri, R. Waugh, M. A. Napolitano, L. M. Forman, M. Appelbaum, P. M. Doraiswamy, and

K. R. Krishnan. "Effects of Exercise Training on Older Patients with Major Depression." *Archives of Internal Medicine,* 159 (1999): 2349–2356.

Bower, B. "Slumber's Unexplored Landscape." *Science News, 156* (1999): 205.

Brown, G. W. and T. O. Harris. *Social Origins of Depression.* London: Tavistock, 1978.

Breggin, P. R. "Electroshock: Scientific, Ethical, and Political Issues." *International Journal of Risk & Safety in Medicine,* 11 (1999):5–40.

Byrd-Craven, J., D. C. Geary, A. J. Rose, and D. Ponzi. "Co-ruminating Increases Stress Hormone Levels in Women." *Hormones and Behavior,* 53 (2008): 489–492.

Carlezon, W. A. Jr, S. D. Mague, A. M. Parow, A. L. Stoll, B. M. Cohen, and P. F. Renshaw. "Antidepressant-like Effects of Uridine and Omega-3 Fatty Acids Are Potentiated by Combined Treatment in Rats." *Biological Psychiatry,* 57 (2005): 343–350.

Caspi, A., K. Sugden, T. E. Moffitt, A. Taylor, I. W. Craig, H. Harrington, J. McClay, J. Mill, J. Martin, A. Braithwaite, and R. Poulton. "Influence of Life Stress on Depression: Moderation by a Polymorphism in the 5-HTT Gene." *Science,* 301 (2003): 386–389.

Chagnon, N. A. *Yanomamo.* New York: Harcourt Brace, 1996.

Chalon, S. "Omega-3 Fatty Acids and Monoamine Neurotransmission." *Prostaglandins, Leukotrienes, and Essential Fatty Acids,* 75 (2006): 259–269.

Chee, M. W. and L. Y. Chuah. "Functional Neuroimaging Insights into How Sleep and Sleep Deprivation Affect Memory and Cognition." *Current Opinions in Neurology,* 21 (2008): 417–423.

Ciesla, J. A. and J. E. Roberts. "Rumination, Negative Cognition, and Their Interactive Effects on Depressed Mood." *Emotion,* 7 (2007): 555–565.

Coan J. A. and J. J. Allen. "Frontal EEG Asymmetry and the Behavioral Activation and Inhibition Systems." *Psychophysiology,* 40 (2003):106–114.

Cohen, M. N. *Health and the Rise of Civilization.* New Haven: Yale University Press, 1989.

Compton, W. M., K. P. Conway, F. S. Stinson, and B. F. Grant. "Changes in the Prevalence of Major Depression and Comorbid Substance Use Disorders in the United States between 1991–1992 and 2001–2002." *American Journal of Psychiatry,* 163 (2006): 2141–2147.

Cordain L., R. W. Gotshall, S. B. Eaton, and S. B. Eaton 3rd. "Physical Activity, Energy Expenditure and Fitness: An Evolutionary Perspective." *International Journal of Sports Medicine,* 19 (1998): 328–335.

Corey-Lisle, P. K., R. Nash, P. Stang, and R. Swindle. "Response, Partial Response, and Nonresponse in Primary Care Treatment of Depression." *Archives of Internal Medicine,* 164 (2004): 1197–1204.

Dement, W. C. *The Promise of Sleep.* New York: Dell, 2000.

DeRubeis, R. J., S. D. Hollon, J. D. Amsterdam, R. C. Shelton, P. R. Young, R. M. Salomon, J. P. O'Reardon, M. L. Lovett, M. M. Gladis, L. L. Brown, and R. Gallop. "Cognitive Therapy versus Medications in the Treatment of Moderate to Severe Depression." *Archives of General Psychiatry,* 62 (2005): 409–416.

Dhondt, T., P. Derksen, C. Hooijer, B. Van Heycop Ten Ham, P. P. Van Gen, and T. Heeren. "Depressogenic Medication as an Aetiological Factor in Major Depression: An Analysis in a Clinical Population of Depressed Elderly People." *International Journal of Geriatric Psychiatry,* 14 (1999): 875–881.

Diamond J. *Guns, Germs and Steel: The Fates of Human Societies.* New York: Random House, 1997.

Dimidjian, S., S. D. Hollon, K. S. Dobson, K. B. Schmaling, R. J. Kohlenberg, M. E. Addis, R. Gallop, J. B. McGlinchey, D. K. Markley, J. K. Gollan, D. C. Atkins, D. L. Dunner, and N. S. Jacobson. "Randomized Trial of Behavioral Activation, Cognitive Therapy, and Antidepressant Medication in the Acute Treatment of Adults with Major Depression." *Journal of Consulting and Clinical Psychology,* 74 (2006): 658–670.

Duncan, S. and L. F. Barrett. "Affect Is a Form of Cognition: A Neurobiological Analysis." *Cognition and Emotion,* 21 (2007):1184–1211.

Dworak, M., A. Wiater, D. Alfer, E. Stephan, W. Hollmann, and H. K. Strüder. "Increased Slow Wave Sleep and Reduced Stage 2 Sleep in Children Depending on Exercise Intensity." *Sleep Medicine,* 9 (2008):266–272.

Eastman, C. I. "Natural Summer and Winter Sunlight Exposure Patterns in Seasonal Affective Disorder." *Physiology and Behavior,* 48 (1990): 611 616.

Egeland, J. A. and A. M. Hostetter. "Amish Study, I: Affective disorders among the Amish, 1976–1980." *American Journal of Psychiatry,* 140 (1983): 56–61.

Freeman C. and R. Kendell. Patients' experience of and attitudes to electroconvulsive therapy. *Annals of the New York Academy of Sciences,* 462 (1986):341–352.

Frodl, T. S., N. Koutsouleris, R. Bottlender, C. Born, M. Jäger, I. Scupin, M. Reiser, H. J. Möller, and E. M. Meisenzahl. "Depression-Related Variation in Brain Morphology over Three Years: Effects of Stress?" *Archives of General Psychiatry,* 65 (2008): 1156–1165.

Gill, D. and S. Hatcher. "Withdrawn: Antidepressants for Depression in Medical Illness." *Cochrane Database of Systematic Reviews,* Jul 18;(4) (2007): CD001312.

Gloth, F. M. 3rd, W. Alam, and B. Hollis. "Vitamin D versus Broad Spectrum Phototherapy in the Treatment of Seasonal Affective Disorder." *Journal of Nutrition, Health, and Aging,* 3 (1999): 5–7.

Goel, N. and G. R. Etwaroo. "Bright Light, Negative Air Ions and Auditory Stimuli Produce Rapid Mood Changes in a Student Population: A Placebo-Controlled Study." *Psychological Medicine,* 36 (2006): 1253–1263.

Golden, R. N., B. N. Gaynes, R. D. Ekstrom, R. M. Hamer, F. M. Jacobsen, T. Suppes, K. L. Wisner, and C. B. Nemeroff. "The Efficacy of Light Therapy in the Treatment of Mood Disorders: A Review and Meta-analysis of the Evidence." American *Journal of Psychiatry,* 162 (2005): 656–662.

Guillemette, J., M. Hébert, J. Paquet, and M. Dumont. "Natural Bright Light Exposure in the Summer and Winter in Subjects with and without Complaints of Seasonal Mood Variations." *Biological Psychiatry,* 44 (1998): 622–628.

Hallahan, B., J. R. Hibbeln, J. M. Davis, and M. R. Garland. "Omega-3 Fatty Acid Supplementation in Patients with Recurrent Self-Harm. Single-Centre Double-Blind Randomised Controlled Trial." *British Journal of Psychiatry,* 190 (2007): 118–122.

Hamet, P. and J. Tremblay. "Genetics and Genomics of Depression." *Metabolism,* 54 (5 Suppl 1) (2005): 10–15.

Hammen, C. "Stress and Depression." *Annual Review of Clinical Psychology,* 1 (2005): 293–319.

Harris, T. "Recent Developments in Understanding the Psychosocial Aspects of Depression." *British Medical Bulletin,* 57 (2001): 17–32.

Health News. "Check Your Vitamin D Intake to Avoid Multiple Health Consequences. Three 2008 Studies Link Low Vitamin D Levels to Depression, Hip Fractures, and Increased Risk of Death." Volume 14 (2008): 9–10.

Henriques, J. B. and R. J. Davidson. "Left Frontal Hypoactivation in Depression." *Journal of Abnormal Psychology,* 100 (1991): 535–545.

Hibbeln, J. R. "Fish Consumption and Major Depression." *Lancet,* 351 (1998): 1213.

Holick, M. F. "Vitamin D Status: Measurement, Interpretation, and Clinical Application." *Annals of Epidemiology,* 19 (2009): 73–78.

Hosseini, M., H. A. Alaei, A. Naderi, M. R. Sharifi, and R. Zahed. "Treadmill Exercise Reduces Self-Administration of Morphine in Male Rats. *Pathophysiology* (in press).

Howland, R. H, B. Lebowitz, P. J. McGrath, K. Shores-Wilson, M. M. Biggs, G. K. Balasubramani, and M. Fava; STAR*D Study Team. "Evaluation of Outcomes with Citalopram for Depression Using Measurement-based Care in STAR*D: Implications for Clinical Practice." *American Journal of Psychiatry,* 163 (2006): 28–40.

Husain M.M., A. J. Rush, M. Fink, R. Knapp, G. Petrides, T. Rummans, M. M. Biggs, K. O'Connor, K. Rasmussen, M. Litle, W. Zhao, H. J. Bernstein, G. Smith, M. Mueller, S. M. McClintock, S. H. Bailine, C. H. Kellner. "Speed of Response and Remission in Major Depressive Disorder with Acute Electroconvulsive Therapy (ECT): A Consortium for Research in ECT (CORE) Report." *Journal of Clinical Psychiatry,* 65 (2004):485–91.

Ilardi, S. S., J. D. Jacobson, K. A. Lehman, B. A. Stites, L. Karwoski, N. N. Stroupe, D. K. Steidtmann, A. K. Hirani, J. A. Prohaska, B. Sampat, and C. Young. "Therapeutic Lifestyle Change for Depression: Results from a Randomized Controlled Trial." Presented at the annual meeting of the Association for Behavioral and Cognitive Therapy, Philadelphia (November 2007).

Ilardi, S. S., L. Karwoski, K. A. Lehman, B. A. Stites, and D. Steidtmann. "We Were Never Designed for This: The Depression Epidemic and the Promise of Therapeutic Lifestyle Change." Manuscript under review (2009).

Karwoski, L. "Therapeutic Lifestyle Change: Piloting a Novel Group-Based Intervention for Depression." Doctoral dissertation, University of Kansas (2008).

Keller, M., J. McCullough, D. Klein, B. Arnow, D. Dunner, A. Gelenberg, et al. "A Comparison of Nefazodone, the Cognitive Behavioral Analysis System of Psychotherapy, and Their Combination for the Treatment of Chronic Depression." *New England Journal of Medicine,* 342 (2000): 162–171.

Kessler, R. C., P. Berglund, O. Demler, R. Jin, and E. E. Walters. "Lifetime Prevalence and Age-of-Onset Distributions of DSM-IV Disorders in the National Comorbidity Survey Replication." *Archives of General Psychiatry,* 62 (2005): 593–602.

Khan, A., R. M. Leventhal, S. R. Khan, and W. A. Brown. "Severity of Depression and Response to Antidepressants and Placebo: An analysis of the Food and Drug Administration Database." *Journal of Clinical Psychopharmacology,* 22: 40–45.

Kimball, S. M., M. R. Ursell, P. O'Connor, and R. Vieth. "Safety of Vitamin D3 in Adults with Multiple Sclerosis." *American Journal of Clinical Nutrition,* 86 (2007): 645–651.

Kirsch, I., T. J. Moore, A. Scoboria, and S. S. Nicholls. "The Emperor's New Drugs: An Analysis of Antidepressant Medication Data Submitted to the U.S. Food and Drug Administration." *Prevention & Treatment,* 5, Article 23 (2002).

Knapen, J., E. Sommerijns, D. Vancampfort, P. Sienaert, G. Pieters, P. Haake, M. Probst, and J. Peuskens. "State Anxiety and Subjective Well-Being Responses to Acute Bouts of Aerobic Exercise in Patients with Depressive and Anxiety Disorders." *British Journal of Sports Medicine* (in press).

Lam, R. W., A. J. Levitt, R. D. Levitan, M. W. Enns, R. Morehouse, E. E. Michalak, and E. M. Tam. "The Can-SAD Study: A Randomized Controlled Trial of the Effectiveness of Light Therapy and Fluoxetine in Patients with Winter Seasonal Affective Disorder." *American Journal of Psychiatry,* 163 (2006): 805–812.

Leiberg, S. and S. Anders. "The Multiple Facets of Empathy: A Survey of Theory and Evidence." *Progress in Brain Research,* 156 (2006): 419–440.

Lenoir, M., F. Serre, L. Cantin, and S. H. Ahmed. "Intense Sweetness Surpasses Cocaine Reward." *PLoS ONE,* Aug 1; 2(1) (2007): e698.

Lipman R. S., E. A. Brown, G. A. Silbert, D. G. Rains, D. A. Grady. "Cognitive Performance as Modified by Age and ECT History." *Progress in Neuropsychopharmacology and Biological Psychiatry*, 17 (1993):581–594.

Lovett, R. "Coffee: The Demon Drink?" *New Scientist,* 2518 (24 September 2005).

MacQueen, G. and P. Chokka. "Special Issues in the Management of Depression in Women." *Canadian Journal of Psychiatry,* 49 (3 Suppl 1) (2004): 27S–40S.

Marcus, G. *Kluge: The Haphazard Construction of the Human Mind.* New York: Houghton Mifflin Company, 2008.

Marshall, T. G. "Vitamin D Discovery Outpaces FDA Decision Making." *Bioessays,* 30 (2008): 173–182.

Masuelli, L., P. Trono, L. Marzocchella, M. A. Mrozek, C. Palumbo, M. Minieri, F. Carotenuto, R. Fiaccavento, A. Nardi, F. Galvano, P. Di Nardo, A. Modesti, and R. Bei. "Intercalated Disk Remodeling in Delta-Sarcoglycan-Deficient Hamsters Fed with an Alpha-Linolenic Acid-Enriched Diet." *International Journal of Molecular Medicine,* 21 (2008): 41–48.

Max, D. T. "Happiness 101." *New York Times* (7 January 2007).

Mayers, A. G. and D. S. Baldwin. "Antidepressants and Their Effect on Sleep." *Human Psychopharmacology,* 20 (2005): 533–559.

McNamara, R. K. and S. E. Carlson. "Role of Omega-3 Fatty Acids in Brain Development and Function: Potential Implications for the Pathogenesis and Prevention of Psychopathology." *Prostaglandins, Leukotrienes, and Essential Fatty Acids,* 75 (2006): 329–349.

McPherson, J. M., L. Smith-Lovin, and M. B. Brashears. "Social Isolation in America: Changes in Core Discussion Networks over Two Decades." *American Sociological Review,* 71 (2006): 353–375.

Mersch, P. P., H. M. Middendorp, A. L. Bouhuys, D. G. Beersma, and R. H. van den Hoofdakker. "Seasonal Affective Disorder and Latitude: A Review of the Literature." *Journal of Affective Disorders,* 53 (1999): 35–48.

Miller, A. H., V. Maletic, and C. L. Raison. "Inflammation and Its Discontents: The Role of Cytokines in the Pathophysiology of Major Depression." *Biological Psychiatry* (in press).

Miller, K. B., B. Yost, A. Flaherty, M. M. Hillemeier, G. A. Chase, C. S. Weisman, and A. M. Dyer. "Health Status, Health Conditions, and Health Behaviors among Amish Women: Results from the Central Pennsylvania Women's Health Study (CePAWHS)." *Women's Health Issues,* 17 (2007): 162–171.

Miyake, Y., S. Sasaki, K. Tanaka, Y. Ohya, S. Miyamoto, I. Matsunaga, T. Yoshida, Y. Hirota, H. Oda; Osaka Maternal and Child Health Study Group. "Fish and Fat Intake and Prevalence of Allergic Rhinitis in Japanese Females: The Osaka Maternal and Child Health Study." *Journal of the American College of Nutrition,* 26 (2007): 279–287.

Moulds, M. L., E. Kandris, S. Starr, and A. C. Wong. "The Relationship between Rumination, Avoidance and Depression in a Non-Clinical Sample." *Behavioral Research and Therapy,* 45 (2007): 251–261.

Mueller, T. I., A. C. Leon, M. B. Keller, D. A. Solomon, J. Endicott, W. Coryell, M. Warshaw, and J. D. Maser. "Recurrence after Recovery from Major Depressive Disorder during 15 Years of Observational Follow-up." *American Journal of Psychiatry,* 156 (1999): 1000–1006.

National Sleep Foundation. *2008 Sleep in America Poll* (2008).

Nemeroff, C. B. and W. W. Vale. "The Neurobiology of Depression: Inroads to Treatment and New Drug Discovery." *Journal of Clinical Psychiatry,* 66 Suppl 7 (2005): 5–13.

Newton, R. P. "The Attachment Connection: Parenting a Secure and Confident Child Using the Science of Attachment Theory." Oakland, CA: New Harbinger, 2008.

Nierenberg, A. A., M. J. Ostacher, J. C. Huffman, R. M. Ametrano, M. Fava, and R. H. Perlis. "A Brief Review of Antidepressant Efficacy, Effectiveness, Indications, and Usage for Major Depressive Disorder." *Journal of Occupational and Environmental Medicine,* 50 (2008): 428–436.

Nolen-Hoeksema, S., B. E. Wisco, and S. Lyubomirsky. "Rethinking Rumination." *Perspectives on Psychological Science,* 3 (2008): 400–424.

Odeberg, H., B. Rodriguez-Silva, P. Salander, B. Mårtensson. "Individualized Continuation Electroconvulsive Therapy and Medication as a Bridge to Relapse Prevention after an Index Course of Electroconvulsive Therapy in Severe Mood Disorders: A Naturalistic 3-Year Cohort Study." *Journal of ECT*, 24 (2008):183–90.

Ogden, C. L., M. D. Carroll, L. R. Curtin, M. A. McDowell, C. J. Tabak, and K. M. Flegal. "Prevalence of Overweight and Obesity in the United States, 1999–2004." *JAMA,* 295 (2006): 1549–1555.

Olfson, M., S. C. Marcus, M. Tedeschi, and G. J. Wan. "Continuity of Antidepressant Treatment for Adults with Depression in the United States." *American Journal of Psychiatry,* 163 (2006): 101–108.

Opbroek, A., P. L. Delgado, C. Laukes, C. McGahuey, J. Katsanis, F. A. Moreno, and R. Manber. "Do SSRIs Inhibit Emotional Responses?" *International Journal of Neuropsychopharmacology,* 5 (2002): 147–151.

Page, M. E., M. J. Detke, A. Dalvi, L. G. Kirby, and I. Lucki. "Serotonergic Mediation of the Effects of Fluoxetine, but not Desipramine, in the Rat Forced Swimming Test." *Psychopharmacology,* 147 (1999): 162–167.

Parker, G. B., J. Crawford, and D. Hadzi-Pavlovic. "Quantified Superiority of Cognitive Behaviour Therapy to Antidepressant Drugs: A Challenge to an Earlier Meta-Analysis." *Acta Psychiatrica Scandinavica,* 118 (2008): 91–97.

Peet, M. "International Variations in the Outcome of Schizophrenia and the Prevalence of Depression in Relation to National Dietary Practices: An Ecological Analysis." *British Journal of Psychiatry,* 184 (2004): 404–408.

Peet, M. and D. F. Horrobin. "A Dose-Ranging Study of the Effects of Ethyl-Eicosapentaenoate in Patients with Ongoing Depression Despite Apparently Adequate Treatment with Standard Drugs." *Archives of General Psychiatry,* 59 (2002): 913–919.

Peet, M., B. Murphy, J. Shay, and D. Horrobin. "Depletion of Omega-3 Fatty Acid Levels in Red Blood Cell Membranes of Depressive Patients." *Biological Psychiatry,* 43 (1998): 315–319.

Penedo, F. J. and J. R. Dahn. "Exercise and Well-Being: A Review of Mental and Physical Health Benefits Associated with Physical Activity." *Current Opinion in Psychiatry,* 18 (2005): 189–193.

Ploughman, M. "Exercise Is Brain Food: The Effects of Physical Activity on Cognitive Function." *Developmental Neurorehabilitation,* 11 (2008): 236–240.

Pollan, M. *In Defense of Food: An Eater's Manifesto.* New York: Penguin Press, 2008.

Post, R. "Transduction of Psychosocial Stress into the Neurobiology of Recurrent Affective Disorder." *American Journal of Psychiatry*, 149 (1992):999–1010.

Praschak-Rieder, N., M. Willeit, A. A. Wilson, S. Houle, and J. H. Meyer. "Seasonal Variation in Human Brain Serotonin Transporter Binding." *Archives of General Psychiatry,* 65 (2008): 1072–1078.

Putnam, R. D. *Bowling Alone: The Collapse and Revival of American Community.* New York: Simon & Schuster, 2000.

Rampersaud, E., B. D. Mitchell, T. I. Pollin, M. Fu, H. Shen, J. R. O'Connell, J. L. Ducharme, S. Hines, P. Sack, R. Naglieri, A. R. Shuldiner, and S. Snitker. "Physical Activity and the Association of Common *FTO* Gene Variants with Body Mass Index and Obesity." *Archives of Internal Medicine,* 168 (2008): 1791–1797.

Rechtschaffen, A., B. M. Bergmann, C. A. Everson, C. A. Kushida, and M. A. Gilliland. "Sleep Deprivation in the Rat: X. Integration and Discussion of the Findings. 1989." *Sleep*, 25 (2002): 68–87.

Rose A. J., W. Carlson, E. M. Waller. "Prospective Associations of Co-Rumination with Friendship and Emotional Adjustment: Considering the Socioemotional Trade-Offs of Co-Rumination." *Developmental Psychology*, 43 (2007):1019–1031.

Rosen, L. N. and N. E. Rosenthal. "Seasonal Variations in Mood and Behavior in the General Population: A Factor-Analytic Approach." *Psychiatry Research,* 38 (1991): 271–283.

Ross, B. M., J. Seguin, and L. E. Sieswerda. "Omega-3 Fatty Acids as Treatments for Mental Illness: Which Disorder and Which Fatty Acid?" *Lipids, Health, and Disease,* 18 (2007): 6–27.

Ruff, C. R., E. Trinkhaus, and T. W. Holliday. "Body Mass and Encephalization in Pleistocene Homo." *Nature,* 387: 173–176.

Russo, S., I. P. Kema, M. R. Fokkema, J. C. Boon, P. H. Willemse, E. G. de Vries, J. A. den Boer, and J. Korf. "Tryptophan as a Link between Psychopathology and Somatic States." *Psychosomatic Medicine,* 65 (2003): 665–671.

Sackeim H. A., J. Prudic, R. Fuller, J. Keilp, P. W. Lavori, M. Olfson. "The Cognitive Effects of Electroconvulsive Therapy in Community Settings." *Neuropsychopharmacology,* 32 (2007):244–254.

Sagduyu, K., M. E. Dokucu, B. A. EddyA, G. Craigen, C. F. Baldassano, and A. Yildiz. "Omega-3 Fatty Acids Decreased Irritability of Patients with Bipolar Disorder in an Add-on, Open Label Study." *Nutrition Journal,* 4 (2005): 6.

Schieffelin, E. L.. "The Cultural Analysis of Depressive Affect: An Example from Papua New Guinea." In A. M. Kleinman and B. Good (Eds.), *Culture and Depression* (pp. 101–133). Berkeley: University of California Press, 1985.

Sears, B. *The Omega Rx Zone: The Miracle of the New High-Dose Fish Oil.* New York: Collins Living, 2002.

Seidman, S. N. "Testosterone Deficiency and Mood in Aging Men: Pathogenic and Therapeutic Interactions." *World Journal of Biological Psychiatry,* 4 (2003): 14–20.

Seligman, M. "Why Is There So Much Depression Today? The Waxing of the Individual and the Waning of the Commons." In Rex Ingram (ed.), *Contemporary Psychological Approaches to Depression* (pp. 1–9). New York: Plenum, 1990.

Simopoulos, A. P. "Omega-3 Fatty Acids in Inflammation and Autoimmune Diseases." *Journal of the American College of Nutrition,* 21 (2002): 495–505.

Simopoulos, A. P. "Evolutionary Aspects of Diet, the Omega-6: Omega-3 Ratio, and Gene Expression." In M. S. Meskin, W. R. Bidlack, & R. K. Randolph: *Phytochemicals: Nutrient-Gene Interactions* (pp. 137–160). CRC Press: 2006.

Stagnitti, M. N. *Statistical Brief #206: Antidepressants Prescribed by Medical Doctors in Office Based and Outpatient Settings by Specialty for the U.S. Civilian Noninstitutionalized Population, 2002 and 2005.* Agency for Healthcare Research and Quality: Medical Expenditure Panel Survey, June 2008.

Steiger, A. "Neurochemical Regulation of Sleep." *Journal of Psychiatric Research,* 41 (2007): 537–552.

Stoll, A. L., W. E. Severus, M. P. Freeman, S. Rueter, H. A. Zboyan, E. Diamond, K. K. Cress, and L. B. Marangell. "Omega-3 Fatty Acids in Bipolar Disorder: A Preliminary

Double-Blind, Placebo-Controlled Trial." *Archives of General Psychiatry,* 56 (1999): 407–412.

Svartberg, M. and T. C. Stiles. "Comparative Effects of Short-Term Psychodynamic Psychotherapy: A Meta-Analysis." *Journal of Consulting and Clinical Psychology,* 59 (1991): 704–714.

Thase, M. E. "Correlates and Consequences of Chronic Insomnia." *General Hospital Psychiatry,* 2 (2005): 100–112.

Tooby, J. and L. Cosmides. "On the Universality of Human Nature and the Uniqueness of the Individual: The Role of Genetics and Adaptation." *Journal of Personality,* 58 (1990): 17–67.

Trivedi, M. H., M. Fava, S. R. Wisniewski, M. E. Thase, F. Quitkin, D. Warden, L. Ritz, A. A. Nierenberg, B. D. Lebowitz, M. M. Biggs, J. F. Luther, K. Shores-Wilson, A. J. Rush; STAR*D Study Team. "Medication Augmentation after the Failure of SSRIs for Depression." *New England Journal of Medicine,* 354 (2006): 1243–1252.

Trivedi, M. H., A. J. Rush, S. R. Wisniewski, N. N. Nierenberg, D. Warden, L. Ritz, G. Norquist, R. H. Howland, B. Lebowitz, P. J. McGrath, K. Shores-Wilson, M. M. Biggs, G. H. Balasubramani, and M. Fava for the STAR*D Study Team. "Evaluation of Outcomes with Citalopram for Depression Using Measurement-based Sare in STAR*D: Implications for Clinical Practice." *American Journal of Psychiatry,* 163 (2006): 28–40.

U.S. Department of Health and Human Services. *Physical Activity and Health: A Report of the Surgeon General.* Atlanta: U.S. Department of Health and Human Services, Centers for Disease Control and Prevention National Center for Chronic Disease Prevention and Health Promotion, 1999.

Vaynman, S. and F. Gomez-Pinilla. "Revenge of the 'Sit': How Lifestyle Impacts Neuronal and Cognitive Health through Molecular Systems that Interface Energy Metabolism with Neuronal Plasticity." *Journal of Neuroscience Research,* 84 (2006): 699–715.

Vieth, R., P. C. Chan, and G. D. MacFarlane. "Efficacy and Safety of Vitamin D3 Intake Exceeding the Lowest Observed Adverse Effect Level." *American Journal of Clinical Nutrition,* 73 (2001): 288–294.

Weissman, M. M., R. C. Bland, G. J. Canino, C. Faravelli, S. Greenwald, H. G. Hwu, P. R. Joyce, E. G. Karam, C. K. Lee, J. Lellouch, J. P. Lepine, S. C. Newman, M. Rubio-Stipec, J. E. Wells, P. J. Wickramaratne, H. Wittchen, and E. K. Yeh. "Cross-National Epidemiology of Major Depression and Bipolar Disorder." *Journal of the American Medical Association,* 276 (1996): 293–299.

Werneke, U., S. Northey, and D. Bhugra. "Antidepressants and Sexual Dysfunction." *Acta Psychiatrica Scandinavica,* 114 (2006): 384–397.

Wu, J., S. Seregard, and P. V. Algvere. "Photochemical Damage of the Retina." *Survey of Ophthalmology,* 51 (2006): 461–481.

Wu, A., Z. Ying, and F. Gomez-Pinilla. "Docosahexaenoic Acid Dietary Supplementation Enhances the Effects of Exercise on Synaptic Plasticity and Cognition." *Neuroscience,* 155 (2008): 751–759.

Young, G. S., J. A. Conquer, and R. Thomas. "Effect of Randomized Supplementation with High Dose Olive, Flax or Fish Oil on Serum Phospholipid Fatty Acid Levels in Adults with Attention Deficit Hyperactivity Disorder." *Reproduction Nutrition Development,* 45 (2005): 549–558.

Acknowledgments

Most of what I know about depression I have learned from my patients. Their courage and determination in fighting the illness have inspired me more than words can express.

Because clinical research is a collaborative process, I am deeply indebted to the many talented students who helped make the Therapeutic Lifestyle Change (TLC) program a reality. First and foremost, I am grateful to Leslie Karwoski for her boundless dedication, intellectual creativity, and administrative skill as the first project coordinator for the TLC Lab; without her heroic contributions, the TLC program could not have come to fruition. I also want to thank Andy Lehman—our longtime lab coordinator—for his rare gift of bringing order to chaos, and Brian Stites for his energetic efforts on every conceivable front. Likewise, I want to express my gratitude to Dana Steidtmann for her steady willingness to step up at every turn and for coining the name of the protocol itself. Thanks are also due to the student cotherapists who served so skillfully on the project—Amyn Hirani, Chantal Young, Jenny Prohaska, Susan Reneau, and Brenda Sampat—and to the other key members of our research team, including April Minatrea, Natalie Stroupe, Eugene Botanov, Matt Gallagher, Brandon Hikaka, Jenny Wurtz, Chris Heath, John Jacobson, Adam Brazil, Sarah Thompson, Mark Brehm, Adrienne Belk, Adriann Farrell, and Christina Williams.

I owe a profound debt of gratitude to Ed Craighead, my mentor in graduate school and beyond, for his unwavering support, and for teaching me much of what I know about clinical research. Additionally, the feedback of my colleagues has served as an invaluable catalyst for improving the TLC program. I am especially grateful to Rick Ingram, Omri Gillath, Nancy Hamilton,

John Colombo, Paul Atchley, Ray Higgins, Ruthann Atchley, and Sarah Kirk at the University of Kansas, and to David Miklowitz (University of Colorado), David Buss (University of Texas), and Scott Lilienfeld (Emory University).

My heartfelt appreciation as well to Harriet Lerner for her generous friendship and insightful guidance regarding the writing process, and for recommending *The Depression Cure* to Jo-Lynne Worley—agent extraordinaire—and her partner, Joanie Shoemaker. I also want to thank Matthew Lohr, my first editor at Da Capo, for believing in the project, and Wendy Francis for her wise editorial role in shepherding the book to completion. Additionally, Christine Marra helped improve the manuscript in countless ways with her editorial production team.

Many dear friends and loved ones—especially my parents—were also kind enough to read early drafts of the manuscript and provide superb feedback, and I cannot thank them enough. Likewise, my beloved daughter, Abby, has shown a maturity and understanding far beyond her years in putting up with my relentless work schedule this past year; her *joie de vivre* has sustained me through many moments of flagging stamina, and I thank God for her every day of my life.

Finally, I am eternally grateful to my wife, Maria, for her love, support, friendship, encouragement, and clinical wisdom, and for serving as such a valuable sounding board during the writing process. Her contributions are reflected on each page of *The Depression Cure*.

Index

Index references in bold refer to text graphics.

About the Author

Stephen S. Ilardi, PhD, is associate professor of clinical psychology at the University of Kansas and the author of over forty professional articles on mental illness. Through his active clinical practice, Dr. Ilardi has treated several hundred depressed patients. He lives with his family in Lawrence, Kansas.

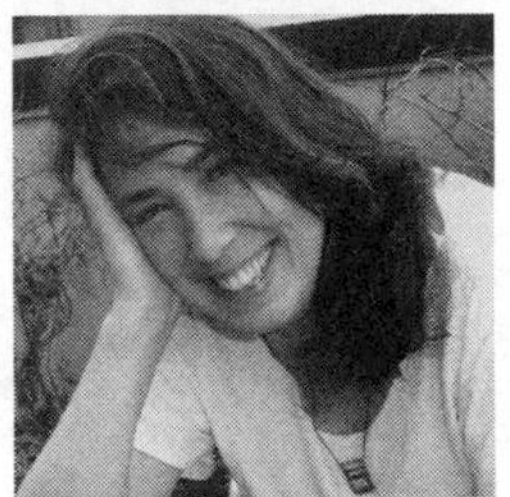

Photo credit: Alice Licht

After the sort of introverted childhood you would expect from a writer, Liz Braswell earned a degree in Egyptology at Brown University and then promptly spent the next ten years producing video games. Finally, she caved in to fate and wrote Snow and Rx under the name Tracy Lynn, followed by the Nine Lives of Chloe King series under her real name, because by then the assassins hunting her were all dead. Liz is also the author of Once Upon a Dream: A Twisted Tale. She lives in Brooklyn with a husband, two children, a cat, a part-time dog, three fish and five coffee trees she insists will start producing beans any day. You can e-mail her at me@lizbraswell.com or tweet @LizBraswell.

A special thank-you to organisations who help save creatures under and around the sea, like the Mass Audubon's Wellfleet Bay Wildlife Sanctuary.

To Elizabeth (the) Schaefer, who started off the series as one of my editors, and continues on as a good friend.

This book is for everyone who helps protect Ariel's ocean – which includes *you*, whenever you eat sustainable seafood and skip the straw!

—L.B.

Prologue

In the foothills of the Ibrian Mountains…

Cahe Vehswo was in the field repairing a wooden fence. It was less to keep the wolves out than to keep the stupid sheep *in*, where the only slightly smarter child-shepherds could watch them.

It was a beautiful day, almost sparkling. The pines weren't yet brittle from the late summer heat and the deciduous trees were in full glory, their dark green leaves crackling in the wind. The mountains were dressed in mid-season blooms and tinkly little waterfalls. The clouds in the sky were ridiculously puffy.

The only off note in nature's symphony was a strange

stink when the wind came up from the southern lowlands: burning animal fat, or rubbish, or rot.

Everyone in the hamlet was out doing chores in such forgiving weather; rebuilding grapevine trellises, chopping wood, cleaning out the cheese barrels. No one was quarreling, yet, and life on their remote hillside seemed good.

Then Cahe saw something unlikely coming up the old road, the King's Road. It was a phalanx of soldiers, marching in a surprisingly solid and orderly fashion considering how far they were from whatever capital they had come. With their plumes, their buttons that shone like tiny golden suns and their surprisingly clean jackets, there was almost a parade-like air around them. If not for their grim, haughty looks and the strange flag they flew.

An order was cried; the men stopped. The captain, resplendent in a bright blue cap and jacket, rode up to Cahe along with his one other mounted soldier, who carried their flag.

"Peasant," he called out somewhat rudely, Cahe thought. "Is this the township of Serria?"

"No," the farmer started to say, then remembered long-forgotten rules for dealing with people who had shiny buttons, big hats and guns. "Begging your pardon, sir, but that's farther along, on the other side of Devil's Pass. People call this Adam's Rock."

"No matter," the captain said. "We claim this village and its surrounding lands in the name of Tirulia!"

He cried out the last bit, but the words bounced and drifted and faded into nothing against the giant mountains beyond, the dusty fields below, the occasional olive tree, the uninterested cow. Villagers stopped their work and drifted over to see what was going on.

"Begging your pardon again, sir," Cahe said politely. "But we're considered part of, and pay our taxes to, Alamber."

"*Whatever your situation was before,* you are now citizens of Tirulia, and pay homage to Prince Eric and Princess Vanessa."

"Well, I don't know how the king of Alamber will take it."

"That is no concern of yours," the captain said frostily. "Soon the king of Alamber will just be a memory, and all Alamber a mere province in the great Tirulian empire."

"You *say* Tirulia," Cahe mused, leaning on the fence to make his statement sound casual. "We know it. We buy their salted cod and trade our cheese with them. Their girls like to wear aprons with braided ties. Perde, son of Javer, sought his fortune down south on a fishing ship and wound up marrying a local girl there."

"Fascinating," the captain said, removing one hand

from his tight grip on the reins to fix his moustache. "And what is the point of all this?"

Cahe pointed at the banner that flapped in the breeze. "That is not the flag of Tirulia."

In place of the sun and sea and ship on a field of blue that was familiar even to these isolated people, there was a stark white background on which a black-tentacled octopus with no eyes loomed menacingly. It looked almost alive, ready to grab whatever came too close.

"Princess Vanessa thought it was time to… update the sigil of house Tirulia," the captain said, a little defensively. "We still represent Tirulia and the interests of Prince Eric, acting for his father, the king, and his mother, the queen."

"I see." Another villager started to speak up, but Cahe put a hand on his arm to stop him. "Well, what can we do, then? You have guns. We have them too to hunt with but they are put away until the boars come down from the oak forests again. So… as long as the right tax man comes round and we don't wind up paying twice, sure. We're part of Tirulia now, as you say."

The captain blinked. He narrowed his eyes at Cahe, expecting a trick. The farmer regarded him mildly back.

"You have chosen a wise course, peasant," the captain finally said. *"All hail Tirulia."*

The folk of Adam's Rock murmured a ragtag and unenthusiastic response: *all hail Tirulia.*

"We shall be back through this way again after we subdue Serria. Prepare your finest quarters for us after our triumph over them and all of Alamber!"

And with that the captain shouted something unintelligible and militaristic and trotted off, the flag bearer quickly catching up.

As soon as they were out of earshot, Cahe shook his head wearily.

"Call a meeting," he sighed. "Pass the word round… we need to gather the girls and send them off into the hills for mushroom gathering, or whatever, for several weeks. All the military-aged boys should go into the wilds with the sheep. Or to hunt. Also, everyone should probably bury whatever gold or valuables they have somewhere they won't be found."

"But why did you just give in to him?" the man next to Cahe demanded. "We could have sent word to Alamber. If we'd just told the soldiers no, we wouldn't have to do *any* of this, acting like cowards and sending our children away into safety…"

"I did it because I could smell the wind. Can't you?" Cahe answered, nodding towards the south.

Just beyond the next ridge, where the Veralean

Mountains began to smooth out towards the lowlands, a column of smoke rose. It was wider and more turbulent than what would come from a bonfire, black and ashy and ugly as sin.

"Garhaggio?" someone asked incredulously. It did indeed look like the smoke was coming from there. From the volume and blackness there could have only been scorched earth and embers where that village had been just the day before.

"I bet *they* told the captain no," Cahe said.

"Such causeless destruction!" a woman lamented. "What terrible people this Prince Eric and Princess Vanessa must be!"

Eric

Eric woke up.

He was having that dream again.

It came to him at the strangest times, when reviewing the menu for a formal dinner with Chef Louis, for instance, or listening to the castle treasurers discuss the ups and downs of dealing with international bankers. Or when his beautiful princess went on and on about her little intrigues.

All right: it was when he was bored and tired. If a room was stuffy and he was sleepy and could barely keep his eyes open.

Or right before he fell asleep properly, in bed – that

moment between still being awake and deep in dreams. The same split second when he often heard angelic choirs singing unimaginably beautiful hymns. He could only listen, too frozen in half sleep to jump up and quickly scribble it down before he forgot.

But sometimes, instead of the choirs, he had this:

That he was not Prince Eric wed to Vanessa, the beautiful princess. That there had been some terrible mistake. That there was another girl, a beautiful girl with no voice, who could sing.

No—

There was a beautiful girl who could sing, who somehow lost her voice forever on the terrible day when Eric fell asleep. He had been dreaming ever since.

There were mermaids in this other world.

He had known one. Her father was a god. Eric's princess was an evil witch. And Eric had touched greatness but been tricked, and now here he was, dreaming.

He looked down suddenly, in a panic. His arms were crossed on his desk over pages of musical notation, supporting his dozing head. Had he spilt any ink? Had he blurred any notes? A rest could be turned into a tie if the ink smeared that way… and that would ruin everything…

He held the papers up to the moonlight. There was a

little smudging, there, right where the chorus was supposed to come in with a D-major triad. But it wasn't so bad.

His eyes drifted from the pages to the moon, which shone clearly through his unglazed window. A bright star kept it company. A faint breeze blew, causing the thick leaves of the trees below to make shoe-like clacking noises against the castle wall. It carried with it whatever scents it had picked up on its way from the sea: sandalwood, sand, oranges, dust. Dry things, stuff of the land.

Eric looked back at his music, tried to recapture the sound and feel of the ocean that had played in his head before waking, aquamarine and sweet.

Then he dipped his pen in ink and began to scribble madly, refusing to rest until the sun came up.

Scuttle

It seemed as if all of Tirulia were crowded into the amphitheatre. Every seat was filled, from the velvet-cushioned couches of the nobles up front to the high, unshaded stone benches in the far back. More people spilt out into the streets beyond. No one was going to miss the first performance of a new opera by their beloved Mad Prince Eric.

It was like a festival day; everyone wore whatever colourful thing and sparkly gem they had. Castle guards stood in polished boots along the aisles, making sure no fights broke out among the spectators. Vendors walked among the crowds both inside and out selling the bubbly, cold white wine Tirulia was known for along with savoury little treats: bread topped with triangles of cheese and olive oil, paper cones filled with crispy fried baby squid, sticks threaded with honey-preserved chestnuts that glittered in the sunlight.

It would all have made a fabulous mosaic of movement and colours and dazzle from above.

And it did for a certain old seagull named Scuttle, who was quite enjoying the view.

He and a few of his great-grandgulls (sent along to watch him) perched on the rail above the highest, cheapest seats in the theatre. While the younger ones kept their sharp eyes alert for dropped morsels, ready to dive down at the tiniest crumb of bread, Scuttle contented himself with just watching the pomp and muttering to himself. Only one great-grandgull remained by his side, trying to understand what he saw in the human spectacle below.

The costumes were lavish, the orchestra full, the sets cunningly painted to look more than real: when a prince produced a play, wealth showed.

And when that prince came out to take his seat in the royal box, arm in arm with his beautiful princess, the crowd went mad, howling and cheering for their royal artist. Sometimes called the Dreamer Prince and even the

Melancholic Prince for his faraway looks and tendency towards wistfulness, Eric looked momentarily cheered by this expression of love from his kingdom, and waved back with the beginnings of a real smile.

Vanessa gave one of her grins, inscrutable and slightly disturbing, and pulled him along to sit down. With her other hand she stroked the large nautilus necklace she always wore – a strangely plain and natural-looking ornament for the extravagant princess.

The orchestra tuned, and began.

La Sirenetta, a Musical Fantasy in Three Acts

In a magical kingdom by the sea, a sad and handsome prince *[tenor]* longs for someone to share his music and his life. While he and his friends celebrate his twenty-first birthday on a decorated yacht, a terrible storm arises. The prince is thrown over the railing of his ship and is almost drowned but for the intercession of a young and beautiful mermaid, who has the voice of an angel *[first soprano]*.

Upon recovering, the prince declares he will marry no one but the beautiful girl who rescued him.

Then a *different* beautiful girl appears *[same first soprano, different costume]*, who, although she has the shining red hair of the mermaid who saved him, is *mute*! So she cannot be his one true love. And yet, as they spend their days together, he slowly falls for her.

But then a rival comes onto the scene. A handsome woman *[contralto]* serenades the prince with the same song the little mermaid once sang and casts a spell over him, causing him to forget the pretty girl with no voice.

[Note: The contralto is a large, full-busted singer, a favourite of the audience. She gets a standing ovation when she appears, smiling slyly.]

Hypnotised, the prince arranges for the two of them to be wed immediately.

In an aside, the princess-to-be admits to the audience that she is actually a powerful sea witch. She desires revenge on the mermaid, whose father, the King of the Sea, cast the witch out of his kingdom years before. By failing to marry the prince herself, the mermaid will have neglected to uphold her end of a bargain, and the sea witch will keep her voice forever.

The sun *[baritone]* then sings about the tragedy of mortal life, which he has to witness every day among the humans below him on earth. He also sings about the peaceful happiness of the immortal mermaids, and how love makes one foolish, but exalted. He drifts across the stage, and, with a clever bit of scenic machinery, begins to 'set' as the ballet troupe comes out for an interlude before the finale: the wedding scene.

The prince and the false princess come out dressed splendidly and singing a duet, but the prince's words are about love, and the princess's are about conquest. The mute girl looks sadly on.

Then, just as the prince and princess are about to recite their final vows, Triton, King of the Sea *[bass]*, resplendent in green and gold armour, appears with a crash of drums. He and the sea witch sing back and forth, trading insults. Finally he raises his trident to attack… and the sea witch points to his youngest, favourite daughter, the now-mute human standing sadly in the corner. With her other hand, she shakes a large painted prop contract.

Defeated, Triton gives in. He trades his life for the little mermaid. The sea witch casts a terrible spell, and with a puff of theatrical smoke the King of the Sea is turned into an ugly little sea polyp, which the sea witch holds triumphantly aloft.

[As a puppet manipulated by the contralto, it even moves a little, which draws a gasp from the audience.]

Triton's daughter turns back into a mermaid and jumps sadly into the sea. The prince and the false princess are married. The false princess sings triumphantly to the little polyp that was once Triton, and talks about how she will keep him forever in a vase in her room.

The moon *[mezzo-soprano]* comes out and sings an ethereal, haunting version of the sun's aria. But hers is about the inevitability and sadness of love, and questions what makes a happy ending. For if the little mermaid had stayed at home and remained a mermaid for all her days, ignorant of love, would that really have been better?

Scuttle

The crowd went mad. If the subject matter of the opera seemed a little fantastic, if the end a little gloomy, if the orchestration maybe just a *tad* simplistic compared to works by more professional, starving musicians, well, it mattered not. Never before had the amphitheatre been witness to such a display of clapping, screaming, stomping of feet and whistling. So many roses were thrown at *La Sirenetta* and the sea witch that they were in danger of suffering puncture wounds from the thorns.

Everyone was already clamouring for an encore performance.

"Perhaps we should," Prince Eric said. "A free performance for all of the town! At the end of summer, on St. Madalberta's Day!"

The cheers grew even louder.

Nobles seated closest to the royal box made a show of appropriately classy, restrained enthusiasm, while keeping their eyes on the prince and princess. Only a fool would have failed to notice certain similarities between the sea witch and Prince Eric's beautiful wife, Vanessa. That night in the great stone mansions, over tiny cups of chocolate and crystal glasses of brandy, there would be much discussion of the thousand possible shades of meaning behind the words in the lyrics.

But the brown-haired princess was grinning and laughing throatily.

"*Eric,*" she purred, "that was positively *naughty*. And *wonderful*. Where do you *get* such *imaginative* ideas?"

She coquettishly took his hand like they were newly-weds and walked out proudly with him into the crowd, beaming as if she were also the mother of a very talented and precocious boy. Her two manservants trailed behind them, looking back and forth at the crowd with suspicious smiles, seemingly ready to kill at a moment's notice should it be required.

Nothing was required; everyone was joyous.

Among the hundreds of people and creatures that were audience to this spectacle, only one was flummoxed by it.

Scuttle stood stock-still, an unusual pastime for him. Two *very important things* had been revealed in the play. And while he was as scatterbrained as a seagull generally is (perhaps more so), the wisdom of his long years made him stop and try to focus on those things in his muzzy mind, to remember them, to pay attention to his quieter thoughts.

"PRINCE ERIC REMEMBERS WHAT HAPPENED!" he suddenly cried out.

That was the first thing, and it was easy.

"Even though he is under her spell!"

Scuttle had been there when the land-walking mermaid had failed to win Eric's heart, the sun had gone down, and he had married Vanessa instead. Scuttle had seen the mighty fight break out between ancient powers, so poorly captured in the paints and papier mâché below. He had seen the ocean waves swell and crash by the power of Triton. He had watched as the King of the Sea traded his life for his daughter's and the sea witch, Ursula, destroyed him. The red-haired girl became a mermaid once more and swam sadly away, voiceless forever. Ursula-as-Vanessa remained married to Eric and now ruled the kingdom by the sea with little or no useful input from her hypnotised hubby.

"Yup, check and check," Scuttle murmured. "And somehow my boy Eric knows this. But how?"

And what was that other thing?

That important thing?

The… *almost-as-important* thing?

Or was it actually *more* important?

"Waves swell and crash by the power of Triton," Scuttle repeated to himself aloud because he enjoyed the sound of his voice and the big, epic words. His great-grandgulls rolled their eyes at each other and flew off. All but one, who sat watching him curiously.

"And the King of the Sea traded his life for his daughter's, and Ursula destroyed him. THAT'S IT!"

Scuttle squawked, jumping up into the air in excitement. He beat his wings and the few lingering spectators covered themselves with their arms in disgust, fearing what the bird would do next.

"KING TRITON IS STILL ALIVE!"

"I'm sorry?" his remaining great-grandgull asked politely.

"Don't you get it?" Scuttle turned to her and pointed at the stage. "If everything else in that show was true, then Ursula still has Triton as her *prisoner*! He's *not dead*! C'mon, Jonathan! We got to go do some investor-gating of this possibility!"

"My name is Jona, Great-grandfather," the younger gull corrected gently.

He didn't seem to hear.

With a purpose he hadn't felt since his time with the mermaid Ariel, Scuttle beat new life into his tired old wings and headed for the castle, his great-grandgull gliding silently behind.

When the king and queen of Tirulia decided that the time had come for each of their children to assume the roles and habits of adulthood, and, more importantly, to move out of the main palace, Prince Eric quite unsurprisingly chose a small castle on the very edge of the sea.

The giant blocks that made its outer walls were sandstone, light in colour and far more evocative of the beach than the granite and grey stone with which other ancient fortresses were built. A welcome addition by Eric's grandfather featured a walkway out to a viewing deck, supported by graceful arches in the manner of a Roman aqueduct. The two highest tiled towers cleverly recalled architecture of more eastern cities; a third was topped by a pergola covered with grapes and fragrant jasmine. The great formal dining room, another modern addition, was finished in the latest fashion with floor-to-ceiling windows.

In fact, all the public and fancy rooms, every single bedroom in the castle, except for the lowliest servants' quarters, had a view of the sea.

This was of great interest to the humans who lived in the castle, the villagers who bragged about their castle and the Bretlandian visitors taking the Grand Tour who stopped to sketch the castle.

But the windows were of *especial* interest to the flying and scurrying members of the kingdom.

It was well known to all the local seagulls where the kitchens were, of course. Their windows were the most important. Boiled seashells, some with tidbits still stuck on; avalanches of crumbs that had gone stale; meat that had been left out too long; fruit that had rotted… All of it got dumped unceremoniously out the windows and into a hidden section of the lagoon. Hidden to humans, that is.

It was also well known that Countess Gertrude, a cousin of Eric's, was much enamoured with anything that flew and could be counted on to stand at her window for hours, enticing gulls, doves, sparrows and even sparrowhawks to land on her hand for a treat.

The Ibrian ambassador, Iase, paranoid and terrified of poison, was constantly tossing whatever he was served out the closest window.

Anything that got dumped out of Princess Vanessa's window, however, was known to be actually bad for you: sharp, and often *really* poisoned.

After a moment's precipitous scrabbling, Scuttle managed to perch himself on the lintel of this last unglazed window, his great-grandgull just beside him.

"Huh. Nice digs," he said, looking around with interest. Then he settled himself in to wait.

Seagulls might be a little scattered and unable to focus, sometimes greedy, and borderline psychotic if it came to fighting over a real prize, but the one thing they *could* do was wait. For hours if they had to: for the tide to go out, for the fishing ships to come back in, for the wind to change, for the pesky humans to leave their middens to those who so rightfully deserved to plunder them for treats.

Jona cocked her head once, observing a chambermaid dumping a chamber pot out the side of the castle, into the sea.

"And humans complain about *our* habits," she muttered.

"Shh!" Scuttle said, keeping his beak closed.

Eventually their patience was rewarded. Vanessa came sashaying in, leaving her two manservants outside.

"I'll see you boys later," she purred. They bowed in unison, almost identical twins in matching uniforms that had costlier jackets and prettier feathered caps than other castle staff.

The princess began to disrobe, pulling off her gloves, her mantle and the wide hat that topped her dark hair. This was brown velvet with golden medallions round the crown and the plumes of rare foreign birds in the band… and she still left it carelessly on her bed. She quietly hummed one of the arias from the opera, one of the *mermaid's* arias, and then opened her mouth wider and belted it out, knocking the seagulls back a little with the force of her musicality.

It did not sound like that when Ariel used to sing.

Oh, it was the mermaid's voice all right, and the tune was dead on. But it was too loud, and the words had no soul, and the notes didn't flow from one to the other harmoniously. It was as if a talented but untrained child with no life experience to speak of had suddenly been commanded to sing a piece about a woman dying of consumption who had lost her only love.

Scuttle tried not to wince. Seagulls of course had no innate musical abilities themselves, as other birds loved to taunt, but the song still sounded blasphemous in Ariel's voice.

Vanessa laughed, purred, and made other noises with her throat Ariel never would have. "Did you enjoy that, mighty sea king? The little song from a lovesick mermaid?"

"I don't see a mighty sea king," the great-grandgull

whispered to Scuttle. "*Maybe she's mad.*"

Scuttle had no response. He frowned and ducked and peered back and forth into every corner of the room that he could glimpse from the window. But there was nothing, not even a small aquarium, that might hold a polyp.

Vanessa paused in front of the overwhelming collection of bottles and trinkets on her dressing table: musky perfumes in tiny glass ampoules, exotic oils in jars carved in pink stone, enough boar-bristled brushes to keep an army of princesses looking their best. The one thing she didn't have, which Scuttle would not have realised, was a maidservant performing these ablutions *for* her. She made a kissy-face into the mirror and then moved on, disappearing from view into her wardrobe. It looked like she was holding something, but it was hard to be sure.

The two birds strained and leant forwards, trying to follow her movements.

"I'm so sorry you missed such a wonderful opera, Kingy," she called from the darkness. After a moment she came back out wearing a bright pink silk robe. Now they could see that she carried a bottle half hidden in her voluminous sleeve. "But I think Eric may put it on again, one more time. Not that you'll get to see it then, either. Such a shame! It was so *imaginative.* It was all about a little mermaid, and how she loses her prince to a nasty old sea witch. The *hussy*."

She paused… and then cracked up, her delicate mouth opening wider and wider and wider, billows of distinctly non-Ariel laughter coming out.

She turned to hold the glass bottle up to regard it in the light coming from the gull-decorated window… and the gulls gasped.

It was a narrow glass cylinder, like that which a scientist might use when doing experiments. On top was a piece of muslin held on with globs of wax. Inside was filled with water… and one of the most horrible things Scuttle and Jona had ever seen.

A dark green mass, gelatinous, with a vaguely plantlike shape filled most of the bottle. One knobbly end kept it rooted on the bottom of the glass. Towards its 'head' were things that looked like tentacles but floated uselessly in the tiny space; these were topped with a pair of yellow eyes. A hideous cartoon of a mouth hung slackly beneath. In a final bit of terrible mockery two slimy appendages flowed down the sides of its mouth, ridiculing the sea king's once foam-white moustache and beard.

The great-grandgull turned her head to avoid gagging.

"It's him!" Scuttle cried, at the last second covering his words with a squawk, remembering that the sea witch could understand the languages of all beasts, same as Ariel.

Vanessa spun quickly and suspiciously.

Jona thought fast. She pecked at her great-grandfather, realistically, as if she were trying to steal a morsel from him.

Scuttle squawked.

"What the..."

"NO IT'S MY FISHY!" Jona screamed. She widened her eyes at him, *willing* him to understand.

Her great-grandfather just stared at her for a moment.

Then he relaxed.

"What? Oh yeah, right," he said, giving her a big wink. "No—my—great-grandgull—that—is—my—fish!"

They both fell off the ledge, away into the air, wheeling and squawking like perfectly normal seagulls.

Vanessa ran to the window but relaxed when she saw just a pair of birds, fighting in mid-air over some nasty piece of something-or-other. With a snarl and a flounce she turned back inside.

"That was some pretty smart thinking back there," Scuttle said, giving his great-grandgull a salute.

"What now?" she asked.

"Now? We go find *Ariel*."

Atlantica

Far, far below the wine-dark waves upon which wooden boats floated like toys lay a different sort of kingdom.

Coral reefs were scattered like forests across the landscape, lit in dappled sunlight that had to travel a long and slow liquid passage to reach them. Long ribbons of kelp filled in for their Dry World tree equivalents. These bent and dipped gracefully in the slightest aquatic breezes, and were soft to the touch, yet tough as leather, sometimes with sharp edges. Finger-like tips reached for the sun, photosynthesising just like their landlocked brethren.

There were mountains in this deep land too, and

canyons. Just as rivers drained the surrounding countryside and flowed downhill in the Dry World, so too different temperatures of water flowed together, creating drifts and eddies. Fissures in the earth erupted with boiling water that blasted out of the hellish depths below, too hot for everyone except the tiny creatures whose entire existence depended on the energy from those vents, instead of on the vague yellow thing so far above.

And everywhere, just as there were animals on land, were the animals of the sea.

The tiniest fish made the largest schools – herring, anchovies and baby mackerel sparkling and cavorting in the light like a million diamonds. They twirled into whirlpools and flowed over the sandy floor like one large, unlikely animal.

Slightly larger fish came in a rainbow, red and yellow and blue and orange and purple and green and parti-coloured like clowns: dragonets and blennies and gobies and combers.

Hake, shad, char, whiting, cod, flounder and mullet made the solid middle class.

The biggest loners, groupers and oarfish and dogfish and the major sharks and tuna that all grew to a large, ripe old age did so because they had figured out how to avoid human boats, nets, lines and bait. The black-eyed predators were well aware they were top of the food chain only down deep, and somewhere beyond the surface there were things even more hungry and frightening than they.

Rounding out the population were the famous un-fish of the ocean: the octopus, flexing and swirling the ends of her tentacles; delicate jellyfish like fairies; lobsters and sea stars; urchins and nudibranchia… the funny, caterpillar-like creatures that flowed over the ocean floor wearing all kinds of colours and appendages.

All of these creatures woke, slept, played, swam about and lived their whole lives under the sea, unconcerned with what went on above them.

But there were other animals in this land, strange ones, who spoke both sky and sea. Seals and dolphins and turtles and the rare fin whale would come down to hunt or talk for a bit and then vanish to that strange membrane that separated the ocean from everything else. Of course they were loved, but perhaps not quite entirely trusted.

The strangest creatures of all lived in a city they built themselves, a kingdom in the depths.

Here no roofs separated the inhabitants from the water above or around them; creatures who could move in any direction had no love of constraint. All was open, airy, or perhaps *oceany*, and built for pleasure and the whimsy of the architect. Delicate fences led visitors into the *idea* of another place. Archways, not doors, opened into other rooms, some of which were above one another. Stairs were unnecessary. Columns, thin and delicate as stalactites in an undiscovered cave, supported 'roads' that soared around halls and were decorated with graceful spires. Everything glowed white from marble or pale pink and orange from coral, or glimmered iridescently like the inside of a shell.

All this beauty was the result of many thousands of years of art, peace and patience, and little to no contact with the rest of the world. If Atlantica was an unimaginable, dreamy splendour to the few humans who had gazed upon it before drowning, it was also unchanged by the centuries; magnificently, eternally the same.

The creatures who built and ruled this underwater world were long-lived and content, with nothing but time and aesthetics on their minds, governed by kings and queens of the same belief.

Or so it had once been.

Now Atlantica was ruled by a queen who had seen another world, and been betrayed by it, and who would live with the consequences – forever.

Ariel

The usual crowd gathered on the throne dais: merfolk of every hue, several dolphins who occasionally flipped up to the surface for a breath, a solitary oarfish, a thin group of sculpin. Primarily the occupants were mer, for the queen was holding court on the Ritual of the June Tide, one of the most important and solemn ordinances of the Sevarene Rites.

And she sorely wished she were anywhere else.

Kings and queens had to address crowds – that was part of the job. Most of the ceremonial aspects could be dealt with by just swimming somewhere, looking regal, nodding seriously and smiling at babies. But when the occasion called for a speech…

… and you couldn't speak…

Annio was chosen to be the acting priest of the Ritual, so it will be he, and not Laiae, who draws from the Well of Hades.

She said this with her hands, carefully spelling out the priests' names alphabetically in the old runes.

Sebastian and Flounder and Threll, the little seahorse messenger, were placed round the outside edges of the crowd, interpreting what she said aloud. They and Ariel's sisters were the only ones who had bothered to learn the ancient, signed version of the mer language, but only the fish and crab and seahorse volunteered to translate.

None of them shouted loud enough, not the way her father had, so not everyone could hear if only one of them spoke for her.

(The one time they had tried to use a conch to amplify Flounder's voice had just been a disaster. He had sounded *ridiculous.*)

In a perfect world, her sisters would be the ones doing it. Those who grew up with her and had similar voices could speak more easily for her, and since they were princesses themselves, everyone was more likely to listen.

But it was too much like work.

And the one thing her sisters tended to avoid, more than the advances of unwanted suitors, was work.

And so Ariel signed, and the interpreters interpreted,

and various parts of the crowds listened to different voices trying to speak for her, and their attention was on the *interpreters,* and their questions were directed to *them*, and it was all a mess.

"Which Annio? The elder?"

"Was my child in the running, my darling Ferestia?"

"But at what hour?"

Her only recourse when everyone started talking at once was to blow loudly on the golden conch she wore round her neck as a symbol of office. She felt more like a silly ship's captain than a queen.

I will send out tablets with the details, posted in the usual public locations, she signed wearily. *That is all.*

After her helpers spoke and everyone thought about it for a moment, it was like waiting for the thunder after lightning, watching the meaning of her words sink in seconds later, the crowd made murmurs both negative and positive, and began to disperse.

Ariel sat back in her throne, leaning tiredly on one elbow, unconsciously assuming the exact position her father always had at the end of an exhausting day. Threll darted from one lingering mer to the next, making sure everyone understood and felt like she or he had been heard. He was a good little messenger, and had proven surprisingly useful in his new role. Flounder was in the back, having a quiet conversation with a fish she didn't recognise.

Sebastian came scuttling over to her, kicking himself up through the water to sit on her armrest.

"Ah, the Saga at the end of the Rites will be *outstanding* this year," he declared, parading back and forth in front of Ariel, claws gesticulating in the air. "So much talent. So much enthusiasm! Nothing could make it better. The sardines are in sync, the trumpet fish are terrific. Everything is perfect. Well, there is *one* thing that could make it better, of course… if only you had your lovely voice."

Ariel raised an eyebrow at Sebastian. Even if she had her voice, she doubted very much if she could have said anything that would have successfully interrupted his monologue. She shifted uncomfortably in her throne. The little crab didn't notice. Although he *could* expertly interpret her signs, read her lips and decipher her moods, it was only when he was paying strict attention.

"Ahh, what a loss that was for de world…" He put a claw on her shoulder and finally noticed her scowl. "Er, of course, in return, we received the best, most excellent *queen* in de world."

The best, most excellent queen in the world tapped her trident, idly considering turning him into a sea cucumber for a few minutes to think about what he had said.

But he was only echoing something Ariel thought about all the time, herself: whether or not she was any sort of decent queen. Since she never should have been queen to begin with.

When she had returned to her sisters five years before, voiceless and deep in despair over what had happened to her, she'd fully expected banishment, punishment, at the very least, severe chastisement. Instead her family did something utterly unexpected: they made her ruler over all of Atlantica. There was no precedent for this; as the youngest child of the mer-king it would normally have taken the deaths of all six older sisters before the crown came to her.

"You're responsible for the murder of our father," they had said. "It's only right that you take on his burdens."

Privately Ariel wondered if it was less punishment for *her* than a relief for *them*. None of her sisters wanted the job. As royal princesses they could sing and play all day, dress up in fancy shells, wear crowns, oversee dances and parades and balls… and never actually have to do any real work. These days she often watched her sisters laughing and singing and wondered at the gulf that had grown between them. Here she was, the youngest, some would say the prettiest, at one time perhaps most *thoughtless* of the lot, and now she sat on a throne, envying them.

The merfolk adored their queen despite her silence and melancholic air. Or perhaps *because* of it. Mer poets and musicians wrote odes and epics to the tragedy of her existence, the romance that had almost caused a kingdom's downfall.

She did not enjoy these.

She did not enjoy the attention of the mermen, either. Once upon a time, as a younger, more innocent thing, she had never even noticed boys. Mer boys, at least.

Now she was *forced* to notice them, to keep an eye on them, to be aware of what ulterior motives they had: to wed the queen, maybe to become king.

Ha, she thought bitterly. *If only they knew what a pain it is to rule.*

She hadn't been even a tide-cycle into her new office before she had begun to understand her father's temper and moods. He had been a firm leader who rarely smiled, presenting the perfect image of an old god: stone-faced, bearded, permanent. Prone to glowering and frowning. She and her sisters always teased him, trying to win smiles from him, trying to get him to steal an hour from his duties to play with them. Mostly they had to content themselves with his presence at official functions, banquets and performances like the one Ariel had skipped – the one that had started the whole thing.

She wished she could tell him she understood. Being a ruler was *hard*. It made one frown, turn pensive, grumpy.

It should have been an easy job; the merfolk and their allies were the happiest, most carefree peoples in the world.

Well, until a tribe of sea bass moved a little too close to the viewing garden of a royal cousin.

Or the shark-magister insisted on expanding his people's hunting rights all the way to Greydeep Canyon.

Or, far more importantly, a reef suddenly turned white and died for no apparent cause. Or the diamondback terrapins couldn't make it to their favourite nesting place because there were houses there now. Or the humans had managed to catch, and eat, an entire delegation from the northern seas. Or the number of fishing vessels was getting too large to ignore, to relegate to the unwritten and ancient Dry World–Sea World laws of yore.

Yet despite these much more pressing concerns, cousin Yerena still complained about the sea bass and her garden and 'their ugly faces'.

It made Ariel irritable just thinking about it.

Besides general grumpiness, there was another more serious similarity between the king and his daughter. Any joy Triton had taken in life, even with his daughters, was constantly shadowed by sorrow over his dead wife.

Any respite Ariel took in her new life was constantly shadowed by her sorrow and *guilt* over her dead father.

And so she ruled, firmly and well, but silently and with much melancholy.

She cleared her throat, one of the few noises she could still make, and was leaning forwards to give the little crab a piece of her mind when Flounder came swimming up.

Her old friend was larger and happily fatter than when they had first set out to the surface years ago. He had a medallion round his neck to show rank; the imprint of the trident meant he was in the innermost ring of the royal circle. But unlike the adorable little helper fish and servant seahorses, he didn't turn his chest into the light or waggle to make the golden disc extra obvious. He remained, despite the years and accumulated wisdom, likeable, down-to-sea-floor Flounder.

"My Queen!"

He swooped in front of her, ignoring Sebastian, and gave the low bow that was required of all but Ariel usually tried to stop, at least from him and Sebastian.

Ariel cocked her head at him: *go on.*

"I've just had some strange, really, really strange, news from a plaice, who heard it from a turtle, who heard it from a dolphin… Wait, I *think* it was the plaice from the turtle.

There might have been another messenger in between. A bluefish, maybe?"

He felt Ariel's impatience before she even displayed it.

"There is a seagull on the surface who claims to have news for your ears only."

Ariel's eyes widened.

She signed carefully, spelling out the name.

Is it Scuttle?

"No, My Queen," Flounder said, trying not to show his own disappointment. "It was hard to make out through all of the… parties involved, but I believe it is a younger one, and a female."

Ariel practically wilted.

Seagulls were useless. Scuttle was a rare bird. Scattered but good-hearted, prone to flights of exaggeration, but a true friend. It should have been *him* coming to visit.

For several years after the day she lost her father, Ariel had tried to return to the land to see Eric and to take revenge on Ursula. But the wily sea witch had used her now very prosaic powers as a *human* princess to set guards all along the coast, officially, in 'case of an enemy kingdom attack, or pirates'. In some cases, close to the castle, guards were literally stationed *in* the water, up to their calves.

With Scuttle's help Ariel had tried to evade the guards,

sneaking in while the gull whipped up a distraction. But it was never enough, and the men were all on high alert for strange, witchy red-haired girls.

After a while, and after much insistence from Sebastian and her sisters, Ariel gave up and returned to her life under the sea permanently. At the very least she could respect the memory of her father by devoting herself to her duties as queen. She had vowed to forget the Dry World forever.

Even Scuttle.

"But… it's a seagull. So doesn't that mean Scuttle *has* to be involved somehow?" Flounder pointed out, trying to cheer her up. "It would be really, really bizarre if some random gull came to talk to you. But I didn't double-check on the origin of the story. I didn't want to break your ban on going to the surface."

Ariel swished her tail thoughtfully.

"Don't even think about it," Sebastian growled. "I know what you're thinking. It's just a silly seabird. Don't even consider it, young lady."

Ariel raised an eyebrow at him incredulously. *Young lady?* In the years that had passed since the duel with the sea witch, she had aged. Not dramatically, but far more than a mostly immortal mermaid should have. There was something about her eyes, they were deeper, wiser and wearier than when she was a young mer who had never been on dry land. Her cheeks weren't quite as plump any more; the angles of her face were more pronounced. Sometimes she wondered if she looked like her mother… aside from her own unreliable memories, the only physical evidence of the former queen was a statue in the castle of her and Triton dancing together. But it was all pale milky marble, no colours at all. *Dead.*

Ariel's hair no longer flowed behind her as it once had; handmaidens and decorator crabs kept it braided and coiffed, snug and businesslike under the great golden crown that sat on her temples, like the gods wore. Small gold and aquamarine earrings sparkled regally but didn't tinkle; they were quite understated and professional. Her only real nod to youth was the golden ring in the upper part of her left ear.

"Young lady," indeed.

She didn't even have to sign, *You cannot talk to me that way any more, little crab. I am queen now.*

Sebastian sighed, sounding old in his exasperation. "I'm sorry for speaking out of turn. I can't help it. Nothing good comes out of you going up there… *nothing ever has.* I just… I just don't want to see you hurt or disappointed again."

Ariel gave him the tiniest smile and tapped him once on the back fondly. Sometimes it was hard to remember that much of Sebastian's attitude was only for show. Underneath, he really did have, what he thought were, her best interests at heart.

But she was a grown-up now, and queen, and her best interests were none of his business. She turned to sign to the little seahorse who floated silently at attention, fins quivering, waiting for orders.

Threll, please tell the Queen's Council that I will be taking this afternoon off. Flounder will be accompanying me. Sebastian is nominally in charge until I return, though no votes or decisions are to be made in my absence.

"Yes, Your Majesty." The little seahorse bowed and zoomed off into the water.

"My Queen, as thrilled as I am…" Sebastian began.

But Ariel was already turned upwards, and kicking hard to the surface.

Ariel

Mermaid queens didn't often have a reason to move quickly. There were no wars to direct, no assassination attempts to evade, no crowds of clamouring admirers to avoid among the merfolk. In fact, slowness and calm were expected of royalty.

So Ariel found herself thoroughly enjoying the exercise as she beat her tail against the water, even as it winded her a little. She missed dashing through shipwrecks with Flounder, fleeing sharks, trying to scoot back home before curfew. She loved the feel of her powerful muscles, the way the current cut around her when she twisted her shoulders to go faster.

She hadn't been this far up in years and gulped as the

pressure of the deep faded. She clicked her ears, readying them for the change of environment. Colours faded and transformed around her from the dark, heady slate of the ocean bottom to the soothing azure of the middle depths and finally lightening to the electric, magical periwinkle that heralded the burst into daylight.

She hadn't planned to break through the surface triumphantly. She wouldn't give it that power. Her plan was to take it slow and rise like a whale. Casually, unperturbed, like *Ooh, here I am.*

But somehow her tail kicked in twice as hard the last few feet, and she exploded into the warm sunlit air like she had been drowning.

She gulped again and *tasted* the breeze, dry in her mouth; salt and pine and far-distant *fires* and a thousand alien scents…

A small gull sat riding the waves, regarding her curiously.

Ariel composed herself, remembering who she was. Trying not to delight in the way the water streamed down her neck; how it dried from her hair, lightening it. Flounder whirled around her body anxiously before popping up beside her.

She signed: *I am told you have a message for me.*

But before Flounder could translate, before she could stop herself, Ariel signed again:

Do you know Scuttle? Where is he? Why isn't Scuttle here?

"Queen Ariel was told you have a message for her," the fish told the gull solemnly. "However, she was expecting her old friend Scuttle. He is the only bird she has ever been close to."

"You are correct to assume it was he who sent me out here. Great-grandfather Scuttle couldn't make it this far," the seagull answered. "How are you breathing?"

It took Ariel a moment to fully register the second part of what the bird had said.

What?

She didn't even have to sign it.

The seagull cocked her head at the mermaid and stared at her, unblinking. "You went from under the water to above water with no trouble at all. Since you live underwater all the time, I assume it's not that you can just hold your breath forever, like if you were a magical whale, say. And you have no gills like a newt. So how are you breathing?"

"You do not address the queen of Atlantica that way," Flounder chastised. Ariel was impressed by how grown-up he sounded, unruffled by the weird conversation.

"Pardon," the seagull said immediately, dipping her head.

Ariel twirled her trident casually, letting the water fly

from it in a hundred sparkling droplets. Although the merfolk accepted her lineage and rights to the crown immediately, there had still been a definite period of adjustment while they still thought of her as the pretty, carefree baby girl of Triton. Some spoke to her far too patronisingly, some spoke to her far too familiarly. And *some* folk of non-mer persuasion (sharks, mainly) had needed several displays of her anger before they acknowledged her authority.

But she didn't think that was what was going on with this odd little seagull. There was no *judgement* in the bird's expression. Just fascination. She had probably never seen a mermaid before. Ariel could have been a sea slug or a demon and the gull would have asked the same question.

What is your name? Ariel asked.

"Jona," the bird said with a little bow after Flounder had translated. "But… if you talk to my great-grandfather at all, he may refer to me, incorrectly, as Jonathan. Jonathan Livingston. He's a little confused sometimes."

Ariel smiled, thinking that sounded exactly like Scuttle.

"Why don't you tell the queen everything, starting from the beginning, Jona?" Flounder suggested.

So the gull told the tale of watching the opera with her great-grandfather, and her great-grandfather's reaction to it. She told of their flight to the castle and spying on

Vanessa, and the revelation of the existence of Triton. She told it succinctly and perfectly: no unwanted description, dialogue, or personal observation. Ariel wasn't sure how exactly she could have been descended from the absent-minded Scuttle. *Maybe an egg got misplaced from another nest.*

Ariel's mind whirled, in shock from the news.

Her father was alive!

... *Probably?*

Good queens did not react immediately to new information, especially if they didn't already have some inkling of what it brought. Snap decisions were rash and led to disaster. Ariel had learnt this the hard way. Not having a voice was an advantage here: she could compose herself while working out how to say what she needed to.

You have really seen my father? Alive?

"I saw a..." Jona struggled for the right word. "... thing in a bottle that the princess spoke to like it was Triton, King of the Sea. And Great-grandfather says the... thing... bore a more than passing resemblance to the entity he once was."

Ariel remembered all too clearly what that 'thing' looked like. It did indeed sound like her father.

"Great-grandfather thought you would be up to another adventure," the gull added, almost timidly. "And I am to let you know that he's in, to rescue your father."

How would we rescue him? Her hands shook a little as she signed. *Impossible... the guards...*

"While I am not directly familiar with the situation as it previously stood, Great-grandfather told me to tell you that the number of soldiers on the beach has been greatly reduced since the two of you last tried to reach Eric. He is not the best at counting," Jona added neutrally, "but when we were there to see if your father was still alive, I saw no more than eight. None of them were in the water, and most looked like they were barely paying attention."

Eight? There had been dozens the last time she tried. And they marched, resolutely, up and down the sands, eyes on the sea. But that was years ago... after Ariel stopped trying, maybe Ursula figured she had given up forever. Maybe the sea witch had turned her attentions elsewhere and let security lapse.

Ariel signed.

"I will take these matters into consideration," Flounder translated, "and will either return here myself in three days or send a messenger in my place."

"Understood," the seagull said with a bow.

"Understood, My Queen," Flounder corrected politely.

"Are you?" the gull asked curiously. "*My* Queen? How

does that work with the Law of the Worlds, that of the Dry World and the World Under the Sea?"

Ariel found herself almost rolling her eyes and making that wide, sighing smile she used to with Flounder.

But the little gull had looked at her, at *her*, while she signed. Not at her hands, or Flounder as he had spoken. There was a friendly heart under Jona's direct and inappropriate questions.

Ariel just shook her head and dove back under the water, signing over her shoulder as she went.

"The Queen says you may call her Ariel," Flounder said. Also, under his breath: "You have *no idea* what an honour that is."

On the way back down Ariel's silence was deeper than usual; it practically echoed into the quiet sea, filling the water around them.

"What are you going to do?" Flounder asked, trying not to sound as anxious as his old self. "We *have* to save Triton. Don't we? But can we?"

Ariel stopped suddenly in the water, thinking. Her tail swished back and forth as she held steady in a tiny current that rippled her fins and tendrils of hair.

Do we even know it's actually true?

Flounder's eyes widened. "But she said… I don't know, Ariel. She seemed like a pretty honest, if weird, bird. And Scuttle!"

It's been years. *Why would Ursula keep him around, alive?*

"No idea. So she can talk at him? All the time? She loves that kind of thing. But if he *is* alive, isn't that great news? Don't we need to *do* something?" Flounder was practically begging, swishing back and forth in the water in desperation.

I don't know… I want *to believe it's true. It's too much to take in. I'm going to go… think for a while.*

Alone, she added.

Flounder didn't need to ask where.

"Sebastian won't like that," he sighed.

Then he tried not to giggle at the very unqueenly thing she signed.

"I'll tell him you've gone to consult some elders or something," he said, waving a fin. "Be safe."

He needn't have suggested that as he swam off; with the trident, Ariel could kill an army or call up a storm that would destroy half the sea. But it was hard to let old habits die. And it was harder still to care for a powerful queen, whose only vulnerabilities were ones you couldn't see.

Ariel

Drifting slowly now, Ariel wound her way through the kingdom to the outskirts of Atlantica.

A few fish stopped to bow and she acknowledged them with a nod of her head. No merfolk were around to bother her. As a rule, most didn't like lonely, dusty corners of the ocean where rocks thrived more than coral.

Eventually she came to the hidden grotto where her collection of things once was. Millions of years ago it had probably vented hot water and lava that provided sustenance for tube worms, which resulted in a perfect, cylindrical series of shelves for Ariel to display her finds on. Then her father had blasted it back to its mineral components. *Which tiny creatures will use again, completing the circle.*

Fine sand, the aquatic equivalent of dust, covered everything in an impressively thick layer. A couple of seaweeds had managed to anchor onto the rubble here and there, and anemones sprouted from the more protected corners.

Ariel looked around at the old destruction her furious father had wrought. She had hated him so much. And then he had… traded his life for hers.

And now he was… alive?

She could hardly let herself believe it. The cries and sobs she couldn't make aloud turned inward into her heart, in spasms of pain.

If he really was alive, Ursula had probably been torturing him all these years. She was not kind to her prisoners.

Or it could be a trap, a complicated set-up to lure Ariel back so Ursula could finish her for good. A strange move to make half a decade after the mermaid had obviously given up, but the sea witch *was* strange.

And all Ariel had was the word of a gull she didn't even know.

Although… despite the short amount of time she had spent with the bird… there was something unquestionably honest about her. The queen had a feeling that if pressed, Jona couldn't lie or exaggerate to save her own life. And despite Scuttle's tendency to misrepresent or fabricate or even believe his own lies, he never really meant it. If he thought there was a chance that Triton was alive, he would do anything in his power to help Ariel save him.

I should do it properly, she thought, hands tightening into fists. She should advance on the human castle with a mer army, and summon the power of the seas, and dash Ursula to bits on the rocks, and drown all those who opposed her, and sweep in and save her father; and he would be king again, and she would have a father again…

… and she wouldn't.

She would never enlist soldiers sworn to protect the mer kingdom to help with a mistake *she* had made. She would never endanger a castle of innocent people just to get back the person *she* was responsible for losing.

Fate was giving her a second chance.

She would take it, but by herself.

She would right the wrongs she had committed on her own.

She would, her heart leapt despite her doubts, find and rescue her father, ask his forgiveness and return the king to his people. Everyone would be ecstatic, her sisters most of all! And she would redeem herself. She might even be a hero. And they would all live happily ever after, under the sea.

But to do this, she would need to return to the Dry World.

She picked up a roundish thing from the ground and shook the sand off. It was the top of an old ceramic jar, once painted bright blue and gold. The humans had so many jars. And amphorae. And vases. And vessels. And kegs. And tankards. So many… things… to put other… *things* in. Merfolk rarely had a necessity to store anything beyond the occasional rare and fancy comestible, like the sweet goldenwine they used to trade for when she was a child. Merfolk ate when they were hungry, almost never had the need to drink anything and rarely had a reason to store food for the future.

She dropped the lid and sighed, drifting over to the rock she used to perch on while admiring her collection. *Things*, so many *things*. Things she never found out the proper use for in her short time on land. Because she had been too busy mooning over Eric.

In some ways, that was the part of the seagull's story that bothered her the most. She could not believe the reaction her traitor heart had when the bird mentioned his name.

Eric.

Eric *remembered* something?

He wrote an *opera* about it? About *her*?

It wasn't just the flattery of it, though. If Eric remembered enough to compose music about it… would he remember her too? A little?

She remembered *him* far too often.

Despite the fact that her life had been ruined because of her pursuit of Eric, when she closed her eyes to go to sleep, her last thoughts were often still of him.

Or when a perfectly handsome, reasonably amusing (and mostly *immortal*, not an irrelevant point) merman tried to win her affections, and all she could think about was how his hair might look when it was dry. Would it bounce, like Eric's?

An *opera*. What were his arias like? What did he write for her to sing?

She smiled, the irony of it not lost on her: she had run away from a concert to pursue a human, and he had written songs for her now that she could no longer sing.

She ran her finger along the sand on a nearby shelf, writing the name *Eric* in runes.

Maybe, just maybe, along the way to save her father, she could pay him a visit.

For old time's sake.

Sebastian

"NONONONONONONONONO!"

Sebastian scuttled back and forth along one of the balustrades that demarcated the edge of the throne dais. It had been grown, as many of the mer objects were, from coral, the original inhabitants coaxed to move on once their job was done.

The crab's toes made little *ticktickltick* noises as he selfrighteously walked one way and then back the other, claws gnarled in the ready position, not even once regarding his audience.

She sighed. While it was, of course, not unforeseeable

that the little crab would respond this way, waiting through his tantrum was not the most efficient use of her time.

As a girl, she would have swum off. As a girl with a voice, she might have argued.

As a mute queen, she could do neither.

She lifted up the trident and struck the ocean floor with it twice. Not to raise any magic, just to get his attention. To *remind* him of who she was.

The little crab stopped mid rant. She raised her eyebrows at him: *Really, Sebastian?*

"Nothing good will come of it," he said, a little sheepishly. "Nothing from the surface ever does."

My father may be alive, she signed. *That is reason enough to try.*

At this the little crab wavered. He clicked slowly along the railing until he was close enough to put a claw on her arm. "Ariel, I miss him, too… but you could be just chasing a ghost."

"Give up, Sebastian," Flounder suggested. "She's already made her decision."

"I think you're encouraging her in this!" Sebastian snapped, aiming an accusing claw at the fish.

Flounder rolled his eyes.

He's not encouraging, he's helping, Ariel said.

"I could help you *more*," Sebastian wheedled. "*I* can go on land for short periods of time."

You're needed down here, to act as my representative. And distraction.

"I am *not* going to get in front of a crowd of merfolk and… *similar ocean dwellers* to tell them that their *queen* has left them to go off on some ridiculous mission by herself! You want to leave, *you* have to be brave enough to tell them."

A single sign: *No.*

She rested a gentle hand on her throat, letting that action speak for itself.

Sebastian wilted. "All right, go. No one has ever been able to stop you from doing anything you wanted anyway, even when it costs you dearly."

For a moment, Ariel felt her old self surface, the urge to grin and plant a kiss on the little crab's back. He was right. She *did* have a habit of swimming in where angels feared to tread. No one could dissuade her once her mind was fixed. And it *had* cost her dearly.

What could it cost her this time?

"Please tell your sisters, at least," Sebastian said with a weary sigh, dropping off the edge and scooting himself along the ocean floor towards the throne. With some quick kicks and sideways crabby swimming he landed neatly on the armrest, the proper place for his official position as the queen's deputy. "I cannot *imagine* dealing with them right now."

Ariel nodded, and then gave him a second nod, eyes lowered: *thank you.*

And then she swam off so she wouldn't have to see the looks he and Flounder exchanged.

Her sisters were in the Grotto of Delights, swimming about, well, *delightedly*; attaching little anemones to their hair, fluffing up seaweed fascinators, rummaging through giant seashells of jewels, pearls and snails. Ariel could barely remember the time before her mother was killed but she was fairly certain that her sisters had been less frantic in their pursuit of pleasure then. Now they drowned their grief in safe, silly things that required little thought and provided constant distraction.

She ran her hand through a shell bowl absently, letting the trinkets slide through her fingers. Mostly they weren't cut or polished the way a human jeweller would treat them: they sparkled here and there out of a chunk of brownish rock. A single crystal might shine like the weapon of a god, but be topped by the lumpy bit where it had been prized out of a geode.

Ariel regarded the stones with fascination. Of course they were beautiful. Yet she still found the bits and bobs from the human world, *made* by humans, far more alluring. *Why?* Why couldn't she be content with the treasures of the sea the way the ocean had made them? What was wrong with them that they had to be altered, or put on something else, or framed, or forced in a bunch onto a necklace, in perfect, unnatural symmetry?

"Oh! Are you coming to the Neap Tide Frolic after all?"

Alana swirled around Ariel, her deep magenta tail almost touching her sister's. Her black hair was styled in intricate ringlets that were caught in a bright red piece of coral, its tiny branches and spines separating the curls into tentacles. The effect was amazing, and not a little terrifying.

Looking around, Ariel realised that her royal sisters were done up more than usual. Once again she had forgotten one of the endless parties, dances, fetes, celebrations and cyclical observations that made up most of the merpeople's lives.

No, I'm afraid it slipped my mind, she signed.

"Oh, too bad," Alana said, making a perfunctory sad face before swooshing away. The sisters had come to expect her absence and no longer even showed disappointment when she declined.

It hurt a little, Ariel realised.

Attina saw her and came over. Despite their extreme difference in age, she was the one Ariel felt closest to. Even if her big sister didn't fully understand the urge to seek out a human prince, or to explore the Dry World, or to collect odd bits of human relics, she always treated her little sister as gently as she could – despite how gruff she sounded.

"What's happening?" she asked, swishing her orange tail back and forth. Her hair wasn't done yet; it was obvious she was devoting all her time to helping the younger sisters with theirs. The only slightly frumpy brown bun was locked in place by sea urchin spikes. "You look… *concerned.* All royal and concerned."

Ariel allowed herself a small smile.

I'm going away for a few days.

"A royal holiday! Aww yeah! You could use it, clearly. I've been saying for ages now you need to relax and kick back for a bit. Haven't I been saying that? Your skin looks terrible. I'm so glad you… oh. *Not* a royal holiday, I can see that now."

Attina said all these things quickly, one after another: revelation, opinion, realisation. When people could speak aloud, Ariel had realised long ago, they spent words like they were free, wasting them with nonsense.

Her sister frowned. "Where are you going?"

Ariel didn't make a complicated sign. She just used her index finger and pointed. *Up.*

"What?" Attina wrinkled her nose, confused.

Ariel waited for the meaning to sink in.

"Oh, *no.*" Her sister shook her head, eyes wide. "You *cannot* be serious."

Ariel nodded.

"No. Nope. No, you don't," Attina said, crossing her arms. "Not again. We lost Dad when you did that last time. You're not doing it again."

The other sisters felt the tension in the water and swam silently up, watching, *hiding,* behind the oldest.

Attina, Ariel didn't spell out the sign; she moved her hand to suggest the robes of a goddess, the sign for Athena, for whom her sister was named. There was an implication of regalness and wisdom; Ariel was appealing to her oldest sister for her best values. *Attina, he may still be alive. That is why I am going.*

Several of her sisters gasped. Tails lashed.

"Nuh-uh," Attina said firmly.

Then she whispered: "Really?"

There's a chance. Someone I trust saw *him, as Ursula's prisoner.*

"Huh," Attina said, crossing her arms again. "Huh."

"Let her go," said Adella, swinging her ponytails.

"She *needs* to go," Andrina, the one closest to Ariel in age, whispered.

"You should go now!" Arista urged, tossing blonde hair out of her face. "Get Daddy back!"

Alana and Aquata were silent, looking at their leader, Attina.

"Can't you send someone…" *Else,* the oldest sister was going to say. But she shook her head. "No, I guess you can't."

I have to do this, Ariel agreed.

"You sure this isn't just a chance to see your little human prince again?" Alana asked flatly.

Ariel felt her face redden. Her left hand clenched round the trident, her right hand clenched in the water, round nothing, around everything, she could throw foam into her sister's face and it would become a poisonous, spiky urchin, or a handful of sharp sand, or a thousand little scale mites.

Attina made her lips go all squishy the way she often did, like a pufferfish before it puffed. She raised a hand to silence Alana. *Not now.*

Ariel reflected, for a moment, how much communication was in sign, even for those who could speak.

"Fine. Good luck. I hope you bring Father back," Attina

said, perfunctorily. "You can go."

Ariel could feel the twists in the water: the oldest sister, who had tried to take over as mother when their real mother died, and never succeeded in that role. The other sisters, who liked the idea of power and ruling and strength and crowns… for someone else. They all just wanted everything the way it had been when Ariel was one of them, when they were all the same.

But Ariel had never really been the same.

I don't need your permission, she signed. *I was merely letting you know.*

"Well!" Attina said, raising her eyebrows.

You made me queen.

"Yes… I suppose we did."

The five other girls flowed and slipped into the currents, their fins flickering sinuously into the depths. Attina swooped and followed behind. "I really hope you do find him," she called over her shoulder.

No one's going to volunteer to come along? Ariel signed, half ironically; with her back turned, there was no way her sister could have known she was saying anything.

She watched them all go back to exactly what they'd been doing before: fixing their hair, gossiping, swirling around each other in a scene that used to delight their father.

Don't you ever get bored with your lives? she signed, even though no one would see it.

Aren't you even a little bit curious?

She mouthed these words, trying to will a sound to come forth. This one time.

Nothing but water flowed out.

It's been over one hundred years since Mother died!

No one saw her. Her hands, useless for communicating, gripped the trident tightly.

She swam off, unheard, unseen.

Ariel

This time she would be prepared. She took a bag, the kind artists used to carry their tools, and packed the few things she thought she would need. Carefully kept clothing, rescued from a trunk sunk when its ship capsized. Waterlogged but not worn. It had been so long since she had been up on land that it took a while before she remembered how to put together a complete outfit. *Dress* and *apron* and *underskirt*... The number of layers of clothing humans wore was insane. Would anyone even notice if she forgot an undershirt or underpants?

Also she had to remember to bring money, every kind

of coin, just in case. Last time Eric had paid for everything. This time, should need arise, she would have to provide it for herself.

Then Ariel settled herself at her dressing table and shooed away the decorator crabs, a little impatient with their crowding presence and constant need to help. She could remove the crown herself, and would not be taking off the golden conch. She shrugged out of the heavy mantle that hung heavily from her shoulders and gave her an older, more regal appearance. It was immediately whisked away by two mackerel who would clean it and hang it properly on a reef to stay wrinkle- and anemone-free.

She pursed her lips and blew on her golden shell, quietly, not enough to arouse alarm. Flounder came swimming out of the depths, where he had been waiting, giving her some privacy.

She flowed her hand across her body, like a tide: *It's time.*

Flounder nodded and swam next to her. Together they rose.

They moved almost as one unit, his body bending back and forth in the middle, her tail pumping up and down in almost precisely the same rhythm. After a few minutes he ventured:

"It's just like old times, isn't it?"

Ariel turned and gave him a smile: so rare, these days. She had been thinking the exact same thing.

When her head broke the surface this time it was less revelatory but still exhilarating. The little gull was almost exactly where they had left her.

Ariel realised she didn't have a sign for *gull.*

"Great," the bird said. "I was really hoping you would come back."

Ariel blinked. *What a weird, banal thing to say.*

"Yes, well, and here we are," Flounder said, a little flippantly. "And by the way, this is a *secret* mission. No one should know about how the queen is leaving her kingdom to pursue matters on land… especially matters involving her father. *Especially* with the sea witch Ursula involved."

Jona stared at him.

"Kingdom? Or queendom?"

"What?" Flounder asked, exasperated.

"The mer are ruled by a queen. Shouldn't it be *queendom?*"

"No, that's… well, I guess so. Maybe. Does it matter?"

"It does if you're the queen," the bird pointed out.

Ariel had to hide her smile; she would have laughed, if she had the voice for it.

"I will fly ahead and find Great-grandfather," the gull said, correctly guessing that her new friends were losing patience, "so we can prepare a diversion for the few guards left at the shore. We should arrange a signal so I know when you're ready to emerge onto dry land."

Flounder watched Ariel's signs carefully and then translated. "A fleet of no fewer than… thirty-seven flying fish will arc out of the water at the same time, heading west."

"All right, I will look for thirty-seven of the silver, flying, hard-to-catch, rather bony, but oh! very tasty fish, flying to the sunset."

"What's that in gull?" Flounder asked, translating Ariel's curiosity.

The bird squawked once, loudly.

It sounded like every other squawk.

Then she took off into the high air without another question or sound.

Ariel jerked her head and she and Flounder dove back under the water. They kept fairly close to the surface, skimming just below it.

She could sense the approach of land, taste when the waters changed, feel when currents turned cool or warm, but it didn't hurt to keep an eye on the shore now and then, and an ear out for boats. The slap of oars could be heard for leagues. Her father had told tales about armoured seafarers in days long past, whose trireme ships had three banks of rowers to ply the waters, you could hear them clear down to Atlantica, he'd say. Any louder and they would disrupt the songs of the half-people, the dolphins and whales who used their voices to navigate the waters.

Even before her father had enacted the ban on going to the surface, it was rare that a boat would encounter a mer. If the captain kept to the old ways, he would either carefully steer away or throw her a tribute: fruit of the land, the apples and grapes merfolk treasured more than treasure. In return the mermaid might present him with fruit of the sea, gems, or a comb from her hair.

But there was always the chance of an unscrupulous crew, and nets, and the potential prize of a mermaid wife or trophy to present the king.

(Considering some of the nets that merfolk had found and freed their underwater brethren from, it was quite understandable that Triton believed humans might eat *anything* they found in the sea, including merfolk.)

Interested and curious sea creatures passed Ariel and Flounder, bowing when they thought to, staring when they didn't. Even without her crown, the queen was well known by her red hair and her friend's constant presence. It was a good thing she had warned Sebastian not to mention her mission; gossip swam faster than tuna.

She stuck her head out of the water and was delighted to discover that she had kept their direction true. They were at the entrance of the Bay of Tirulia, just beyond where spits of land on either side had been extended with boulders by the Dry Worlders to keep their ships safe. Inside these two arms the sea grew flat. On the southern side of the bay, the land was rocky and grey like southern islands where octopuses played and olives occasionally fell and floated on gentle waves. For a very brief stretch, in the middle of the shore near the castle, the rocks gave way to beach. North of that were tidal flats where the sea became land more slowly, gradually invaded by grass and rich brown tuffets of mud where all sorts of baby sea life began: mussels, clams, oysters, crabs, eels and even some fish. Beyond that were the marshes proper, brackish water that mixed with a river that went, Eric had once claimed, all the way to the mountains.

And between the mermaid and the shore were the ships.

Small fishing boats with bright blue eyes painted on their prows to ward off bad luck. Fast and sleek whalers. Tiny coracles for children and beachcombers, for puttering around the marshes and low tides, for teasing out the eggs, shrimp, shellfish and tastier seaweed eaten by the poor but prized by the rich.

Towering over all of these were mighty ocean-faring tall ships, giant white sails unfurled, ready to cross the open water and come home again laden with spices and gold, chocolate and perfumes, fine silks and sparkling salts.

Ariel regarded these last vessels with a twinge of jealousy. They carried their human riders farther away than she had ever been, to places she had only heard of in legend. They probably sailed right over the heads of the Hyperboreans, without even realising it. It seemed unfair somehow.

Then she noticed one tiny boat, no more than a rowboat, really, that floated apart from the rest. It was by itself and farthest out, right at the edge of the bay, closest to her.

A person sat hunched over in the prow of the boat, gazing gloomily out to sea. Ariel frowned, squinting to see better. She was tempted to paint over the blurry details with her imagination: an eye-patched pirate or peg-legged old sea captain, chewing on a pipe stem, dreaming of his glory days and looking out for a storm that would never come.

But there was something about him… his hair was a little too glossy and black. And though he sat bent over, the curved angles of his back seemed still sleek with the muscle, sinew and fat of youth. His hand reached up to pull his coat tighter in a strangely familiar gesture—

Ariel gulped. If she had a voice she might have yelped.

It was Eric.

Without a splash she sank beneath the waves: soundlessly, immediately, eerily, like any sea creature that didn't want to be seen. No drama, no excited tail thwap.

She hovered just below the surface, blinking slowly, heart pounding.

"Ariel…?" Flounder asked, nervous at her behaviour.

She looked at him, chagrined. She made the sign, spelling out the runes:

Eric.

"WHAT?"

She held up a finger, translatable into any language: *one moment.*

Keeping her motions small and efficient, she swam closer to the boat, round the back and silently poked her head above the water. There were, of course, sharp-eyed sea widows and captains, girls on the shore hoping to see something great and boys who wanted a prize for spotting a whale or its ambergris. But on the whole, humans were oblivious to the quiet world around them. She counted on that, and the sailor's eyes on the horizon, to keep her invisible.

It was indeed Eric.

His eyes were still the same dreamy sky blue, or sea blue, right before the sea becomes the sky. But they no longer looked prone to crinkling up in smiles of confused delight. Now they stayed wide, focused on things she couldn't see, miles and hours and worlds away from the bay.

His face was thinner, his appearance paler than that of a man who liked spending his days on a boat should have been. Still too healthy to be *haggard*, but not carefree.

His hair was much longer, caught back in a loose ponytail.

Although he had a worn, salt-faded cape over his shoulders, Ariel could see the trappings of rank beneath it: a crisp white shirt, several golden medallions, an unbuttoned but very fine and tight waistcoat. Below a fancy, wide belt of almost military lines he sported an *incredibly* well-tailored pair of trousers that obviously did not give as much freedom of movement as the old Eric would have liked. His boots were worn and seemed like an afterthought, like the cape, thrown on at the last moment. For disguise, or to protect the better clothes.

He kept staring across the ocean as if waiting for something. The tiny boat was anchored, Ariel realised. As if he had been there, or expected to be there, for a while.

"It's so nice out here, isn't it, Max?" he murmured. "It's so quiet. You can almost hear… almost hear…"

Ariel's eyes widened. She saw the tuft of an old furry

ear lift up above the side of the boat.

Hesitantly Eric pulled something out of his pocket. At first Ariel thought it would be a pipe, it seemed appropriate for someone of Eric's current age and station. But as he placed it to his lips she realised that it was a tiny instrument. Smaller than the recorder he used to carry around with him, and fatter. More like an ocarina, the instrument humans used to play in the days they still talked to animals and merfolk.

He took a breath and waited for a moment.

Then he played a few notes. Quietly and slowly.

Ariel's heart nearly stopped.

It was the song she had sung after she rescued him, the song that had burst unbidden out of her heart as he lay there, unconscious. It described the beauty of the sea and the land and the mortality of humans and the wonder of life. It had poured out of her like life itself.

Hearing it again was the sweetest pain she had ever experienced. Far deeper even than having her tail split in two for legs. It coursed through her whole body, hurt and recognition and pleasure all at once.

He played only the first dozen notes, then trailed off. *Listening.*

Waiting.

Ariel opened her mouth, willed the notes to come out. She closed her eyes and tried to squeeze them from her heart, from her lungs. Didn't love break all spells? What was the good of it otherwise? *Please, please, Old Gods. Let me sing… just this once…*

But all was silent.

"Mmrl?"

Max's little questioning noise caused Eric to blink, and Ariel to curse.

"No, I know I didn't use it in the opera," Eric said as if he were answering a much more coherent question from the dog. "I know, it would have been perfect. But it didn't seem right somehow… I needed to save it for… for…"

He blinked suddenly and smiled at himself.

"That sounds ridiculous, doesn't it, Max?" He grinned and scruffled the dog's ears. Ariel dipped lower into the water, melting at his smile. Still! When he smiled it was like the whole world was smiling, his lips pulled the sky like a rainbow, the sun danced in laughter. She felt utterly helpless and stupid. Queen of the Sea! Brought to her fins by one silly smile.

Eric sighed. "Thanks for joining me on these little expeditions, Max. I know they wear you out. But out here, it's almost like I'm… clearheaded. Or slipping deeper, into another dream. One or the other. They're the same. Oh, I don't know."

He sighed, clenching his hand round the ocarina in frustration. For a moment Ariel thought he was going to hurl it into the sea, as he had his recorder so many years before. But he brought it to his lips and played the dozen notes again, letting them die into the breeze.

Ariel didn't try to finish the tune this time. Tears leaked out of the sides of her eyes and trickled down her cheeks, joining the briny sea.

Finally Eric put his ocarina away. "Come on, let's head back before the missus decides we've been out on our walkies too long." He pulled the anchor and took up the oars, expertly turning the little boat round with no wake and little effort.

As the prow swung out closer to Ariel, Max began to shuffle to his feet.

"Mmmrrl?"

He tried to look over the side of the boat, sensing that something was off.

Ariel dipped low into the water. She doubted the dog could see very well now, much less through the matted locks over his eyes. He put his nose to the air, sniffing… but Eric was rowing away, back towards shore.

Ariel watched them go, the old dog and his master on the tiny, tiny boat – the man who once commanded a ship as large as a castle and the heart of the sea king's daughter.

Ariel

Flounder stuck his head up out of the water next to her.

"That sure was Eric," the fish said. "Wow, he looked so different."

Ariel signed absently: *I'm sure he'd say the same about you.*

"Hey," Flounder said a little shyly, a little proudly, swaying back and forth in the water to admire his own belly. "I have an official position in the castle now. I *have* to keep up my weight!"

Ariel smiled.

But these were all just words meant to diffuse the tension and emotional weight of the moment. They didn't mean anything. Flounder was really asking if she was all right, and saying that he was there for her.

So little actual communication was represented by words that were said aloud, she had realised upon losing her voice. Often the real meaning lay underneath and unspoken.

Sometimes people forgot that she wasn't deaf as well as mute, and then the conversations got really interesting.

They scooted together just below the surface. The water turned and began to stink of organic matter, tar, things alien to the ocean. While the overall smell was a little much for a mer, human activity and refuse often meant extra food for the fish who dared to live so close to the shore. Covering every stony and wooden surface underwater were razor-sharp barnacles; ebon black bouquets of mussels; clusters of soft purple velvety tube worms, all mouth and utterly harmless. Crabs braver and less artistically inclined than Sebastian endlessly clambered up and down piers and shipwrecks. Sometimes one would wave to her and then drop to the ocean floor, unable to hang on with one claw, and tirelessly begin the climb again.

The way to the castle was a bit of an obstacle course between the trawling nets that scooped up everything on the floor of the bay, regardless of its edibility, and the raw sewage that leaked out of giant pipes hanging over the water. They had to swim a broad way round the marsh: water billowing out from a drainage creek was an unhealthy bright yellow. The seepage blossomed and flowed into the sea as pretty as an octopus's ink, but it burnt Ariel's scales. What were the humans *doing* up there?

When they made it to the blessedly cleaner waters near the castle (built a bit removed from the commercial centre of town, specifically to avoid the bad airs and plagues), Ariel spun through the currents like an otter, shaking out her hair and ruffling her scales free of filth. Then she and Flounder popped to the surface and looked around.

There were exactly eight guards posted along the beach and at the entrance of the lagoon where she had once saved Eric. Easily a third as many as the last time she had tried to approach the castle. One was trimming his nails with a small knife; another had his boots off so he could rest his feet in the sand. Not a single man was taking his job seriously.

And why should they? The foreign princess of the castle had ordered soldiers to guard the beach against the incursion of… an unspecified pelagic threat. Possibly a mermaid. Who on earth *would* take that seriously?

Maybe… maybe this really will work this time.

A squawk drew Ariel's attention skywards. Seemingly

innocent, a half dozen shining white seagulls soared picturesquely above the beach. Well, one had greyish underwings and a grey tuft of unlikely feathers sprouting on his head. Another, smaller than the others, trailed the grey one – Scuttle and Jona.

They were ready, waiting for the signal.

"On it," Flounder said, gliding off.

Ariel waited in the water while he sought out a flying fish and conveyed her orders. Just a few moments later she felt the shimmering vibration of the school swimming in unison, above and below the water, where worlds collided.

They were beautiful. Silver and winged, they took to the air as easily as they sped through the water, like the material world meant nothing to them: space, objects, water, air, time, light – they were all the same. They made the noise of a thousand large locusts or of the strange crackles before lightning strikes.

A couple of the guards looked up curiously.

And then the gulls attacked.

Ariel had to turn away, remembering that what they did was for her and that she should be grateful. She hadn't been quite sure what to expect when Jona had suggested a distraction; she figured it would involve eyes and soft human parts and clawing and maybe the dropping of sharp shells on their scalps. What they chose to do was far less violent but devastatingly more effective.

In any case, it made Flounder almost choke in laughter.

The guards ran. At first crazily, back and forth, around and around, trying to escape the stinking, terrible hailstorm. The smarter ones immediately made for the shelter of the castle and the cliffs.

"Go!" Flounder said, recovering himself.

With a few quick leaps Ariel porpoised herself into much shallower water. Using all her strength she forced herself upright so she was standing on her tail. Then she waved the trident and became a human.

That was it.

That was *all*.

Her father could have done it years ago. Long before all the terrible things began.

Before she had even met Eric.

He could have turned her into a human for a day, or several days, and let her explore life on land until she tired of it, or became scared, or grew lonely, or missed him.

Once she had met Eric, Triton could have saved her the trouble of selling her voice and her life, and then *his* life, for the chance to fall in love with the boy. She would have been able to walk on her own two legs, and say things with her own voice, like "I'm the mermaid who saved you. Yep, I know that song, because I wrote it. Let me sing it for you."

And she could have sung. And they could have fallen in love.

She and her father could have worked out a deal like the Old Gods: Proserpine and Hades and Ceres. She could spend some of her days on land, the rest of her life in the sea. And then everyone would have been, well, if not deliriously happy, then at least satisfied that it was the best they could all work out.

But… the slightly older Ariel added… *who knows what really would have happened?* The trident's power rose and fell with the sea and the moon. She could have stayed human for only a few days a month; a week, maybe two at best. Would that have been enough to sustain a relationship?

Would it have turned out that human princes were just as boring as merprinces?

Ariel dismissed the old familiar thoughts and focused on the matter at hand. She scooped the human clothes out of her bag and dragged them on as best she could. They were thick and coarse, and her now-human skin was tenderer than the scales of a mermaid tail. The shoes, crusted with old barnacles she had to scrape off, would have to wait until they had dried out on land for a while. She shook the trident and it changed, shrinking. Its surface glittered even more golden, as though the metal became more refined the more tightly together it was pushed. Finally it was in the palm of her hand and shaped like a comb. Countless tines replaced the initial three, each with a tiny spike on its tip that minutely replicated the barbs. She admired it for half a moment and then slipped it into her hair, above her right ear, wedging it in place among her intricate braids.

Keeping one eye out for the guards and her hands close to the ground in case she slipped, Ariel clumsily made her way through the shallows to a sheltered part of the lagoon. It was like the first walk of a baby sea turtle in reverse: tentative claws in the sand, a burst of warmth from the sun on her face after incubating in the earth for so long. The dragging, terrified walk to the water. The land and sky full of danger and death, the ocean full of safety and warmth. All this was the same; she was just doing it backwards.

It was hard thinking things and keeping track of her feet at the same time. Sand *felt*. Pressure on the skin of her feet *felt*. The breeze kept whipping away her breaths in little gasps. Salt, which surrounded her normally, dried in white patches on her skin and stung her lips like acid.

She stumbled, pitching forwards.

With the will of a queen, she forced, she *ordered* her left foot out to stop the fall. Tail muscles recently converted to thighs screamed at the strangeness of the motions.

She paused, taking a breath, knowing her body would recover. It wasn't as if she were walking on iron blades that cut deep into her soles with every step, though that's what it felt like for a moment. This was beach sand, always described by humans as soft and inviting. If she fell, it wouldn't be the end of the world.

The noise of gulls and guards drifted on the wind to her.

"*Stupid bird…*"

"Get offa me!"

"RUN!"

But as she rounded the edge of the escarpment that began the sheltered area, everything shut off like a spell: the wind, the sting of the wind on her face, the noise of the guards, the constant *feel* of the air pushing against her skin. Without realising it consciously, Ariel wound up in the lagoon with the rounded rock that stuck out of the sea where she had first brought Eric, where the water was warm and slow and shallow.

And it was silent.

Ariel slumped down into the sand and let out a sigh that was almost a sob. She took several deep breaths now that she didn't have to fight the breeze for them. She closed her eyes and tilted her head towards the sun. Years ago her desire to win Eric had been so strong that she had forgotten all the other reasons she wanted to walk on the land: to feel the sand and the warmth of Helios directly on her skin.

It was just as amazing as she had always imagined it.

But Ariel was spending too much time caught between sea and land in the little lagoon. She was there to find her father, not enjoy herself.

"I followed your footprints," came a voice from above.

Ariel turned and watched the seagull execute a delicate landing on the stone with such precise control her feet touched the surface just as she slowed to a stop.

"Think of that," Jona said. "I followed a *mermaid's footprints* in the sand. That should be part of an epic poem. Or a book. Or something."

Ariel raised an eyebrow at the gull.

"It's something that shouldn't exist," the gull went on, explaining helpfully.

Ariel rolled her eyes. *I get it. I'm not stupid.*

Flounder popped his head out of the water. "Wow, that was amazing. It went right according to plan!"

Scuttle landed heavily on the stone next to his great-grandgull, more like a bomb of feathers than a professional flier.

"You bet your gills it did!" Scuttle crowed. "You shoulda seen them. They ran like we were the plague! Like we were terrifying multiarmed giants! Like we were—"

"Gulls making a mess everywhere," Flounder finished.

"Well, you say potato," Scuttle sniffed.

If you're all done, Ariel signed, *I think I have a castle to get to.*

"The queen thinks it's time to go," Flounder said.

"Phase two, I gotcha," Scuttle said, winking.

"You'll… you'll keep an eye on her, right?" Flounder asked softly.

"Aw, you bet we will," Scuttle promised. "She's like family. We'll watch over her like hawks. No, not like hawks. They're too snooty. Like albatrosses. No, they're so *difficult.* Like… lions!"

"We'll make sure one of us has an eye on her at all times," Jona translated.

"But right now…" the old gull wheezed a little. "I may take a breather, you know? These bones ache more than they used to. The kid here can take care of things for a bit. I'd trust her with my life."

In answer, Ariel scruffed him under the chin and kissed him on the beak.

She then turned to both gulls and bowed, clasping her hands together.

Thank you both for everything.

Scuttle tried to imitate the gesture. It came off as far less impressive, but was twice as endearing. Jona cocked her head and regarded him with a glittering right eye: if Ariel had to guess, she would have said that the younger bird was smiling, perhaps fondly, at her great-grandfather.

"Good luck. We'll be up above," the gull said, and waited for just the right wind to sweep her like a kite up into the sky, slowly and methodically. Scuttle flapped hard and took off like a shot.

"Be careful. *Please*, Ariel," Flounder begged, sounding like the old Flounder.

Ariel gave him a smile.

Then she made her way to the castle.

Ariel

She decided to avoid the stone staircase that led directly from the beach into the castle; that was for the enjoyment of the prince and his household only. She remembered joyfully racing down its steps to the sunset beach, then belatedly noticing maids and footmen carefully skirting the edge and going round to the back of the complex.

She followed her memory, circling round the north side of the castle. Right before the wet, compact sand petered out into a lush estuary, the well-trodden path of the commoners who worked in the castle became visible. Hidden from the amazing views and picturesque scenery of the bay, scullery maids scoured out pots with rags and the bristly stalks of local horsetail plants. Housekeepers beat carpets draped on the stunted, hearty little bushes and pines that lived too close to the salt water that was life to the sea and poison to the land. Scullery maids and boys dumped baskets of rubbish onto a growing midden.

Right there.

In the middle of the rich, clean water that fed and drained the shellfish nursery, where seashore birds made their nests, where eels and elvers and minnows made their lives.

Ew.

There was no formal sign for that.

Ariel wrinkled her nose and turned away.

As she passed more servants and messengers and peddlers and couriers, she wondered if anyone would recognise the mute girl from years before. She hadn't aged the way humans did. Her face did look different, but was it different enough? Her hair was tightly bound against her head. She wasn't wearing the pretty blue dress with its fitted bodice and was definitely missing the giant, floppy, pretty-as-a-picture bow the maid Carlotta had put in her hair.

Was she imagining it, or were people looking sideways at her? Were they trying to take her in without seeming to stare? Did they notice her? Was she just being paranoid?

She didn't have a plan if someone stopped her. She had nothing more to go on than *sneak into the castle and find her father.* Either she had enough confidence as queen that she felt she could deal with whatever was thrown at her, or she literally had no way to plan for the unexpected and so didn't. *Probably the latter,* she thought with a sigh. Still the same old Ariel, swimming in where sharks feared to paddle.

On the other hand, I could always return to the other plan – calling up the waves to more forcibly rescue Father...

She held her breath at the main gate, but none of the guards looked at her twice.

None of the guards.

She looked around, suddenly realising what should have been obvious if she hadn't been so nervous: there were many, many more guards than when she had last been there. *Here,* in the castle, not at the beach where they once were. And not just guards, either; there were real soldiers patrolling the halls. Men and boys in keen military dress, shined boots, shined buttons, sabres hanging from their sides and caps cockily perched on their heads.

There were other people too. Richly clad men and women walked in slow, carefully paced pairs and trios, talking in low voices, checking fancy pocket watches, smiling to other pairs and trios they passed with smiles that disappeared immediately after. Men in poufy shirts with questionable expressions, dour and shifty. Women in bustles and long-flowing gowns that trailed behind them like jellyfish tendrils, looking at each other shyly from behind fans or boldly from under giant hats.

Someone almost crashed into Ariel, pushing a small wagon with an open chest loaded up on it. Laid carefully over sawdust and packing on the top were – *guns.* She remembered seeing the castle guards carry them, present them, occasionally shoot them. Muskets with cruel bayonets, shining and black and freshly oiled.

While she was staring, Ariel was knocked from behind by a self-important man with florid cheeks and weak eyes. He strode past her without apologising and was followed by a servant carrying what looked very much like a small chest of gold.

What is going on here?

Tirulia was a sleepy little kingdom, and this seaside castle was the unofficial capital of its most carefree, bucolic quarter. Eric had no real duties. His parents were still alive and actively ruling, at least they had been the last time she was here. He had no particular desire to take over as king. He had a real desire to sail. He was young, he was enthusiastic, he loved music and the sea and wind in his hair. Everything that she loved too, but flipped to its Dry World version.

This castle no longer felt like him. It felt… foreign.

Confused, Ariel tried to reorient herself and keep walking, undistracted by what was apparently the new normal.

When a washerwoman walked by, unable to see directly in front of her because of the pile of freshly dried linens blossoming like an anemone out of the basket she carried, Ariel swiped a couple from the top. She carried them in front of her as importantly as if they were a chest of gold, and no one even glanced at her.

I'm becoming as tricky as a human. So quickly! She thought with light irony as she marched into the next room…

… and then immediately hid behind a cabinet.

Standing there stiffly, giving a footman the sort of quiet, gentle-but-severe dressing down that could be done only by the Bretlanders, was Grimsby, Eric's manservant and closest confidant.

Much like a mermaid, he hadn't aged at all since the last time she had seen him. But perhaps that was because he had already been old when they first met and didn't have that many more changes to make before his final transmogrification. His light blue eyes did seem a little wearier, also like her own.

He finished with the footman, sending him off red-faced and chagrined, then headed with slow, solid steps down the hall. The energy of this new castle swirled around him; servants, visiting nobles' servants, the visiting nobles themselves, the men and women with the money… and though he was a true Bretlandian butler who rarely let his feelings show, Ariel watched him trying *not* to disapprove of it all with his clear and tired eyes. He moved like a shepherd of comb jellies, trying to urge them through a foreign school of quick-swimming minnows, neither affected nor scared by them, only vaguely concerned.

Ariel found herself holding the skirts of her dress tightly, almost like a timid girl.

She wished she could go to him. In his own way, Grimsby had been extraordinarily kind to her in her short time on land. Gently guiding when she did the wrong thing, leading silently by example rather than chastising aloud.

She wanted to grab him, to pull him aside and find out what was wrong. Why did he seem upset? What had changed? Did it have to do with all the activity in the castle?

But… even if she did manage to get him alone… they couldn't talk.

She couldn't talk.

And she highly doubted he could understand a sign

language based on an ancient and, to him, foreign language.

She watched Grimsby go, his exit immediately camouflaged by skirts and jackets, scurrying and bustling, and felt something tighten within her. They could have meant something to each other, had things worked out differently.

She took a deep breath, willing the knot in her heart to go away.

The Queen of the Sea had a mission. She had come to find her father. Anything else she would deal with later, if at all. For now, she had to figure out where her father was being kept.

Think logically, she reminded herself. The gulls had told her that they'd seen Ursula getting dressed, primping, while talking with Triton. With a feeling of nausea she faced the obvious: as Vanessa, the sea witch was married to Eric. The two would either be sharing the same room or adjoining apartments in the royal tower. Ariel knew where that was.

She straightened up, held her linens out and marched forwards, trying to set her face into the blank stare of a maid. It was easier than it would have been the first time she had come on land, when she had no cause to do anything aside from stare around with wide eyes, drinking in the strange world and its goings-on. She had never even considered trying to blend in before; there *was* no strange or different in the world of the mer. It never occurred to her that people would notice or not like her if she stuck out and acted odd.

She brushed aside this slow-moving slipper shell of a thought to another corner of her mind, and wondered if there was a possibility of catching another glimpse of Eric.

The stairs were a little tricky, 'up' was a strange movement for her still-new legs and feet, and she made it as far as the first hallway before she was discovered.

"Hey, you! Who are you? You're not supposed to be upstairs!"

It wasn't one of the now-multitudinous soldiers; it was a rather pretty but shark-eyed maid. Ariel didn't react; she just stood there, unsure what to do. She couldn't even make up an excuse for being there, or at least make it be understood.

The maid grabbed a passing guard. He didn't seem to have any interest in either one of them and tried to continue his rounds, but the maid sort of *shook* him at Ariel.

"*Hey!* She's not supposed to be up here. She could be a spy!"

The guard grunted in displeasure but started toward Ariel.

The Queen of the Sea dropped her laundry and ran.

Ariel wondered vaguely how her new legs would react to this new situation.

Just fine, apparently.

She ducked between footmen, dodged through couples, threw herself round corners. There was a second stairway she remembered, towards the back of the residency tower, which the chambermaids used. The one she probably should have chosen to begin with. She put a hand out to the sandstone wall to steady herself as she began her first descent with new legs. The firmness and familiarity of the rock gave her courage. She urged her feet down the steps like ceremonial dolphins pulling her golden chariot in a circuit race.

"Halt!" came a voice from behind her, along with the sound of polished boots striking stone.

Ariel panicked and practically fell onto the landing. She wasted a moment trying to decide whether to continue down another narrow flight to the sub-basement where the wine cellars were, along with another exit to the outside. But that was probably what the soldiers expected her to do.

She plunged ahead instead, towards where she remembered the grand ballroom was.

There was less chaos here, and fewer people. But just as Ariel thought she had escaped the last of them, she saw someone looming, blocking her escape at the end of the painted hall.

Carlotta.

The friendly maid who had tried to show Ariel the proper way to bathe. Who had taken it upon herself to pick out an outfit for the mermaid and show her how to dress nicely. With the floppy bow. Who hadn't been upset when Ariel made a fool of herself using human things the wrong way, who had only found it delightful, and a wonderful curative for the often moody prince.

Carlotta's black hair was still thick though shot through with grey, and in its usual bun, and not under the bright red kerchief Ariel remembered. Her bodice and new little hat were starched white cotton, pure and strict. But the strangely formal uniform upset Ariel less than the look in Carlotta's eyes when she saw the mermaid bolting towards her.

Surprise.

Realisation.

Suspicion.

Their moment of glowering silence was interrupted by voices down the hall:

"Where did she go?"

"Did you see her?"

"You check downstairs, I'll check this floor."

They would be upon her in a moment.

Carlotta reached out and threw open a small door: a broom cupboard, its edges cleverly concealed in the overly ornate golden mouldings.

She raised an eyebrow at Ariel.

The mermaid decided, for no reason she could logically explain beyond the past kindness shown her, to trust the scowling woman.

She dove in, trying not to wince as the door was slammed behind her. A cloud of dust rose from the brooms and rags and other cleaning implements. A distinct odour of mould and dry rot assailed her nose.

She tried not to sneeze, holding her face and nose with both hands, pressing her palms into her cheeks.

Queen of the Sea, she thought. *Look at me now.*

Voices outside the cupboard, muffled but loud:

"Carlotta, have you seen a maid? She wasn't authorized to be upstairs, and…"

"Oh, you don't mean the pale one, about yea high, skinny as a bean?" Carlotta sounded exasperated and very, very believable.

"Yes, with the blue skirts…"

"Blast that girl. She's new. Not gifted with much besides her girlish figure, I don't mind saying. You know, up here."

Ariel frowned despite knowing it was a lie. She could practically see Carlotta tapping her head in illustration.

"I told her the wash was for Lord Francese's *manservant*, not the lord himself. And then she disappeared. Should have known."

"There is a problem of security in the castle, Carlotta. The spies..."

"If that girl's a spy, I'm the pope," Carlotta snorted. "She's just a pretty dumb thing from the country. I'll give her a good talking to when I find her and lock her in her room without supper."

At this, the guard laughed. "You've never withheld a meal from anyone, or anything, in your life. You'll probably scold her and then force five rolls on her to fatten her up. But you've got to talk to her. Princess Vanessa..."

"Say no more. It will be resolved, or she will go."

"Thank you, Carlotta. I'll inform my men."

Ariel waited for the clicking footsteps to fade, then waited some more.

Just when she thought it might be safe to open the door a crack, it was thrown wide open. A serious, annoyed-looking Carlotta filled the entire frame and blocked most of the light.

"Come with me," she ordered, in a tone she had never used on Ariel before.

The Queen of the Sea meekly obeyed.

They went through the ballroom, over the beautiful inlaid floor covered in meaningless brown and golden curlicues. Ariel wondered what it would be like to glide over the slippery polished boards, music swirling around her. She had only danced with Eric once, on a cobbled plaza to an amateur violinist, but even that had been incredible.

The ceiling was a frescoed masterpiece: a sky with little fluffy clouds at the edges, winged cherubs peeping out among them. Giant glazed windows let in sea light, sparkling off the water as well as from the sky. Circling very deliberately was a single white gull, who managed to keep her head pointed at the castle wherever she was in her revolutions. *Jona.*

Carlotta hurried on through the great room into a white corridor at the end and pulled Ariel into a small space lined with benches and tables. It looked like a staging area for servants to plate hors d'oeuvres and wine before bringing them out to hot and thirsty dancers, very much like at the palace in Atlantica, but this one had a ceiling, and the tables were all at one level. Under the sea, you could swim to whatever height you needed. *How limited humans are.*

But she didn't have time to ponder such things. Carlotta stood in front of her, arms crossed.

"It's you!"

Ariel nodded and shrugged. *Well, obviously.*

"Where have you *been*?" Carlotta demanded. "Where did you go?"

The mermaid winced. How could she explain?

"Eric loved you. You two would have been so happy together..." the maid continued accusingly. Ariel wondered if she had been spying on them any of the times they almost kissed. "And then you just... disappeared! And he married that horrible, horrible Vanessa, and now she's ruining the kingdom and he's... he's not the prince he was. Not the boy he was. That boy's gone. Where did *you* go?"

Merfolk and humans and fish and *all* those who spoke seemed to be the same: they wasted language, throwing out words like chum, hoping some of them would land accurately and truthfully convey what they were thinking or feeling. Ariel paused, carefully weighing and measuring the other woman's words while she figured out how to answer.

Eric married Vanessa. This was an objective fact; Ariel had seen that happen.

Vanessa is ruining the kingdom. Interesting! So the changes in the castle were probably due to her.

Eric is not the boy he was. Also interesting, and terrifying. He was still under the spell Ursula cast to put him under her power. That would certainly explain the haunted, hunted look on Eric's face when she had seen him earlier. He probably knew *something* was wrong, but not precisely what.

Ariel pursed her lips. Then she mimed a formal walk, hands together.

She drew her hand gracefully down her hair, indicating a veil.

She put her hands together again: flowers.

Vanessa marrying Eric.

"The wedding, yes, yes, the wedding. They got married," Carlotta said, impatiently.

Ariel tapped her head, pointed at the maid.

"I remember it! What do you mean? *Think* about it? It was just the wedding on the yacht. Beautiful. Hideous. At the same time. There was nothing…"

Ariel shook her head. She tapped her head harder. She rotated her other hand: *Come on, there's more.*

"What are you trying to say…? They were married, and Max ruined the lovely cake, and oh…" Carlotta's vision went cloudy; she stopped focusing on the girl before her. "He ruined the cake because… he was scared. There was a storm. No, the sky was clear. No, but there was lightning. Lightning… from… a man in the water. A man with a beard, and a crown, naked… like Neptune himself…"

Carlotta frowned, rubbing her head.

"What is this nonsense? Why is it coming to me now, clear as day? Clear as a picture: the man in the sea wasn't drowning. He was throwing lightning. And Vanessa… he and she were… *fighting*? They were fighting like… titans, from the old stories. There was magic. All around.

Dangerous and violent. And then you, and then he… and then you and the naked man were gone. Both gone. But Vanessa stayed…"

She sat down heavily on a stool. Her skirts puffed up around her, almost as if in sympathy. "I… haven't thought about that in years. I know I've thought it before, or dreamed it before. I haven't wanted to. It's like it *hurts* to remember. I couldn't remember."

She looked up at Ariel.

"Some funny business about Vanessa, isn't there?" she ventured. "That man, he was your father, wasn't he? He really was Neptune, or someone out of the Old Testament. A patriarch. He wasn't evil, I never felt that for a moment. And then you disappearing… into the sea. Eric acting strange and moony around Vanessa. She isn't… she isn't a good… person, is she?"

Ariel shook her head very slowly. *No.*

"She isn't like… us, is she?"

No.

"And what does that make you, then?"

Ariel hesitated. Would knowing the truth put Carlotta in danger? She already knew half of the truth. The *main* truth. That Vanessa was not a good person. That there had been a battle. And all the strange and terrible things that had happened on her prince's wedding day. So how would knowing this little extra bit make a difference, really?

Ariel looked around the room, searching for the answer. She didn't have a sign for it.

Finally she put her hands together and moved them sinuously forwards, cutting the air like water.

Carlotta stared at her, mouth open like a gaping fish.

Then she shook her head.

"You know what? Forget I asked. I don't think my tired old brain could deal with it right now anyway. The important thing is that Vanessa *is* bad, really bad, which is fairly obvious if you just see what she's doing…"

While pleased that Carlotta had come to the same conclusion she had, Ariel was intrigued by this news. She reached out and tapped the maid's shoulder and shrugged obviously. *What* is *she doing?*

"Well, she has us at war with our neighbours. Look at Garhaggio," Carlotta said with a snort, throwing her arm out at the window as if the village were right there, visible. "Never had a problem with them before. Never had much to do with them at all aside from occasionally getting their nice cheese in. It *is* a nice cheese, though. I love it, the fancy white rind. They say it's the mountain spring water."

Ariel tried not to look impatient.

"… I'm just a senior housemaid, I know!" Carlotta said, seeing her face. "I don't know about politics and wars and international policy. All I know is that Garhaggio was burnt to the ground. By *us*. By Tirulia! So no more cheese. And there is a conscription for able-bodied boys here. So, I suppose, we can burn down more cheese-making villages that won't bend the knee to Tirulia. And yet we're friends with *Ibria* now? We've been on uneasy terms with them for over two hundred years!

"Strange, sneaky-looking men and women roam the castle, and they all have Vanessa's ear. And yet the princess also thinks everyone is after her. So everyone thinks everyone *else* is a spy and hopes for a reward by turning his neighbour in. Vanessa is turning the kingdom upside down, and no one trusts anyone else, and we're nearly at war with everyone around us.

"And you're back," Carlotta finished with conviction.

Ariel looked at her sideways. She couldn't figure out where the maid's look of satisfaction came from as Carlotta resolutely crossed her arms and nodded like she understood.

The Queen of the Sea started to tilt her head. *Yes. I'm back. And…?*

"And you're here to set everything right, aren't you?"

The mermaid blinked her large aquamarine eyes.

"With Vanessa and Eric and all. You're going to make things like they were," Carlotta said, somehow perfectly mixing the utter belief of a five-year-old with the stern voice of an adult who knew Ariel would *do the right thing.* "You're going to defeat her, or make Eric fall in love with you, or something. Maybe you'll make him forget that you *and* Vanessa ever existed… I don't know or care about the details, although you did seem like a nice enough girl at one time."

Ariel put her hands up and started to shake her head.

"Don't you start with that," Carlotta said, putting her hand up. "I may not be a scholar or a wisewoman, but it wasn't until *after you showed up* the first time that all of this happened. Whatever your role, you had some hand in this, in the destruction of Tirulia and our way of life… and *Eric.*"

Ariel's queenliness faltered for a moment at his name. Everything else was just supposition, theory, people who had nothing to do with her. But Eric, that sad, ageing sailor on his lonely boat…

Carlotta was right. He was an utterly defeated man.

And despite Ariel's mix of bitterness and wistfulness about the realm of humans and her misadventures in the Dry World, *none of what happened afterwards would have happened at all without her interference.*

Not that she would take *any* blame for the chaos Ursula had wrought: the Queen of the Sea would not be held responsible for the evil sea witch's doings. But the truth was that Ursula would not be there, causing havoc, if it weren't for Ariel.

The world, both wet and dry, spun for a moment as Ariel thought about this. Although the humans had complete dominance on the planet, although they controlled all land and nature and everything around them, *she*, a little mermaid, had introduced a foreign element that threatened to utterly destroy the kingdom of Tirulia. Like a single pathogen infecting a coral reef. She wondered how far it would spread if she simply… found her father and left. Would Ursula stop with this one kingdom, or would her mad quest for power and glory continue until she took over all human lands?

Ariel's plan was to find her father, restore the trident to him and leave.

Perhaps her plans had to be amended somehow.

She nodded slightly.

Carlotta sighed. "Thank you."

Somehow the maid intuited the squall that had just risen and dispersed in Ariel's mind, and seen through her large eyes to a calm decision made underneath.

"And now, were you trying to sneak in the castle for the reasons of this mission?"

Ariel nodded, again, feeling somehow foolish.

Carlotta laughed.

"And did you think doing it in the dress of a long-drowned princess, a visitor to Davy Jones's locker, would somehow fool us?"

Ariel looked down at her outfit. She now saw the worn shades of blue that striped and stippled the garment in uneven strengths. The strangely frayed hems, threads dried in all positions, used to the freedom of the sea and not to hanging in proper ragged fringes, straight down. The circles and whorls of salt she had thought sparkled so prettily under the sun. Her shoes, decorated with dead barnacles, which had a sad elegance about them.

"You're seeing it now," the maid said with a sigh. "And your *hair*, of course."

Ariel put a hand to her locks in surprise. Her hair, while healthy, thick and long, was hardly an unusual colour. There were merfolk families who had tresses the blue of waves, the green of gems, the purple of poisonous molluscs.

Once again Carlotta read her correctly.

"Maybe red is normal for… wherever you're from," she said quickly, skipping over any thoughts that she didn't want to acknowledge, "but here it's very, very distinctive. The people up north sometimes have it… and right now, everyone is suspicious of northerners. Come with me and we'll get you dressed up right, with a headcloth to cover your hair. And then you can save us all. Is it a deal?"

Ariel nodded, and Carlotta nodded, and no more words were needed.

Ariel

There were fairy tales, known even to those who starred in those fairy tales, about human girls who worked for merwitches or mermaids in return for their help. The mermaids in the story would be so charmed by the good little girls that they not only help but also bedeck them in gems and pearls, and brush their hair with jewelled combs, and let them choose whatever gowns they desire out of a treasure trove of goods that were lost at sea.

This is a very strange, upside-down version of that story, Ariel decided.

Carlotta searched for the plainest, oldest, most

unremarkable shift she could manage, a maroonish thing that was more bag than dress. It acquired a little shape once a suitably stained apron with braided ties had been fitted round Ariel's waist. They didn't even bother with stockings, just a pair of ugly boot-like slippers. The final touch was a rusty grey headscarf the maid expertly knotted at the nape of Ariel's neck and pulled down close round her braids, making sure it stayed there with a strip of dishrag she tied at the back of her head, above her ears.

Like a crown.

"All right, that'll do, though maybe you'll want to smear a little bit of dust on your cheeks," Carlotta said, eyeing her professionally.

Ariel looked down at her outfit. When she had been in the Dry World the first time they had outfitted her with a pretty little dress that the maid had thought was appropriate for a beautiful girl of no readily apparent station: she could have been a student or a modest princess. The mermaid tried not to smile, amused at the difference.

Then she thanked the woman the only way she could, managing it awkwardly without the supportive, thick feel of the water around her: she bent at the waist and bowed her head, giving Carlotta the respect that normally only another member of royalty received.

"Hmm," the maid said, suddenly a little unnerved. She made as if to curtsy, then patted down her hair. "Something's different about you, girl. You're not the same little strip of a thing who came dancing into our castle, making our prince smile… you've changed. Somehow. I don't know how, exactly."

Neither do I, Ariel thought back.

Now she could search for her father properly. In her new outfit Ariel felt invisible, like she was wearing a magic cloak that allowed her to go anywhere unseen. Carlotta had given her a tray with some random food scraps on it, heels of bread, a goblet, some small fruit knives, that made it seem like she could have been on her way from anywhere in the castle. For a moment Ariel wondered if there *were* any spies from the north, or anywhere else, posing as servants. Apparently it was quite easy to go unnoticed if you dressed the part, kept your head down and acted servile.

The one time a guard stopped her, Ariel just gestured the tray at him. That was enough: he grabbed a heel of the bread, leered at her and ushered her on.

Ariel had to fight the urge not to gag. Was he really eating what he *knew* were someone else's scraps? Did these 'advanced' humans, with their machines and fires and carriages with wheels, know nothing about the spread of diseases? Surely there was a land equivalent of the unseen, tiny sick-fishes that surrounded and lived in those who were ill…

Thinking about this kept her from growing nervous as she approached the main royal apartments.

Two girls passed her, gossiping.

"Not me. I *love* how many baths she takes. It means I get a half watch to myself practically every night…"

"Sure, but is it worth it overall? My aunt is paying *twice* as much tax this season as she did last… while our princess bathes in expensive oils and burns through wood in the middle of summer!"

"But she doesn't bathe in the oils *or* hot water. That's the strange thing. Her baths are always cold and usually with mineral salt."

"Whatever! She's stealing from the poor of this kingdom to finance her stupid army and her stupid baths!"

"Shh! Keep your voice down!"

Ariel chanced a look at the girls as they passed, trying to guess their ages. Would she have been friends with them if she were human? Or was she, despite her looks, already too old? Did losing your voice and the love of your life and having to run a kingdom change you in ways more dramatic than mere years?

From the moist air that hit her a moment later it was obvious that Ursula was in the middle of one of her fancy baths right then. *Good.* It gave Ariel time to search the bedrooms.

She knocked tentatively on the royal couple's apartment door. The way a servant might, or a nervous ex-lover.

No answer.

Disappointed and relieved, Ariel pushed the door open with her back and shoulders the way she had seen other servants do, so she didn't need to use her tray-encumbered hands. And once she was in…

She sighed in relief.

She had never been in Eric's room; humans had very odd notions of appropriate behaviour. But if she had to guess, this was still Eric's room, and *only* Eric's room. No girly or princess-y things at all.

There was a bookshelf stuffed with maps and scrolls and folios of music. There was a drum from a foreign land. There was a portrait of the prince and a much younger Max, all smiles and sunlight. There were piles of arcane metal apparatus; tubes with thick glass lenses, pyramids with pendulums hanging from the apex of delicate golden crosspieces, things that were almost recognisable as rulers. There were several toy, *model*, ships.

There was a soft, puffy pillow on the floor that was obviously for the dog, but there was dog hair all over the foot of the bed.

There was a heavy desk under a small window, buried under endless sheets of music paper, inkwells, pens.

There wasn't a single hint of anyone besides Eric in the room. Nothing of a tentacled sea witch with questionable taste in decor, nor of a human princess with human-princess belongings. There was nothing soft, brightly coloured, pastel, glittery, flowery, no random scarf tossed over the back of the bed, no velvet or silk shoe kicked halfway under it. Nothing that wasn't shipshape, masculine and Eric-y.

Ariel wanted to stay and poke through things, try to get a glimpse of the boy she had loved. But her time was limited.

There was a doorway that connected his bedroom to an adjacent one. She tiptoed in. This was Vanessa's room.

The royal couple was living side by side. Not together.

Not together.

Ariel didn't really want to unpack her feelings around this, but she couldn't help picking at them, like taking a stick and seeing what was in a crevasse of dead coral. Surely she hadn't hoped for Eric to stay… single? After all these years? To remain as he was in her memory?

Surely she couldn't *blame* him for having any feelings

for Vanessa. The witch had cast a mighty spell on him. It wouldn't be his fault if he did everything she said, fawned over her, slept in the same room as she.

None of these logical thoughts explained away the joy that she felt. Somehow Eric had managed to keep a portion of himself separate from his beglamoured wife; somehow he knew something wasn't quite right.

Ariel allowed herself one tiny, triumphant pull of her lips into the ghost of a smile, then stepped into what was very obviously Vanessa's domestic demesne.

There was a ridiculous bed shaped like a scallop, or maybe a deep-sea clam. The ridges were wide and deep but far too precise and symmetrical for either creature. Its plaster shell was open, so the bed was in what would have been the bottom half of the mollusc; the top half stood upright as a decorative backdrop hung with golden lanterns and convenient little shelves for knick-knacks. The whole thing was upholstered in purple silk the colour of a deadly Portuguese man-o'-war.

The rest of the room, crowded by the bed though it was, was further filled with mismatched and disturbing treasures. There were statues of twisted and tortured heroes, their faces distorted in agony. Covering one entire wall was a painting of squiggly, squirming humans in some sort of fiery cavern. There was pain on their faces but glee on the visage of the one who was tormenting them – he was red and bearded and had a trident like Triton's.

Triton himself didn't appear to be anywhere obvious in the room. Ariel moved farther in, picking up and putting down the disgusting little pieces of bric-a-brac. Among all the horror was an ironically delicate dressing table covered in mother-of-pearl, and, intriguingly, all manner of exquisite little glass bottles. Scents from the east, oils from the west, attar of roses, nut butter, extract of myrrh, sandalwood decoctions, jasmine hydrosols… everything to make someone smell exquisite.

Or to mask whatever it was she really smelt like, Ariel thought wryly.

Or were the oils and butters for more medicinal reasons, for the cecaelia's skin? Ariel found herself looking at her own hands, rubbing them over each other lightly. Last time she had only been in the Dry World for a few days. Was it, literally, drying? Was it difficult, or painful, for creatures from the sea to remain for months battered by void and air, despite their magic?

Ariel shivered. Magic didn't make everything simpler. Crossing the thresholds of worlds was no minor thing.

But none of the bottles looked like it contained a polyp.

Father? she asked silently. *Where are you?*

Footsteps rang in the hallway outside.

Frozen, Ariel waited for them to pass.

But they didn't. They came *in*... to Eric's apartment.

The mermaid looked around. If whoever came in knew that Vanessa didn't like heels of bread or drink wine at that time of day... the jig was up.

The intruder continued to pad around maddeningly. There were accompanying sounds of things being lifted, patted, folded. A maid, straightening or cleaning... Ursula's room would be next.

What should she *do*?

What would she do if she were the old Ariel and a shark were hunting her?

Without a second thought, the Queen of the Sea folded herself down as small as possible and hid under the dressing table.

Less than a second later the maid came into the doorway.

Ariel saw padded cloth house shoes and closed her eyes, willing invisibility.

As if the person standing there knew Ariel's position and were bent on drawing out her torture as long as possible, she *continued* to just stand there: neither leaving the doorway, nor entering Vanessa's room.

Ariel felt the strange sensation of sweat popping out on the back of her neck. It was thoroughly unpleasant, and tickled besides. She had to fight down an urge to scratch, or move, or stretch. *I am a queen*, she told herself as the itch became maddening. *I am not ruled by my body.*

"Max!" the maid called out. Ariel could just see her skirts move as she put her hands on her hips. "Max, where are you? Dinnertime! C'mon, you silly thing. You can't have gotten far..."

There was no impatience in her voice, only love for the old dog.

But Ariel was so angry with the servant's existence she wanted to turn her into a sea cucumber. *Just for a few minutes.*

"Well, I know you wouldn't want to be in *here*, the *princess's* room," the maid said, her final words heavy with meaning. She spun and left, going all the way back out to the hallway. *"Maaaax..."*

Ariel breathed a heavy sigh of relief. She unfolded herself carefully, avoiding hitting her head on the ornate edge of the dressing table.

Whew! That was ridiculously, painfully close.

She proceeded into the dressing room, where Vanessa kept her ridiculous assortment of clothes: bright-coloured gowns with tiny, corseted waists and laced bodices that dove deep to expose vast amounts of décolletage. Wraps and shawls and jackets and hats with jewels and goldwork and more often than not the feathers, and sometimes the entire body, of some poor, exotic and thoroughly dead bird.

She felt the silk of one long pale-rose sleeve. It was expert workmanship and utterly beautiful and thoroughly disgusting that such labour had been wasted on the evil woman. In a fairy tale, Ursula would be the wicked, lazy girl who wound up with dried seaweed and empty shells. *And maybe shrimp crawling out of her throat.*

She noticed something funny about a button on the sleeve just as she was about to let it drop: it was etched like scrimshaw, with lines so fine and thin they must have been made by a master, or a creature of magic.

The design was of an octopus.

Not a friendly one, like many that Ariel knew; this was elongated and sinister, with strangely evil eyes.

Ariel's own eyes darted around the room like a barracuda distracted by sparkly things. It was immediately clear, once she knew what to look for, that every piece of clothing and accessory had the octopus sigil somewhere on it: the diamond brooch on a collar, the buckle on a belt, a hidden embroidery on the more traditional Tirulian dresses.

Whatever her motivations were in staying among the

humans she'd married into, Ursula had not forgotten her origins or her true self.

But there was nothing in the wardrobe that could have been her hidden father; not a bottle or a jar or even a repurposed shoe. Maybe there was a hidden panel somewhere, or maybe the sea witch kept him locked up in a real dungeon, downstairs.

And then, along with a current of moist, soapy air…

… came a voice…

Her voice.

In the trailing end of a song.

"*… up on the land, where my lover walks. But I can only pine from the foamy waves…*"

Her voice.

She hadn't heard her own voice in years.

The day when Ursula first took her payment, it had felt like Ariel's very soul had been sucked out of her body. The young, silly merthing she was then hadn't even realised it. Like a ghost she went on with her quest, her desires, intent on her prize, not even realising she was already dead to the world.

Okay, perhaps it wasn't quite that dramatic, Queen Ariel corrected herself gently.

But seeing Vanessa wed Eric, and her father killed,

and realising she would never get either man, or her voice, back… a part of her *had* truly died that day.

And now that witch was using her voice to sing in the bath.

Ariel wouldn't let the rage that was coursing through her veins control her. She *wouldn't.* She was a queen, and queens didn't lose control. Not for sweat, not for rage.

It was no easy task; like sweat, this kind of anger was a new experience.

She had been sad. She had been melancholy. She had cursed her fate as a voiceless monarch, railing against her lot quietly. Once in a while she had a burst of temper when she wanted to be heard and no one would listen, when people were shouting over her and ignoring her hands, as if because she had no voice she had nothing to say.

This was like nothing she had experienced before. It was like lava, burning through her skin and threatening to consume her whole.

Without thinking she moved towards the direction of the sound.

"… *heartless witch of the sea…* ha ha!… *heartless, heartless indeed, ensorcelling me…*"

The air grew moister, but not with the accompanying clouds of steam one expected from a luxuriously royal bath.

"Oh, let him see me for who I am, for without a voice, my face alone must speak for me..."

This was a pretty, wistful aria, but Vanessa let the last note quaver just a little too long, seeing how long she could keep the vibrato going. Then she broke into a peal of laughter that, despite being in Ariel's voice, sounded nothing like the mermaid.

Ariel pushed the far door open a crack. Some previous king or queen had designed the royal bath to look as dramatic as possible, almost like a stage, perhaps so he or she could soak while members of state gathered around asking for decisions. There was even a sort of viewing balcony or mezzanine that the hall led to, above the bath; this held a few cabinets to store bath-related bric-a-brac and a privacy screen for robing and disrobing, although despite the plentiful storage, Vanessa's morning clothes were thrown carelessly over a chair. Wide and ostentatious spiral stairs led down to the bathtub itself.

"*If I could dance with him but once, I know he would love me... One waltz in the sand; I would be free...* I don't know, it's really not so great. Not much to write home about. The sand, I mean. It gets positively everywhere and feels nasty in your foldy bits."

When Vanessa stopped singing and lapsed into her own

editorial comments, the cognitive dissonance was almost overwhelming. Ariel's voice was higher than the sea witch's and lacked the burrs and tremolos the cecaelia was fond of throwing in when she was being dramatic. Yet still the tone and nuance was all Ursula.

Ariel edged silently out onto the mezzanine and peeped over the side.

Vanessa was clearly enjoying the bath. Her brown hair flowed around her in slippery wet ringlets that very much brought to mind the arms and legs of a squid. Great quantities of bubbles and foam towered over the top of the tub and spilt out onto the floor, slowly dripping down like the slimy egg sac of a moon snail.

Vanessa was splashing and talking to herself and playing in the bath almost like a child. Ariel remembered, with heat, when *she* had been in that bath, and was introduced to the wonders of foam that wasn't just the leavings of dead merfolk. The whole experience had been marvellous and strange. Imagine the humans, kings of the Dry World, keeping bubbles of water around to bathe and play in. There was no equivalent under the sea; no one made 'air pools' for fun and cleanliness.

For just a moment, so quickly that Ariel could have dismissed it as a shadow or a trick of the light and bubbles if she didn't know better, a tentacle snaked out of the water, then quickly back in, like it had forgotten itself for a moment.

Unthinking, Ariel reached for the comb hidden in her hair. True, the trident's power wouldn't work on dry land. But she didn't need its power. With barely a thought to nudge it in the right direction, the comb melted into fluid gold and reformed into something with heft: a three-pronged dagger, deadly and sharp.

If she had been human born and raised, she would have attempted to hurl it into the witch's heart. She had a perfect view and the advantage of height.

But she had been raised in a watery world where friction was a constant enemy. Except for the strongest, no one ever *threw* things across or up; stones slowed down and sank almost immediately.

Ariel crouched down, preparing to sneak and then run, driving the dagger into the witch's flesh with her own hands.

She lifted one delicate foot…

"What's that?" Ursula suddenly demanded.

The mermaid froze.

"Did you hear…? Was that a…"

Ariel put her back flat to the cabinet that was right behind her, sucking in her stomach and trying to shrink.

There was splashing, frantic. It sounded like far too

many appendages or people were in the water for it all to be one person.

"No one is supposed to interrupt my baths!" Ursula shouted.

Ariel could tell by the change in pitch that the sea witch was standing up now, possibly on six of her legs.

The mermaid tried to slide along the cabinet towards the dressing room door, but the revolting carved-ivory handles and drawer pulls kept tangling in her ugly dress. One particular thread pulled tightly across her legs until she couldn't move.

Ariel gritted her teeth and forced her hip slowly out, and the string popped with a heart-wrenching *twang*.

She stopped breathing.

"Vareet! Vareet!" Ursula called out. "What is that? Go investigate!"

What if she just got up and ran? Would Ursula be able to see who it was? Would they send the guards after her? Would she be able to make it out in time?

Ariel worked muscles that were still new to her, stretching and bending her foot, trying to silently move her thighs so she could crab-walk to the door.

"Maaaaaaax…" came a lilting voice from the distance.

The same infuriating maid from before.

"Ugh," Ursula swore, strangely echoing her own feelings. "If that stupid dog comes in here I'm having it muzzled. And *Max* too."

There were more splashing and sloshing noises; the sea witch was settling back down into the water. Ariel could once again hear her own voice, muttering and grumbling to herself. A pail of water was poured, a tap turned, the tub refilled.

Relief and disappointment and continued fear competed like braids in a lock of hair hanging from Ariel's soul. She fell back against one of the cabinets. *What am I doing?* She was nothing like the warrior merfolk some of her ancestors and relatives were. She never cared enough to train for the Mer-games and win the golden crown of sea heather. Cousin Lara, with her mighty spear, was better made for this sort of thing.

Ariel was here to find her father. And so far, she had failed. She had been utterly distracted.

She should go back and thoroughly search Vanessa's room while she had a chance. If ancient plays, poems and songs taught nothing else, it was always one of these two repeating themes: one, don't ever fool around with a god's wife or husband, and two, revenge always leads to sorrow. And while she had never been the most diligent student as a princess, she loved a good story.

She dipped her hand and the dagger turned into a comb once more. She set it carefully back in her hair.

How much more time did she have to search the bedroom? Had that interruption lengthened or shortened Vanessa's bath ritual?

Ariel risked another peep to see if she could tell.

Ursula appeared to be lounging carelessly in her bath again, full-on Vanessa, no tentacles in sight.

The mermaid could now see that standing close to the tub was a little maid waiting in attendance, maybe eight years old. Though her body faced the bath and Vanessa, she kept her eyes directed out at the sea, through the windows. She hugged a giant fluffy towel tight, ready for the moment Ursula decided it was time to get out.

She was biting her lip.

It was obvious she knew something about Ursula's true nature, how could she not, as bath attendant? She must have seen things even more terrible than tentacles…

Ariel said a silent prayer for the poor girl and prepared to tiptoe back.

But just as she reached the door, something glittery caught her eye from the frumpy pile of Vanessa's hastily cast-off clothes.

She gulped, for once glad she didn't have a voice to

vocalise whatever it was that came up from her heart.

The nautilus.

Ursula's totem of power, the necklace she wore everywhere. *The token that held Ariel's voice.*

Barely able to believe it was true, Ariel ducked down and crawled over to the chair.

With a gesture that was less 'regally acquiring what was rightfully hers' and more like the crazed swipe for a sea bean by a starving mer, she snatched up the nautilus and held it to her chest. Dazed and in shock from her find, of *having it in her hand*, she rose and stumbled back to the door.

The little maid spotted her.

Ariel's mouth went dry and her heart sank.

She stared at the girl, and the girl watched Ariel with large, hollow eyes.

Realising how strangely ironic it was, Ariel put a finger to her lips.

Please.

The little girl glanced over at Vanessa in her bath.

"*My dark and villainous plans, how they unfurl* – no, wait. Was that how it went? I can't remember..." Ursula sang and muttered to herself, heedless of her maid.

Please!

Ariel threw the word through her eyes, across the space

between her and the little girl, praying for her sympathy.

The little girl gave the faintest nod.

Ariel put her hands together as best she could, clutching the nautilus and bowed her head.

Thank you. If ever I find a way to repay you, I swear I shall.

Not that the little girl would ever know, but the gods would.

Ariel crept to the door… and then bolted out of the castle.

Ariel

She pounded through the castle as fast as she could, new heels hitting the stony floors with surprising force. Faces were a blur as she sprinted to the exit.

"Woof?" came from somewhere near the ground at one point.

Max! Your dinner is ready! she thought, and mentally promised to pet him later, if there was a later. She risked looking up to see if Eric was there with him, but he wasn't.

As soon as her feet touched sand she redoubled her pace, making for the hidden lagoon. Several guards looked after her curiously, but not too curiously; she was behaving like a scorned lover or someone who had been in a fight with a friend. In a castle full of enemies and noble spies, a scampering maid drew little interest from people with better things to do.

The hot sun hit her back like a reproving shove. At that moment she hated everything about being human. The long skirts of her dress tangled in her new legs and chafed her skin. Her stupid boots were clumsy in the sand, like she was stepping into holes and pulling her feet out of sucking, grabby mud.

But soon she was in the blessedly quiet cove where the wind was still and the noises of humans and their activities far off and easily forgotten. She sank down onto the sand like she would have as a mermaid: tail folded under her, leaning to the side a little, one hip up, the other down. The instinct to flip her fin impatiently went nowhere; the thought travelled down her spine and stopped where her legs split.

She opened her tightly cupped hands and looked at what lay in her palm.

The nautilus shell was exquisite, brown and white and perfectly striped. The maths that lay like a dazzling creation spell over all who lived in the sea showed clearly in the spiral, each cell as great as the sum of the two previous sections. Everything in the ocean was a thing of beauty and numbers, even in death.

Mermaids could live for a long time, but their bodies became foam that dissipated into nothing when they died.

The poor little mollusc who lived in this shell had a very short life, but his shell could last for centuries.

Ariel sighed and brushed her fingers over it, feeling strangely melancholy despite the triumph she literally held in her hands. Years of being mute could be swept away in a second. Years of frustration, years of silent crying, years of anger.

And then what?

If she destroyed it, what would it change?

Ursula would immediately know she was back. That she had been in the castle, practically under the sea witch's nose.

And then what would happen to Ariel's search for her father? This was more complicated than a simple diversion; this could set everything back and make her whole task harder.

Queen Ariel held the nautilus and considered thoughtfully.

But the little mermaid didn't think. She acted.

Before she realised fully what she was doing Ariel had smashed the nautilus on a sharply faceted rock.

It didn't break like a normal shell. It shattered like

a human vessel. Shards flew in all directions equally, unhampered by gravity or luck.

Ariel pitched forwards.

She choked, no longer breathing the air of the Dry World. Her arms flailed up like a puppet's. Her torso whipped back and forth, pummelled by unseen forces. Something flew into her mouth, up her nose and suffused her entire body with a heat that threatened to burn. It rushed into her lungs and expanded, expelling whatever breath she had left, pushing blood to her extremities, pushing everything out that wasn't *it*, leaving room for nothing else.

Ariel collapsed.

It was over.

It was like the thing, whatever it was, had been absorbed by her body and had now dissipated into her blood and flesh.

She took a breath. Her heart started beating again.

She hadn't been aware it had stopped.

She coughed. A few grains of sand came out.

And then she sang.

Eric

His hands were raised, trying to draw more out of the violins with his left while holding back the percussion with his right.

He fumbled.

It was like a pile of books had fallen from a high shelf onto his head, and, having broken his skull, somehow managed to directly impart their contents into his brain.

It was like a sibling had snuck up behind him, and, thinking he was prepared, expecting him to get out of the way, whacked him with a wooden baton. The *crack* on the head was twice as painful as it should have been, the simple blow compounded by shock that a sister would strike so hard. Feelings and pain were utterly mixed.

It was like he were suddenly afflicted by a grievous, mortal fit of the body: as if his heart or kidney or some other important organ had seized up and failed.

He experienced the wonder of taking a first breath after the terrible pain receded with a clear-headed, deep relief that presaged either death or recovery.

Eric blinked at the orchestra and singers before him. Instruments faltered. A hundred pairs of eyes looked back at him expectantly.

He saw, as if for the first time, the plain yet comely smile of the second soprano, the brown mole on the likeable brow of the basso profundo, the L-shaped smudge on the copper timpani. A veil had been drawn away.

He was Prince Eric, and he was conducting a practice session for an opera.

Not sailing a pleasure ship or playing his recorder to himself, or, more appropriately, running this part of his parents' kingdom, which was his duty, his chore, his right.

Something was very, very wrong.

He gulped.

But the people before him waited on his very fingertips. For now *they* were his kingdom. They needed their prince.

He would deal with personal revelations later.

And so he conducted, and when the soprano sang he winced, and tried not to think of another singer with hair as bright as fire and eyes like the sea.

Ursula

Vanessa stood in the tub slowly drying herself, starting with her face. She always left the lower half of her body in the water as long as possible.

She sang quietly, luxuriating in the gradual process. The one thing the humans did right, at least the *princesses* did, was take the proper time and care in making themselves presentable to the world.

Her little maid stood attentively nearby.

"Mmm, something-something, and I shall be Queen of the Sea, mm-hmm... keeRACK!"

Suddenly the princess heaved violently. It felt like her

uvula had been pulled violently out through her lips. Like her mouth had been turned inside out. Like the meat and blood of her lungs were following close behind.

She coughed, certain that blood was going to spray out. But there was nothing on the piles and piles of white, sweet-smelling bubbles that filled the tub. No scarlet spittle, no physical proof of the massive change within her.

"My *voice*," she said, the words coming out in a low-pitched growl. The tenor of a much older, much larger, much… *different* woman.

"MY VOICE!" she screeched, pretty red lips squared and askew. She clenched her hands into fists, shaking with rage.

Her maid looked concerned, obviously unsure what had caused this outburst. She waited nervously for orders.

Vanessa, princess of Tirulia, clawed her way out of the tub and stalked up the steps, white foam trailing off her like smoke. Naked and not cold. Vareet, unnoticed, hurried after her with another towel. The princess dug desperately through the pile of clothes she had taken off so carelessly before and threw them every which way in her panic.

"Where is my necklace?!"

But of course it was gone.

She spun to focus her wrath on the tiny maid, who tried to hide behind the giant towel she still held at the ready. Not that her mistress hadn't lost her temper before, of course; she had *many* times, when no one else was present. But this time seemed particularly bad. Vanessa's teeth bit into her bottom lip; she didn't even notice the tiny droplets of dark blood that welled up. Her cheeks sucked in under high cheekbones until her face looked like a skull. Her eyes were wild and the whites seemed almost yellow, and sickly.

"WHERE IS MY NECKLACE?" the princess demanded again, tapping her chest to indicate where it used to hang.

Vareet shook her head, terrified.

"*BAH!*"

Vanessa drew her hand back. For a moment it seemed like she really would strike the girl. But the sea witch wasn't dumb; the maid had been within her sight at all times. She had nothing to do with the missing nautilus shell or its obvious destruction.

It could have been a simple sneak thief, of course. It could have been some sort of accident. But it wasn't. It was…

"The *hussy*," Ursula growled, rolling the words out.

She paused her rant, savouring the sounds. Her stolen voice had been fun to play with, worked wonders on others and caused pain for the one from whom it was ripped. That was more than enough. But… she rather enjoyed hearing her real voice again. It was a voice with depth, with command. With character and *substance.* It was so *her.* Not at all like that bubbling, perfect-pitched, whiny little merthing.

"The hussy is *back*," she repeated.

Vareet took one timid step backwards, obviously torn between terror at this strange change in her mistress, and fear of her mistress herself.

"She was in here, somehow, and stole my necklace, and destroyed it."

Vanessa looked round, at the door to her changing room that led to her bedroom… but there was no evidence of anything out of place.

"This is a problem," she said, fingering her throat. "A disturbing development I need to deal with immediately, and *permanently.*

"GUARDS!"

Ariel

She sang.

Wordless hymns of the sea: immediate, extemporised passages about waves and sunlight and tides and the constant, beautiful pressure of water on everything. The glory of seaweed slowly swaying, the delicious feeling that foretold a storm in the Dry World and turbulence below.

The music came out of her without pause, driven by years of observing, seeing, listening, enjoying, experiencing the world and unable to express it. The wonder and sadness of being alive. The joy of being a mermaid; the pain of being the only one like herself, the only mermaid who had been mortal, temporarily, and then lost everything.

When she finally stopped, her eyes were closed and her hands rested on her human lap, and she felt the dry, human sun and imagined wet things.

She opened her eyes.

The silence was now deafening in the lagoon.

She had the voice of the gods, some had said. The sort of voice that could lure landlubbers to sea and sailors to their deaths, a voice that could launch a thousand ships. She had the voice of the wind and the storm and the crash of the waves and the ancient speech of the whale. She had the voice of the moon as it glided serenely across the sky and the stars as they danced behind. She had the voice of the wind between the stars that mortals never heard, that rushed and blew and ushered in the beginning and end of time.

She sat for a moment quietly, remembering how it sounded but enjoying the silence.

The songs were from the old Ariel. Perhaps the new Ariel too.

She coughed and tried again, cocking her head and effecting a stern look.

"Just *do* it, Flounder; I need the tax audits by the third tide so we have something to present to the council.

"Sebastian, I don't care about the gala or its details. I'm

sure it's all fine in your very capable claws.

"And with the cutting of this ribbon, I hereby declare the Temple of Physical Arts open to all!"

Ariel smiled, then threw back her head and laughed, but it was brittle.

She picked up a shard of the nautilus and sighed.

Her voice had been such an important part of her life before. The merfolk celebrated her for it. Her father excused her occasionally questionable behaviour because of it. Eric loved the girl who rescued him, because of her singing…

But…

… she'd never really enjoyed singing for anyone else. In fact, she hated audiences. She sang because she liked to sing. She just… *felt*… something, and had to sing it. If she were happy, or sad, or angry… she would go off by herself and sing to the coral, sing to the seaweed, sing to an audience of sea snails or tube worms (who listened, but never commented). Most of her mergirlhood had been spent swimming around, exploring, singing to herself. Making up little stories in her head and then putting them into song.

Ruefully she remembered the concert that Sebastian had so carefully planned, which she had missed, which her dad had punished her for, which led him to set the little crab on her case, and so on…

She hadn't been deliberately disobedient. She just… forgot.

Sometimes people thought she was a snob because of the way she acted. But she wasn't *trying* to be a diva, she was just a young mer whose head was full of fantasies.

And by taking away her voice, Ursula had stolen what Ariel treasured most: the only way she knew how to express those stories.

Without spoken language, and no knowledge of signs, back then, she wasn't able to tell Eric what had happened to her or how she loved him. She wasn't able to tell her father not to trade places with her. She wasn't able to rule her kingdom without the help of a fleet of people to interpret and speak for her.

She had lost a means of communicating her desires, her commands, her wishes, her needs, her thoughts.

"How do you feel?"

Ariel looked up, suddenly aware of the gull who was perched quietly on a nearby rock, watching her with a curious, beady eye.

"Jona," Ariel said, relishing the sound of the name. "How long have you been sitting there?"

"I spotted you the moment you came out of the castle. But it looked like you needed a moment to yourself. I was going to interrupt if you kept on with that singing."

"*That* singing? Why?" Ariel asked archly. Her hands signed as she spoke, too used to the process.

"Well, you were getting a little loud."

The mermaid blinked at the gull.

Then she began to laugh.

She laughed so hard she began to have trouble breathing. Great, pealing gulps of laughter and air: it felt *good* to laugh and have it actually come out, not just be a silent recognition of something mildly amusing.

"I… beg your pardon?" Jona said, a trifle offended.

"Oh… it's just…" She breathed deep, trying to control herself, not wanting to. "I was *just* sitting here thinking about singing, and how much everyone loved to hear me sing, and how I was celebrated for my voice, and how someone fell in love with me for my voice, and you…" She lost it for a moment again.

Jona turned her head back and forth, trying to get a good look at the mermaid with one eye, then the other. "I mean, well, it was… nice. I just meant that you were going to call over the guards."

"'Nice'? You've heard better?" Ariel asked, half-joking, half-curious.

Jona opened her beak for a moment, closed it, choosing

her words carefully now that it was obvious she had offended. "Your singing is extraordinary; it is epic; it has something in common with the very forces of nature, like the wind and the sea itself.

"If you were to ask me how I felt about it personally, however, I would say I prefer the cries of my own kind, or the mindless trill of a sandpiper, or the sad call of a plover. They're more accessible."

Ariel put her hand to her face to stop the next peal of laughter. She snorted instead.

"What?" the bird asked, confused.

"I like you, Jona," she said, scruffing the bird under her neck. The gull closed her eyes and leant into it.

"ARIEL! You're SINGING!"

An explosion of grey and white feathers landed on the beach next to them. As soon as he recovered himself, Scuttle threw his wings round her in a gull-y embrace.

"I am," she said, stroking his head.

"Oh, it's *so good* to hear you," Scuttle said with a sigh. "It does my old heart… it's just the best."

Ariel smiled. There was something specifically beautiful about what he had said: *It's so good to hear you.* He didn't say anything about her singing, just that it was good to hear her voice. He was genuinely pleased just that she had her voice back – whatever she chose to do with it.

This is a friend.

And… wait a second… she didn't have to just think these thoughts any more.

"Scuttle," she said aloud. "It does *my* heart good to talk to you."

"You're so queenly now, listen to you. So noble and regal and genteel and all. So does this change the Big Plan?" Scuttle asked, elbowing her with his wing and giving a conspiratorial wink. "You're still gonna look for your father, right?"

"Of course. But now… I've effectively… alerted… Ursula to my presence. I'm a fool. I should have waited before destroying Ursula's necklace."

She shook her head and sighed, picking up the leather band that had held the nautilus. Now a golden bail and a bit of shell were all that was left. For reasons she couldn't put into words, either aloud or in her head, she wrapped the strap round itself twice and slipped it onto her wrist. Maybe it would remind her to not be so rash in the future.

"I dunno, Ariel," Scuttle said. "What else would you have done? Left it there? Your *voice*? That would take the will of a mountain or something. You couldn't just leave it there with Ursula. *No* one could have."

"No, I don't… suppose I could have. I don't know."

"Did you manage to look around at all?" Jona asked. "Maybe get a hint of where she might be hiding him?"

"Only a little. He's probably in her bedroom… or *was* in her bedroom. I didn't see any bottle or anything immediately like what you described when I was there, and now that she knows I'm back she'll probably hide him somewhere else. At least I have an ally in the castle. Maybe even two! There's a little maid who didn't reveal me to Ursula, and also Carlotta, who was so nice to me the last time I was human. She's aware that *something* happened the day Eric and Vanessa were wed. She also told me that a lot has happened as a result of that day. Ramifications, bad ones, for people besides me and my father."

"Oh yeah? With Ursula as Vanessa, running the kingdom?" Scuttle asked. "I mean, you hear things as a bird, you know. But it's hard to tell when humans are happy or unhappy. Especially when you're just trying to pick through their rubbish."

"What I don't understand is why Ursula would stay. Married to Eric, I mean. And *here*." She indicated all the Dry World with her hands. "What does she want? I thought her only desire was to beat me and get revenge on my father. She did that. This isn't her home…"

Scuttle shrugged. "I don't know, Ariel. She's evil, right? Who knows why she does anything? To make more evil, maybe? Or maybe she just likes it here. Whatever is going on in her crazy head, we gotta take her down, that's what we gotta do. We'll eighty-six her, get your dad back, get the prince and everyone lives happily ever after."

"I don't know about *all* of that," Ariel said with a smile. "I don't think I can be responsible for *everyone's* happily ever after." *Even my own. Get the prince*? It was an intriguing thought, but one for later. *Duty first.* "… I think it would be difficult to, um, 'eighty-six' a princess and a sea witch, especially now that I've lost the element of surprise. Let's focus on getting my father back, and then see what else we can do afterwards."

"You don't want the prince any more?" Jona asked curiously.

Ariel looked at her in surprise. Had the bird read her mind? "Excuse me?"

"The character of you really seemed to pine after the character of him in Eric's opera, *La Sirenetta*," Jona said with a shrug. "And Great-grandfather always told the story of the two of you, and you *gave your voice away to win him…*"

"It was a long time ago. I was young, he was handsome and exotic. I don't think, in reality, there's much of a possibility of a long-term relationship between a mermaid and a human."

It was so much easier to speak quickly first and then decide later if it was truth or lies. She was already losing the thoughtfulness that came with being silent. Ariel scolded herself mentally.

"Better ease off," Scuttle said to his great-grandgull in what he probably thought was a helpful whisper. "She seems a little touchy. Still an open wound."

Ariel took a deep breath and stood up. "Well, I don't think I can go back to the castle right now. Everyone saw me rush out."

"What will you do?" Jona asked.

"While I'm waiting for things to die down a bit, I'll go see for myself what mess Ursula's rule over Tirulia has created. If Carlotta is right, it makes my task even more urgent. I can't have humans dying because of a princess I, however inadvertently, gave them. I need to go to town, where the people are, and listen to what they are saying."

"Absotively," Scuttle said. "Having a sea witch for a princess has got to have some bad, you know, reiterations."

"*Repercussions*, I think you mean, Great-grandfather," Jona corrected politely. She stretched her wings. "I should go alert Flounder of your status change, regarding your voice."

"Thank you, Jona," Ariel said warmly. "Please tell him to meet me in this cove four tides from now for an update. And make sure he *fully understands* not to tell anyone else at all yet."

"Anyone?" Scuttle asked, surprised. "Not even old crabby-claws?"

"*Especially* not Sebastian. Not yet. I already feel bad enough getting my voice back, and not my father. I can't bear the thought of explaining that to him right now. Also, if everyone knows that I can talk again, it's just more pressure, to get me back, to have me stay and rule. It would be hard to escape and look for Father a second time."

"But you wouldn't be telling everyone, just Sebastian," Scuttle pointed out.

"Once Sebastian knows, the entire kingdom will hear about it within hours," Ariel said with a wan smile. "He's as bad as a guppy with gossip."

Eric

He made his way back from rehearsal to the castle with the uncomfortable feeling that he was hiding something.

It was not unlike the time he had caught his first really sizeable sea bass. The old fishermen on the docks had cheered when the eight-year-old princeling ran home as fast as his little legs could carry him, holding his prize aloft.

But then, realising he had a catch of serious merit, Eric was suddenly convinced that his mother and father, the king and queen, would yell at him for such plebeian pursuits and forbid him from cooking and eating the dinner he had caught for himself like a real man.

He hid the fish under his shirt.

The sea bass (known commonly as the wolf fish) had extra-sharp fins and spines and scales, all of which cut into the boy's flesh as it struggled.

Little Eric arrived at the castle desperate and bleeding. He went straight to the kitchens, where he collapsed into a puddle of tears, cursing his own weakness.

(The king and queen, as any parent could guess, were delighted with the skill and determination their son had shown. They gave Eric a really solid lecture on the importance of knowing what common people did to earn their dinner, for he would be ruling a kingdom of fisherfolk some day. Then the cook oversaw the bandaged, once-again cheerful Eric as he fried up the fish himself. It was presented to the royal family on a golden platter, and everyone lived happily ever after that day.)

This was *also* not unlike the time when, as a young teen, he had fallen in love with a stray puppy that did not at all fit the royal image of a hunting hound. This too, he stuffed under his shirt and carried home. Guilty and tortured, he snuck Max into his bedroom and fed him the best bits of purloined steak from dinner.

He was of course found out.

"It's not a Sarenna imperial wolf mastiff," his father

had said with a sigh. "We kings of Tirulia have always had those. For *centuries*."

"At least it's not a fish this time," the queen had pointed out lightly.

But little Eric and older Eric and even now oldest Eric never had a *truly* terrible secret. Those two were the worst ones he could come up with when trying to compare what he felt now to something similar in his life.

What was it, exactly, he was hiding this time? It wasn't tangible, like a fish or a puppy.

Clarity?

Was that a terrible secret? Why did he feel the need to hide it?

He tried to mimic the way he usually walked home, but all the Erics, little, older, and present Eric, were terrible liars. It was just one of the many reasons the prince refused to be in his own shows, even in a bit part. He knew his limits.

He looked up quickly, guiltily, askance, expecting things to appear different. More colourful. More detailed. More truthful. More meaningful.

But all the houses he passed looked the same; the flowers and plants were the same colours as the day before.

Yep, that grain storehouse is still the same. Same dry rot round the windows, same mouldering timbers…

Wait a moment, that looks really bad. I'll bet it smells terrible up close. Isn't that where we keep the surplus grain? In case of blight or disaster? Good heavens, is it leaking*? That could ruin everything. Why is that being allowed? I'd better look into that…*

Oh, look, it's that girl from the market who sells the sea beans. What's she doing here? I used to know her mother… what was her name? Lucretia.

My word, look at that enormous guarded wagon driving up to the castle, with so many soldiers around it! What on earth are they delivering? I want to say… munitions? Yes! That's it.

Wait, munitions? But why? I can't quite… why do we need…? This is all so bizarre.

Then it hit him.

There hadn't been a *physical* change to himself or his sight; the veil or whatever it was, the charm, had been lifted from *in*side his head. It was like an old net, full of slime and dead shellfish and falling apart and utterly useless, had enshrouded his brain, and had just now been extracted by some clever doctor. He could think for the first time in years. He could react to the things around him. Generate opinions. Hold on to thoughts. *He* had changed, not his eyes.

That was reassuring, and having figured that out made him feel a bit better and more in control. He strode confidently into the castle. Grimsby was waiting just inside and in one fluid, habituated movement helped the prince spin out of his academic robe and into a very neatly tailored day jacket, dove grey with long tails.

"Thanks, Grims," Eric said, continuing on to the lesser luncheon room and fluffing up his cravat. All he *wanted* to do was grab his old manservant, out of sight of the guards, and grill him about the past. He was the only one in the castle Eric could trust. But that would look odd, and until he got the lay of the land, he preferred to play along like still-bewitched Eric.

Princess Vanessa was already seated at the delicate golden table where they would dine together after meeting with the Metalworkers' Guild. Thank goodness he didn't have to greet her and take her arm and lead her in. He had very, very mixed feelings right now, but all the ones around her induced nausea.

"Good afternoon, Princess," Eric said politely. She extended a gloved hand and he perfunctorily kissed the back of it, extending his lips so that only the furthest, tippiest bit, the part that often got chapped at sea, barely brushed the smooth fabric.

He noticed, and was unsure if this was the result of his new state of being, her dress: she wore an unusually demure pale blue day dress with less bustle than usual and understated lace ruffs at the wrists. Also a giant woolly muffler wrapped round her neck and shoulders. Oh, it matched, of course; it was a beautiful, expensive shade of blue and was fringed with the sort of exotic imported feathers that had long skinny shafts and little bouncing dots of colour at the top that flashed in gold and iridescence. They obscured most of Vanessa's face.

More luck, Eric thought.

"Bit of a nasty cold," she whispered huskily. One delicate gloved hand went to her throat.

"I'm so sorry," he said, settling down into his own seat. Parched from the dry air in the practice hall, he picked up a carafe and began to pour himself a glass of *cava*.

Then he stopped. Did he really want to be foggy headed? At all? After this… awakening?

He reached for the crystal decanter of water instead.

Vanessa watched him silently.

The suited and dour captains of the Metalworkers' Guild stood before them, the symbol of their station gleaming here and there on their persons: silvery cane handles, the shining tips of their boots, simple rings, sashes with obscure buckles on them.

"If we may, Your Highness…" A short and stocky man stepped forwards. He had a luxurious, well-trimmed beard, and if it weren't for his modern tricorn hat, he would have looked exactly like a character out of one of Eric's fairy tale books, one of the fair folk who actually dug the precious metals out of deep mines. "We don't want to delay your lunch any further."

"Very considerate," Vanessa hissed. Without her normal, lilting tone, it sounded exactly as snarky and sarcastic as she probably meant. The man's bushy eyebrows shot up, but of course he said nothing about it.

"T-to put it plainly," he stuttered, "we… of course… support any and all military actions as planned and carried out by you, of course… it does keep us busy, after all. All the musket barrels… and mechanisms… and cannons… no shortage of work!"

Eric frowned. How much *work* did Tirulia's metalworkers have, precisely, involved in the crafts of war? The only reason there were fortifications in the city at all were because Roman governors and then medieval kings had liked the surroundings for their holidays by the sea.

"The problem is *supplies.* Your… strategies have unfortunately angered some of our trading partners. And the pass in the north is now unsafe for shipping, especially cargo that could be seen as military."

"I thought our mountains had some of the finest mines in the world," Vanessa whispered, asking the question before Eric could pose it himself. His father had first shown him the location of the mines and quarries on a parchment map when he was a lad. The ink in which mountains were sketched, in little upside-down 'Vs', was a dull black for iron and metallic orange for copper. That had fascinated young Eric, although he had wanted to put a dragon in there as well.

"What, Your Highness?" the man said, leaning closer. "I'm sorry, your voice..."

"MINES," she croaked. "FINE MINES. WITH COPPER."

"Absolutely, Princess," the man said. His eyes had darted briefly, questioningly, to the prince before resettling on her.

Eric started to feel relief at this close call of being noticed, then realised something: *no one paid attention to him any more.* No one had in years. And that 'relief' that he now seemed to be accustomed to? What was that? Wasn't he crown prince? *Shouldn't* he be dealing with the head of the guild and all his boring business himself? That was his duty!

The man was still talking.

"… and if we didn't have to make bronze or pewter, or things out of tin, we would be set. Steel has its uses, but there are other things to be made besides weapons, and those other things need other metals."

"What things are those?" Vanessa hissed. Maybe if she were speaking normally, with her large eyes and eyelashes aimed at the men, it would have come out as *Teach me, I'm an innocent young girl who relishes your older-man wisdom.* But there was a strange cognitive disconnect because of the husky whisper: almost like she was a much older woman poorly play-acting the role of young ingénue.

While Eric was pondering this, he also was puzzled by *what* she said. *What things are made of* metal? Didn't she have eyes? Didn't she live in the castle and use the objects within it?

"Well… Your Highness…" the man said awkwardly, looking around for support. "Most people in the kingdom, even wealthy folks like myself, tend not to eat off golden spoons and forks." He indicated the royal couple's place setting with a tip of his head. "Or burn candles in silver candelabra. Pewter, bronze and tin make all the tools and useful things for the rest of us – they have for thousands of years. And since we don't have tin in our mountains, we must trade for it. And we can't right now."

"Well, then," Vanessa whispered thoughtfully. "We must go to the place it is found and take it for ourselves."

The man blinked at her. *"Bretland?"*

She looked at him slyly out the corner of her eyes, gauging his reaction. Eric watched her tawdry performance, horrified and yet fascinated.

"You want us to… invade the *Allied Kingdoms of Bretland*?" the man asked again.

"Never say never," the princess purred.

"Excuse me? I'm sorry, I couldn't hear Your Highness."

"I *said*, 'Never say never.' "

"Beg your pardon?"

Eric wanted to leap up and announce that this ridiculous meeting was over. That Vanessa should not even *suggest* the, incredibly stupid, unheard-of idea of military aggression against one of the world's greatest powers to a civilian, much less without discussing it with him first.

But…

While he wasn't a *very* skilled chess player, his mother had told him that the most important thing in gamesmanship was this: you could never be completely sure of the other person, so never make a move until you were sure of *yourself*.

And he wasn't. Not yet. Not until he had some time to think and figure things out.

"I think this merits more discussion," he said aloud. Which was perhaps more than he had said in a while, but so wishy-washy no one could accuse him of acting forthrightly with thought and opinion. Vanessa did shoot him a quick sidelong glance, but that was all. "Your concerns about tin and, I assume, aluminum, will be taken into consideration. Thank you for your time, gentlemen."

The group of men, somewhat startled at the prince's words, all nodded and made quick bows both to him and then the princess, and shuffled out. The head of the guild gave Eric one last, appraising look before following.

Eric steeled himself for a tense and obnoxious lunch with his princess…

… but once again, the prince was saved.

"My dear, I'm afraid I must be off to bed now with this nasty cold. One must take care of illnesses before they grow serious," Vanessa hissed, indicating her throat. "So sorry to leave you alone."

"That's quite all right. I pray you feel better," Eric said, trying not to joyfully reach for a leg of quail before finishing his sentence.

He was nothing if not courteous.

Ursula

Good, little Eric swallowed the whole 'cold' thing.

She strode down the hall to her bedroom, Vareet and her manservants trailing like eddies in the wake of a very large ship. Her mind raced. *This* was what it was like to be a queen. *Er, princess.* This was what it was like to actually rule and wield power and make decisions and get things done. Real monarchs didn't shy away from their problems; they dealt with them head-on and then either beat them into submission or used them to further their own objectives.

Every stumbling block is a stepping stone.

She laughed to herself, remembering the first time she

had heard that saying, from one of the especially sycophantic Tirulian nobles. At the time she had no idea what it meant. Because obviously if there was a *stumbling block* in the ocean, you just swam over it.

She checked out herself askance in one of the large gilt-framed mirrors that lined the eastern hallway. Getting her gait just right was one of the hardest things about being on land. Imperial, regal, yet simpering and attractive. She wished in retrospect she had chosen a slightly older, more imposing human body. But of course twits like the prince needed something young and pretty to fall for. Absolutely no respect for or appreciation of maturity and wisdom. And pulchritude.

But honestly, she didn't have that many bodies to choose from. This sad sack of a human with gorgeous brown hair that the sea witch now wore had wanted to be one with the ocean… and Ursula had been only too glad to give her what she wished.

The transformation was a fairly permanent one, its origins invisible to all but the wearer. She had been wise to keep that body's essence around for all those years. Some might have said she had a tendency to hoard, but Ursula knew everything had a use eventually. For an emergency, or as the Dry Worlders said in their ridiculous way, "a rainy day."

Vanessa adjusted her muffler. It was uncomfortable and itchy and made her sweat and possibly break out. Human skin was so temperamental, exposed to naked air, too moist, too dry, far too parched, pimples and rashes and exfoliation… was this true with all Dry World creatures? Or just mortal ones?

Ursula, focus.

She went into her bedroom and headed directly to the dressing table, where she pulled off the ridiculous muffler and threw it to the floor. Vareet dashed over and immediately picked it up, shaking it out and dusting it. The sea witch coughed and touched her neck lightly, dabbing it with a silk powder puff. Then she leered into the mirror. For a moment she could almost see her true self. She grinned, delighted with her remembered appearance.

"Good to see you, old girl," she purred in her real voice, enjoying every syllable. "So tell me. *Where is the little hussy now?* Did she crawl back to the sea, or is she hanging around, hoping for a chance to reunite with Prince Dum-Dum?"

Anyone watching would have just seen a reflection of Vanessa, checking her teeth, running a hand through the top of her hair.

The transformation and accompanying charm and memory spells were some of the biggest, most interesting cantrips she had ever cast. She had done her sorcerous best in the three days Ariel pranced about on land. There was a lot there to be proud of. Still, it was a bit hasty and thrown together, and now its weakness showed, especially the mass-forgetting bit.

And was Eric regaining his will? He had acted a little odd at lunch, but sometimes it was hard to tell with humans. *Especially dumb ones.*

But if the day of the wedding began to grow clearer in the memories of those who had witnessed it… well, Ursula knew enough about mer and human behaviour to know that it would amount to nothing. Mermaids? Witches? Sea gods? There was an opera about it already, for heaven's sake. People who saw the show would confuse that with reality, and people who hadn't actually been on the boat would think anyone who said otherwise was mad. No, Ursula wasn't worried about the staff, the servants, the peasants, the nobles, the riff-raff.

Only Eric and Ariel.

A quick tempest of a rage crossed her face, deranging it for a moment into a hideous snarl of lips and eyes and teeth.

Eric and Ariel. Whether apart or together, they were determined to screw up her life.

The game had begun! Or… continued from years before.

Ariel had made the first move, and it was a good one.

Well, she would put an end to that. Now it was *her* move.

"FLOTSAM! JETSAM!" she snarled.

Both servants were in front of her less than a tail slap later. Upon seeing them Vareet quickly betook herself to the wardrobe, perhaps on the pretext of hanging up the muffler, and peeped out timidly. *Ridiculous little idiot.*

Speaking of hiding, she would have to do something about old Kingy now. He wasn't safe from theft any more…

… and maybe it was finally time to do *that thing* with him. The thing she had kept him around for, all these years, besides the fun of gloating. Just in case. Maybe it was time to set certain *other* plans in motion. Being a princess was fun. But there were greater stakes to play for…

"I want this castle put on high alert," Ursula snapped. "I want a meeting with a captain of the guard. I want watches doubled, tripled. I want *everyone* to know about a certain red-haired enemy of the state. I want a reward put out for a sighting and another for capture. I want dozens of men on the beach again, men in front of every low window and for every maid to be told exactly what she looks like."

"Absolutely, Ursula," Flotsam said with a grin.

"About time, Ursula," Jetsam said with a sneer.

Vareet said nothing.

The bright bit of beach outside her window caught Ursula's attention. A slow smile spread over her face.

"And," she said slowly, "I think… a warning… might be in order…"

Ariel

She watched the two birds fly off. She knew that one of them, or another winged friend, would remain silently near her at all times, above her, keeping an eye on things.

What a strange ability to have in this two-dimensional land! To be able to break the barrier of *height*, to ascend and descend at will above their fellow Dry World creatures. Yet even for seagulls it was an effort. If they didn't keep gliding or flapping, they fell.

I need to keep gliding and flapping, Ariel thought as she picked out the path to town, *or I'll fall too.* Right now she was neither a creature wholly of the sea or the land. She should be ruling the waves. She should have been married to Eric, ruling the little kingdom. She should have been swimming free in the ocean, singing and playing with her friends and dreaming. But here she was instead, doing none of those things.

The town rose over the next crest, and so did her heart at the sight. Houses and shops as pretty as a scene out of a play. Tiny dark temples filled with smoke and clingings and clangings and noise and laughter and shouts. *Life.* The quick, speedy movements of a people who ferociously enjoyed their short time under the sun.

Ariel stepped quickly past the first great pier that stuck out into the bay: fishing ships were unloading net after net of catch, and she really didn't want to witness that. By ancient law the rules for the World Under the Sea and those for the Dry World were different, but that didn't mean she had to witness the more distasteful aspects of their differences.

And speaking of differences, the changes in Tirulia from the last time she had been there were immediately apparent.

Three guards, no, *soldiers*, stood in a boyish cluster at the front of the docks, puffing their chests out, smoking and bragging to a trio of girls who seemed so familiar Ariel could almost see them swishing their tails while flirting. They were rosy-cheeked with blushes as the boys regaled them with tales of their exploits.

"… they put up quite the fight, let me tell you. But that

didn't stop Andral and me from gettin' them all out..."

"... aye, we torched the place good. Not a barn left standing..."

"... orders. Got the chief of the village myself, I did..."

"See what I got? Pretty, ain't it? It was just lying out, practically *begging* to be took..."

Put up a fight? *Torched* the place? For Tirulia? Seizing people in the mountains, burning villages to the ground? Looting?

As Ariel looked around she noticed even more soldiers wandering among the crowd. Some had an extra medal on their lapels, some had bandages where their hands once were. New recruits wore their uniforms with an air of cockiness, finding every excuse to touch their caps when a lady looked their way. One scratched the back of his head with the muzzle of his gun.

Ariel shuddered. Eric had taken her to see a ten-gun salute at the castle; it was a tradition that honoured Tirulia's connection with the sea and the old sea gods they used to worship. An explosion of modern fire and gunpowder was thought to be pleasing to the occasionally warlike Neptune.

But the gunshots were utterly terrifying, especially because they didn't come from the clouds or the waves or the sky or the rocks, the proper places for thunder.

Ariel had thrown herself to the ground under a cannon

and covered her ears until Eric had taken her into his arms and told her it was all right. That had almost made it all worth it.

And here was a man scratching his head with a gun. There were men with guns all over the market. Carlotta had spoken truly – this was not the same peaceful and sleepy seaside town it was half a decade before.

The place wasn't completely transformed, however. Past the soldiers was the usual line of stands and carts displaying vegetables, fruits, cheese, dried meat. Customers haggled over prices while eyeing great stalks of leafy things.

There was also an amazing scent of freshly baked… *something*.

Baking wasn't a thing under the sea. When Ariel lived at the castle with Eric she had tried breads, cakes, pies, rolls and sweets, and found them all mystifying (though delicious). They were like nothing she had ever eaten before and sometimes came to her plate still warm, which was also an odd way to eat food. Eric had bought her twelve different kinds of pie at a fancy shop in town and laughed as she had a bite of each, swooning.

That was the old Ariel. The one who dove right into town life and interacted a little too closely with a puppet show, poking at things in shops that were for display only, dancing to music that was probably just for listening to. Now she stood back and watched. Was this the result of age, and experience, and time? Or of not having a voice for so long? Had quiet observation just become a habit?

Maybe this would provide an excuse for her to gather more information.

Observation is all well and good, but only if it leads to a thoughtful plan of action!

She followed the delicious aroma until she came to a small bakery. In front of it a young man with red hair, not half as bright as Ariel's, was setting out savoury pies.

She pulled out her little satchel and went through the things in there: gems, pearls, coins, bits of mismatched and sea-changed jewellery that could be useful. Two coins looked like the same kind she had seen other people use; with those in her palm she cautiously approached the stand. She felt like she moved slower than when she was younger, as if the water on the Dry World had become heavier and thicker.

"Excuse me," she said, and it was still strange to hear her voice. The man looked up from his pies to give Ariel his full attention. There was a streak of flour in his red hair and a tired but pleasant smile in his eyes. So much plainer than Eric... *but still, so much more interesting than a merman!*

"How much are the..." She fought for the right word to speak aloud, which had no equivalent underwater. "That?" she pointed.

"Onion and cheese pie's a *real*," the man said.

Ariel held out her coins.

The man looked at her, raised an eyebrow, then carefully chose a single green coin.

Ariel tried to memorise it: the size, the colour, the smell. *One* real. *Made of the metal that tastes like blood.*

The baker, still mystified but too polite to say anything, picked out a good-looking pie and handed it to her.

"Thank you," Ariel said, trying to make her words sound normal.

Then she bit into the pie.

It was all those tastes she remembered from before. Fatty, doughy flour crust. *Cheese.* Spices and flavours that spoke of foreign Dry World places. And, she supposed, the overwhelming taste of *onion*. Green, and not unlike certain seaweeds. But stronger.

The baker just watched her as she chewed and enjoyed.

Ariel stopped. Didn't people eat the things they paid for?

She looked around and saw that no one else was gulping down their treats immediately. There went the old Ariel again. *Impulsive.*

"Ah, this is wonderful," she said quickly, sounding interested; as if she were eating it only to compare with other pies she had in the past. "Very unusual."

"It's my pickled *calçots*," the baker said triumphantly. "It is the wrong time of year for those, so I preserve them in the early spring, when they are harvested. A special treat, for an… unusual lady. I haven't seen you around the market. You must not be from Tirulia?"

"No, I'm from… farther south."

"The *ocean*, then?"

She began to choke, possibly on an onion. Or calçot.

But before she could come up with a suitable reply the baker was already talking again. "One of the islands, or the continent of Alkabua, I suppose."

"Oh, but I've been here before," she said smoothly, as if he were right in his guesses and therefore it didn't merit more discussion. "Tirulia has changed a bit since the last time I visited. There seem to be a lot more soldiers."

"Oh, aye." The baker's look soured. "Prince Eric, or should I say, Princess Vanessa, is much more hungry for war than the king and queen ever were. Of course there's always been the fight over water rights or passes through the mountains or a particularly fine hillside for vineyards… but this is a whole new cursed thing, and it's bad business, I don't mind saying."

"Why are you so against what the princess is doing? Specifically, I mean?"

The baker looked at her as if she were mad. "War is *war*. Fighting and death and more food for the soldiers and less for everyone else. Twenty-three Tirulian boys are dead and buried already. And still more boys flock to join the insanity, lured with promises of pretty uniforms and gold for their families. Have they been coming around and spending their new pennies on pies for their sweethearts? Certainly! Win for me! But rather less of a win for their dead comrades."

"Oh…" Ariel began, unsure what to say.

"And that won't be the end of it, I'll bet you *reales* to sweet buns, sister. There are already shortages because the trade routes are getting cut off. And we will lose more than our fair share of soldier boys, families, mothers, fathers, babies when the other countries decide to hit us back."

Ariel studied the baker: what was his age, really? He seemed young, but spoke with a strange authority on the subject. Like a mermaid suddenly made queen.

"You seem to know a lot about war," she ventured.

"My parents moved here from up north, where those kingdoms are always fighting. Kings and queens and princes and princesses like a giant bloody game of chess where no one cares about the pawns.

"*I* got out. I was nine. My oldest brother didn't. Enjoy your pie and treasure peace, while it lasts. You won't miss it until it's gone."

And with that, the pie maker turned his back on her.

Ariel was a little flummoxed. She was queen; no one ever turned his, her, or its back on her. To someone who couldn't speak aloud, that was the most effective, and devastating way to end a conversation with her.

Then she remembered her voice.

"Your pie was delicious. I will think over your words. Have a nice day."

The pie maker waved over his shoulder: not upset, just busy. He was speaking his mind to a customer who would listen and held nothing against her.

Ariel wandered away with mixed feelings. On the one hand, everything the baker said was troubling.

On the other hand, she was exploring a whole new world, successfully, *by herself.* She was getting to observe a completely different way of life, and it wasn't just about breathing air; it was how families and people worked, and how food was made, and customs and actions and habits, and it was all *fascinating.*

Of course she knew that a ruler's actions had an effect on the people, but up until now, she had thought only of the *direct* effect. She wouldn't send merguards to storm Eric's castle, for instance, because she didn't want to put their lives at risk. But… would she have thought of how sending soldiers into battle might impact bakers, down the line?

Was this something her father understood, and which had tempered his own decisions?

Father.

She hadn't forgotten her quest; she had just become distracted for a moment.

She ate her pie and made her way back through town, heading once again towards the beach. She passed the cart with the puppet show she had rudely interrupted years ago; sitting in the back was the man who made the puppets, carefully painting a lush set of eyelashes onto one of his manikins. *Fascinating.*

Of course merfolk had plays and costumes and costume balls, and dolls and temple figurines that boys and girls played with, making them 'talk'. But nothing was as rehearsed and polished as what the human did. Why didn't the mer have *that* art? Were the two peoples so different?

For there were obvious similarities between them that could not be denied. The tendency towards ridiculous monuments that commemorated unlikely events, for instance. The mer had a mural the size of a reef illustrating the division of the two worlds, embedded with gems and bright coral that hurt the eyes to look at. The Tirulians had an ugly fountain in the square where she and Eric had once danced. Neptune was carved into the face of the bowl, along with some utterly unrealistic dolphins. The Tirulians believed that the sea god had a fight with Minerva over who would be the patron god of Tirulia, and that he had won by creating this font of undrinkable salt water that was somehow channelled up from the sea.

(All wrong, as the mute Ariel couldn't explain to Eric at the time. Neptune had *lost* the fight, because he'd made a useless salt spring while Minerva/Athena had made the olive tree. Oh, and it took place in *Athens*, because, well, Athena.)

Besides monumental art and kings and queens, humans were very recognisably similar to mer in their normal, everyday lives. The women over there, heads bent together, were obviously gossiping. The men over there, heads bent together, were obviously discussing something they thought was *very important* and that they had great influence over, but which, of course, was also just gossip. A mother breastfed her baby, a beautiful fat-faced thing with the cutest feet.

How many other races were there on Gaia, more similar than different? Who would get along if just introduced properly? All they needed was a voice: the right voice, an understanding voice, a voice of reason that spoke everyone's language.

Ariel felt she had something there, the wisp of an idea, when something caught her eye and distracted her. Like a flash of sunlight that somehow manages to make its way, unobstructed and successful, to the sea floor and sparkles on a glistening white structure there.

Apples.

A tower of them. Bright red, red like blood, red like precious coral. Shining in the light. Some were half-green, which was both disappointing and yet more entrancing: did they *taste* different?

She would buy enough for all her sisters. Wouldn't that be a treat! Several for herself now, and a sack to present upon her return.

Not even realising she was salivating, Ariel approached. The vendor was old enough to be a great-granny, but large and strong-limbed, and her black eyes sparkled, full of intelligence and interest in the world around her.

"I would like those, please," Ariel said, pointing to the apples.

" 'Those'? Which ones?"

"All of them, please."

The woman laughed. "All of 'em? That's a pretty penny, girl. I'm expecting that poncy little buyer from the castle over here in a moment, I'm going to haggle her up good. What could *you* offer me?"

Wordlessly Ariel pulled out her little satchel again and poured its contents into her hand. This time she let the pearls and gems spill out with the golden coins: surely treasure enough to buy all the fruit.

The old woman's eyes widened.

"I'll take this," she said, choosing a gold coin, "and this," she said, choosing a pearl. Then she took her large hand and closed up Ariel's hand with the rest of the things. "And you just put that away. I'll get you a sack."

The woman rummaged around her stand and managed to fish out a dirty but sturdy burlap bag. With a sweep of her arm she guided the apples into the sack like a magician; not a single one spilt. She shook them down and then tied it with a piece of twine.

"Don't know how useful it will be, underwater, but it should hold for a while," the woman said.

"Thank you, I… what?"

"It's a marvel… your kind *do* like fruit of the land."

"I haven't the foggiest notion what you are talking about," Ariel said with great dignity.

"Those coins haven't been used in two hundred years," the woman said, nodding her chin at Ariel's satchel. "And those pearls and gems didn't come from no stronghold, no stolen purse. By the smell of 'em, they came straight from Davy Jones's locker."

"I… found… a chest… when I was walking… on the beach… and…"

As queen and as girl, as someone who could sing like the gods and someone who had been mute as a stone, one thing about Ariel had never changed: she was a terrible liar. Most of the time it didn't even occur to her to lie.

Which, now that she thought about it, would have made things a *lot* easier with her dad.

"Oh, a treasure chest found on a beach, like a pirate left it there," the old woman said, nodding seriously. "To be sure."

Ariel tried to think of something else.

The old woman leant forwards.

"Your secret's safe with me, seachild. I would give you all my apples in return for a favour some day instead, if I didn't need the money."

"What would you ask for?" Ariel asked, too intrigued to bother pretending further.

"I'd ask… well, if no emergency popped up to use it on, like 'I wish for someone to save my grandgirl from drowning' or something, well…" The old woman looked faintly embarrassed. "I'd ask to see *you*, in your true form, swimmin' out to sea. If I could see that, I'd know *all* the tales were true, all the good ones and bad ones. That there is more to the world than I see with my old brown eyes every day, and I'd die a happy woman, knowing there was magic."

Ariel was silent, overcome by the woman's words. The mermaid had probably been a little girl at the same time as this old woman. And the woman would die, happy or not, many hundreds of years before the Queen of the Sea had to begin contemplating her own mortality.

Ariel put her hands on the woman's and squeezed them.

"There is magic," she said softly. "There is always magic. Even if you can't see it."

The old woman looked at her for a long moment. Then she laughed. "Ah well, ye already paid, so no favour's necessary. But it sure would be nice to see you anyway, I've never inked a mermaid from real life! And I do them all the time... used to, leastways..."

"Inked?" Ariel asked curiously. "Are you an artist?"

"An artist of the skin. Argent the Inker, at your service!" She pushed up her sleeves and showed Ariel her arms. They were dark and freckled with even darker spots, scars and other spots of varying shades without a name or purpose. But in the places where the skin hadn't aged or stretched or sagged so much were some of the most incredible pictures Ariel had ever seen.

A ship with its sails billowed, a fat-cheeked cloud puffing wind to speed it along. A single wave, curled and cresting with foam flying off, so full of life and movement

Ariel almost felt it on her cheeks. A fish caught mid jump, honestly, in an unlikely contrapposto of tail fin and lips, but still, seemed to glitter in the light.

Everything was a single shade of dark blue; Ariel's mind filled in the colour without her even realising it. The fineness of the lines was almost unimaginable from such a mortal creature; all the pictures were as detailed and delicate as scrimshaw.

On skin.

"I've never seen anything like this," Ariel breathed. Of course sailors drowned, and sometimes their bloated bodies sank to the bottom of the sea before scavengers tore them up. Often they had tattoos: blurry, dark images of anchors and hearts and words like *Mum*. Nothing that bore any resemblance to what she saw now.

"I was quite famous, before my eyes started to go," the woman said proudly. "Sailors, captains, people from all over the world would come to see me, them that could afford it. As far away as Kikunari! Oh, I did some amazing things… an entire circus for a girl in Lesser Gaulica… ah, well. Now I'm selling apples to make ends meet. At least I have my little house and orchard by the sea. And my own teeth. There's them as have far less."

"What a fascinating story," Ariel breathed. She could

already hear the song in her head: something about an artist in a shack by the ocean, whose pictures came alive off her arms and kept her company… porpoises that dove into the waves, gulls that flew off her skin and into the air and…

… and squawked?

Ariel jumped. A real gull had broken her reveries: it had landed on a roof nearby and was flapping its wings and making noises at her. *Jona.*

"I must go," she said, throwing the sack of fruit over her shoulder as gracefully as she could. Things in this world were *heavy*. "But I will see you again."

"I pray you do," the woman said softly.

The mermaid smiled to herself as she walked away, wondering when the woman would find the satchel of gems and coins that she had left on the stand where the apples had been.

Eric

He gnawed on his quail leg contemplatively, thinking about the strange meeting with the metalworkers, and of misty fantasy mountains, and of how much simpler life would be if he were a sailor, or a metalworker, or a real prince who went out and found dragons.

Suddenly he leapt up and strode out of the room, feeling something akin to panic.

The halls were filled with strange people. He didn't remember it being like this before… before he was married. Some looked at him, *the prince*, suspiciously. Men in dark breeches and boots barely gave him a passing glance and whispered behind gloved hands. Representatives from eastern districts walked with broad steps and wore more traditional garb, loose shirts and broad leather belts. These gave the prince a nod at least. Women with waists so tiny and tight it was hard to see how they could breathe minced along in skirts too wide to easily fit through doors.

"Who *are* all these people?" Eric asked, more confused than ever. "When did they all start showing up in my castle?"

But of course, it all started when *everything* that was bad had started…

"… the night of my wedding." He paused, consciously directing his thoughts to that day. He replayed memories that were so dusty and unused they sprang up clear and glossy, unmarred by use or the merciful editing of time. Each moment played like… a play.

There really was *a mermaid. And a mer… uh, man?* La Sirenetta *was all real?*

A pair of soldiers walked by, and didn't even bother to salute the prince.

Am I mad? Eric wondered, feeling like a ghost as real life played on around him.

"Excuse me, I need your signature here, Your Highness." A stalk-thin man held out a small board with a paper neatly tacked to it, and a quill. *He at least sees me,* Eric thought dryly. "The dynamite from Druvest. I hate to bother you, but the vendor must get back on the next boat."

"Dynamite? The… explode-y stuff?" Eric winced at how stupid he sounded. But he couldn't think of any other way of asking.

"Yes, Your Highness. It's part of the new munitions order. Much more exciting than the bill for oats from Bretland I signed in your name last week, if I may say so. All new technology! What a world we live in."

"Yes, what a world," Eric repeated darkly. "No, I will not sign this now. I need to review our accounts first. No more orders for anything military without my review."

The man started to protest but saw the look in Eric's eyes. He chose instead to bow and back away. "Yes, Your Highness."

Eric sighed. He had read about dynamite, of course, and the idea *was* exciting, like firecrackers but bigger.

Much, much bigger.

And without the pretty coloured sparkles.

When had Eric agreed to such an order?

Why did he know that those two who hurried by him now, the ones in red jackets from Eseron, were there to discuss a potential alliance, allowing Tirulia to trade up through the northwest in case their land grab directly north failed?

For how many years had he been under the spell? Five? Six?

Air. He needed air. Sweet sea air.

The prince stumbled through the halls, desperately trying to undo his buttons, trying not to knock into anyone. *Everyone*. He ripped off the jacket and threw himself onto the first balcony he could find.

The sunshine and brisk, stinging breeze from the ocean had an immediately salutary effect. He took big gulps, leaning against the railing. When he closed his eyes he could imagine he was on a ship, surrounded by the water and gulls and a sail snapping in the wind.

When he opened his eyes he could see the gulls and the sea… but all that snapped were the banners flying above his castle.

And these banners no longer sported the beautiful Tirulian sailing ship that Eric had loved since infancy; now they were imprinted with a terrible, grasping octopus thing.

While his wi—*the princess* had been ordering munitions and seizing land and preparing invasions and changing their flag and who knows what else, he had done… what? *Nothing*. He hadn't put up a fight at all when Vanessa took over the day-to-day tasks of ruling. He had merely… grown bored, hanging around the castle with no responsibilities. And his ocean jaunts were strictly limited now; Vanessa didn't like him risking his life at sea. Or, perhaps, venturing out of the radius of the spell or hypnosis or whatever it was.

So he had begun to try his hand at real composition. Little movements, tiny concertos, even a ballad here and there. And all of Tirulia loved it, all of Tirulia encouraged him, even Vanessa. And thus he found a role and a purpose again: the Mad Prince, glamoured and dreamy, who wrote music while his wife ruled.

He found himself looking at funny spots in the sea, brown and black just under the water. Seals? Or mermaids?

He thought about Ariel. *Really* thought about her, for the first time in years. With the added insight of clear memory: the old ocean god hurling lightning, Vanessa hurling insults and waving a contract. The polyp. The sad, voiceless mermaid swimming away.

If Eric had just listened to his heart and not someone else's singing, none of this would have happened.

He *had* fallen in love with the voiceless red-haired girl. He was just too stupid and obstinate to recognise it. He loved everything about her. Her smile, the way she moved, the way she took delight in everything around her. She was impulsive, unmannered, willing to get dirty, a little strange and extremely hands-on. *And* beautiful. So different from all the princesses and ladies his parents had introduced him to.

If he had just married her, he would be… married to that girl. Who was a mermaid.

He blinked at the thought. *Imagine that!* He, Eric, who always loved the sea, could have married a child of the sea.

Would she have stayed human? Would she have eventually returned to the water, leaving him heartbroken? That happened in a lot of fairy tales. Sometimes after having a child.

Would their children have tails?

And what about his father-in-law? Imagine having *him* in the family, a mighty king of the sea!

He could have had all the adventure a prince could ever want just by staying home…

His thoughts slowly turned course, souring a little.

But if Ariel was a mermaid, what was *Vanessa*? Pretty and ostensibly human… but then again, Ariel had looked just like a human too.

Eric couldn't remember Vanessa looking any different. His princess had just appeared, walking on the beach. And then she met Eric… and sang… and married him… and then… all was grey.

He was like a fairy tale creature come out of a long sleep

to find everything changed, moved on without him – despite being awake the whole time.

The door to the balcony opened but Eric didn't bother looking around: he knew from the way it was carefully, precisely manipulated that it was Grimsby.

"Master Eric, are you feeling all right?" he asked, his tone absolutely neutral.

"Grimsby, what is that ship they are building there?" Eric asked, pointing towards town. The dry docks, which he often liked to watch from his spyglass if he couldn't get down there himself, were a strange mass of activity, like ants where you don't expect them. It was the peak of summer fishing; all energies should have been bent on catching summer flounder. Only after they been dried and salted properly, only after the autumnal equinox and harvest festival, should the town go back to the business of repairing nets and building ships… before the winter flounder and cod fishing seasons began.

"That is the *Octoria*, the first of three warships commissioned for the glory of Tirulia." Grimsby said it delicately, as if he had wished to clear his throat before answering but didn't get the chance. He busied himself with pulling out his pipe and preparing the bowl, possibly to give his hands something to do.

"I approved this?"

"You signed the order, Prince Eric, but I believe it was Princess Vanessa and her advisers who originated the plan and wrote up the decree." The butler frowned at his pipe, then went to tap it on the balcony and empty the old ash out into the water.

"Don't," Eric said distractedly, putting a hand out to stop him. "People live down there, you know."

Grimsby's eyes widened in concern, but he decanted the pipe onto the balcony floor instead, sweeping the ash into a corner with his foot.

"It's for the invasion of the north?" Eric asked, nodding at the warship.

"An alliance with Ibria requires that Tirulia provide the sea power, Your Highness."

Both men were silent for a moment. Eric stared out to sea; Grimsby looked at Eric, his pipe forgotten in his hand.

"She is going to bring us to war with the whole continent before this is over," the prince swore.

"Oh, I hardly think so, sir," the butler replied mildly. "Unless you conscript literally every citizen of Tirulia, you will be dealing with a civil uprising long before then. Sir."

Eric blinked. Grimsby's cold blue eyes and stalwart face gave no indication if he was being serious or flippant. The man never offered his uninvited opinion on affairs of the kingdom, much less made jokes about it.

"I came out to say that I had lunch delivered to your study since you and the princess left before you had finished, Master Eric," he added after a moment, finally putting the pipe away in his pocket. "So you may take it in private while you work on your music after your walk, as you are accustomed."

"Lunch? Compose? *Walk*?" Eric looked at him, aghast. "There's too much to do to have time to eat or... play around with music! I don't know where to start! Bring me the decree I signed for the warships, and the original order for dynamite, and *any* official correspondence with Ibria! At once!"

Grimsby's face broke out into a warm smile, like a beach that mostly sees cold rain and the pummel of waves but wants to prove it is entirely possible for it to enjoy the sun, if only given a chance. "I... *felt* there was something different about you today.

"Welcome back, Master Eric."

Ursula

After attending to her maquillage, Ursula put her muffler back into place and nodded approvingly at her 'public' face in the mirror.

"Everything is arranged with the guards, Mistress," Flotsam hissed.

"Excellent. Now all I need to do is figure out *this* mess." She pointed at her throat, not bothering to whisper. No one was around who mattered. With a wave, she dismissed Vareet. The little maid scampered off, hopefully to make sure the rest of the royal apartments were being cleaned properly. That stupid dog's hair got *everywhere*.

"Perhaps a new voice would help? A new... *donor*?" Jetsam suggested.

"That's not a bad idea," Ursula said thoughtfully. "Not a bad idea at all. I'll get right on that, later. So much to do... throwing the little redheaded twit off the trail of finding her father... cementing our relationship with Ibria so I can proceed with our military plans... but right now I have to deal with a *petitioner.* Ridiculous, really."

Her receiving room was little more than a large study with a few bookshelves and a partially hidden door in the back that led to the library proper. Taking up most of the space was a large naval-style desk strewn with the books she was currently reading, sheaves of notes, a log for meetings and a small burner for the teas and tisanes she told people she enjoyed for their... *medicinal properties.*

Which was not entirely a lie. While being princess gave her a different kind of power than she was used to, power over *people* rather than mystical forces, well, call her old-fashioned, but magic was still magic. Its potential for destruction surpassed everything else.

And she had none in the Dry World.

So she set to work researching magic of the *land.* Among the many occult trinkets she kept hidden were bloodstained crystals; the tongues of several extinct beasts;

a curvy, evil-looking knife with a shiny black blade and several books bound in strange leather that did not smell very good. They explained many things, from the proper sacrifice of small children to the use of certain herbs.

In one of these she ran across a particularly interesting spell known as a *circuex* that could potentially and permanently imbue her with magic that she could wield in the Dry World. Unfortunately it was a bit messy and bloody, involving lots of sacrificial victims and it required one very rare component. *Fortunately* this component was something she just happened to have, because, as said, she was a bit of a hoarder.

She played with the new golden chain round her neck and considered.

No, not yet. Casting the circuex required an awful lot of work and commitment. And an end to her fun with Tirulia! She had such plans for the little nation. Maybe she would pursue the matter later. For now she would work with her rather prodigious *non*-magical powers: manipulation, deception and all the gold in the coffers of the kingdom.

And as for the kingdom, right then she had to deal with more pressing princess duties. She settled herself primly into a tiny, very ornate golden chair with delicate curled legs that ended in the sweetest little tentacles.

Flotsam took a polished brass urn from a shelf and carefully tapped out leaves that resembled ashes more than tea. Jetsam decanted water from a crystal jug into a tiny copper kettle and set it on the burner. How he lit it would have been unclear to any human watching the scene.

One never knew when a tea like this would be needed…

"You may let in the first," Ursula announced grandly, only remembering to whisper at the end.

"Lucio Aron, of the St. George Fishermen's Cooperative," Flotsam said snidely. Ursula tried to not roll her eyes. She was a *princess*. She did not have time for fools such as this.

A small man with clothes noticeably shabbier than the metalworkers' came in, bowing as he went. He clutched his cap and seemed generally uncomfortable.

"Thank you for seeing me, Your Highness." One hand went from his cap to his moustache, a plain, albeit thick, salt-and-pepper affair. His brown eyes were almost fully shaded by woolly eyebrows. "I wish my daughter could have come. She loves all the… royal things, you know. Princess things. Gowns, teacups, golden spoons. She's even mooning over several of the Drefui boys, sons of the duke, you know. I told her, 'You'll always be *my* princess, but don't set your sights above your station.'"

"What is it you want?" Ursula whispered, barely able to contain her irritability.

"Beg your pardon?" he asked, leaning forwards.

"What," she whispered as loudly as she dared. "Do. You. Want."

"Oh." He blinked, surprised at what he saw as an odd change in the conversation. He took his cap off and twisted it in his hands, dark skin cracking into white lines round his knuckles and wrists and palms and scars. "It's just… we need a new fishing trawler, Your Highness. I mean, I would like *us* to get it, of course, but one of the other companies would be better than nothing. We've been short one since the *Chanderra* sank."

"We're in the middle of a number of military campaigns," Ursula whispered haughtily. "I can't be throwing money around willy-nilly."

Lucio leant forwards, nodding as if he understood.

Everyone was silent.

He obviously hadn't heard a word she said.

"She said she's not going to buy you a new ship *because the funds are being spent on war,"* Jetsam hissed impatiently.

Lucio blinked first at him in confusion, then at Vanessa.

"No, no, you misunderstand, Your Highness. We have the funds. It's just that the shipyard is busy working on your warships full time. We were wondering if maybe… you could take a break… or… maybe establish another shipyard. Yes! Another shipyard. That would be good. For everyone."

Ursula's eyebrows shot towards the ceiling.

"You want me to *what*?" she whispered. "Waste time with another building project for, *what*? So you can *fish*?"

"Yes, Your Highness. So we can fish. That is what we do."

He was obviously terrified… but it was also obvious that he had a cause and a belief he was committed to, and he wouldn't back down.

Ursula hated people like that.

"I think. As a princess. I know. What is best. For my people," she whispered, slowly and clearly.

"But…"

"Your audience is over," Flotsam added swiftly.

Ursula whispered something that none of the three men could understand. All leant forwards in confusion.

"Your *daughter*," she said, letting a little of her real voice come through.

The fisherman looked understandably startled.

"Yes?"

"What is her *name*?" she said.

"Julia," he said, first seeming confused, then saying her name again with pride. "*Julia.* A beautiful, but sometimes naïve, girl."

Good.

Ursula *loved* people like that.

Flotsam took the fisherman by the elbow and steered him out.

The sea witch wondered for a moment how, with all their fables, stories and morality plays, humans still fell into the same old traps. It was kind of amazing. With their pathetically short lives they repeated the same mistakes of previous generations, almost as if they were all one endless being. Why tell a stranger the real name of someone you love? Why brag to a person in power about the beauty or skills of your son or daughter? Why offer up any information, or any need, when it could be used against you?

"Send in the next," Ursula said with a chuckle. The meeting with the fisherman had put her in a surprisingly good mood after all.

"Iase Pendrahul of Ibria," Flotsam announced.

With rather more sureness than she liked, the ambassador, spy, sauntered calmly into the room. *Now* that's *a powerful gait,* the sea witch thought. His skin was clear and his cheekbones high, his hazel eyes lit from within like an ember you thought you had put out. Thick, curly brown hair attacked the air around his head, barely contained in a riotous ponytail.

"My dear Iase," Ursula whispered indicating the only other chair, a stool, really, with no back, set there for the express purpose of making the other person feel lesser.

Yet the representative from Ibria took it and sat arrogantly at ease.

"I've heard you have a cold. A thousand blessings on your health," he said, touching his heart.

"Forget about it, it's nothing," she whispered. "Let's talk about our alliance."

"We can talk, or at least *I* can," he said with a smile that didn't reach his eyes, "but I do not see any advantage to our siding with you. Your fleet is still short three of the warships you swore to provide, six, I believe, was the original promise. Your land skirmishes have been of questionable success at best. Burning down defenceless villages isn't really much of an accomplishment, I'm fairly certain Gaius Octavius would agree with me on that one. Ibria is wealthy enough. We have no reason to spend resources on a war that doesn't directly lead to our advantage."

"Oh, but it will," Ursula whispered, putting a hand on his arm.

Iase stared at her fingers with distaste.

"I'm sorry, what?" he asked.

"It will," she hissed louder.

"You'll forgive me, Your Highness, but you have given me no proof of that. I see no reason to make deals with a princess who dresses prettily but lacks any strategic ability."

"You refuse to deal because I am a *woman*?" Ursula

growled, perhaps a little loudly, in her own voice.

"On the contrary," Iase said, patting her hand and then removing it from his arm. "I have had many dealings with fine women I respect. Including at least one pirate captain. It is *you*, personally, Princess Vanessa, whom I am hesitant to entrust the resources or future of my country with."

The two were silent for a moment, looking into each other's eyes. His were steady and dark; hers glittered strangely.

Ursula wished she were underwater. She wished she had her tentacles. She wished she had her *old* necklace. She wished she had anything she could smite him with, frankly, a large piece of coral would have done nicely.

First she lost her stolen voice, and with it the charm and *forget* spells that made dealing with the humans around her easier. *Now* it looked like she was losing a potential, and very powerful, ally. Not only would this be a severe setback for her war plans, but her failure would be the talk of the court. She would look weak and pathetic and incapable of mustering the help they needed to conquer their neighbours. And the weak were devoured. It was the way of the world.

"Thank you for your honesty," she finally whispered.

"I beg your pardon?"

"Oh, never mind. I need some tea for my throat. Join me?" She indicated the bubbling teapot: this gesture was perfectly clear, even if what she said was not. Flotsam was suddenly at the desk, laying out a pair of beautiful Bretlandian teacups, golden spoons, a fat little jar of honey and some lemon slices.

"Don't mind if I do," Iase said carelessly. "Feel a tickle in my throat myself."

She put the pretty gold strainer, not silver, no no, never silver; when prepared properly the metal had the power to negate certain desired effects of a potion, over his cup and poured, and over her cup, and poured. Strangely grey liquid came out, neither opaque nor completely translucent. It was precisely the same colour at different depths.

Each person doctored the drink the way he or she liked: lemon, two lumps… Ursula put a candied violet in hers, one that had a silver dragée as its centre.

"Good for the throat, eh?" he asked, holding the cup up to toast her. "To life!"

"To friends," Ursula whispered over the rim of her teacup.

He raised his cup again before bringing it to his mouth, but waited until she sipped before taking a draught himself.

She watched him, the grey liquid pouring over his lips and into his mouth… and he swallowed…

Ariel

On the fourth tide she was back at her lagoon as promised.

Flounder leapt into the air, flipping himself like he hadn't since he was small.

"Ariel!! *Talk! SAY SOMETHING!*" he cried.

She smiled, feeling her cheek tug to one side the way it used to when she was indulging her best friend. She closed her eyes and put her hands in a student-y clasp, reciting:

"There was a young guppy from Thebes, whose fins would often grow—"

"Ha-*HA*!"

Flounder leapt into the air again.

She laughed too, and ran into the water to hug him, unconcerned about her clothes. They were uncomfortable and hangy and close anyway, much heavier than what mer chose to wear. Flounder cuddled and leapt and nuzzled her like a puppy before recovering himself.

"Tell me all about it!"

So she did. And it was strange, telling a story with her mouth. She let her hands do some signing. It would have been uncomfortable keeping them still.

"Wow," Flounder said when she was done. "That's all… crazy."

Jona dropped silently from the skies and landed on a nearby rock with the delicacy of something that wasn't a seagull. "What did you learn in town?"

Ariel sighed and sat down in the shallow water. A warm breeze picked up the tendrils of her hair that were sticking out of the head cloth. She wrapped her arms round her knees, feeling young and exposed.

"I learnt it is the wrong season for calçots. I learnt about tattoos.

"I learnt that Ursula is using Tirulia as the jumping-off point for her private empire, seizing land from neighbours who probably aren't strong enough for reprisals and that she is antagonising other, larger powers. I learnt that the town is full of soldiers. I learnt that twenty-three of them have died in her crusade and yet dozens more boys go to join up because of the promise of gold for their families and the gold buttons on their uniforms."

Flounder gulped. Jona let out an avian hiss.

"And all I can think of are these two things. One, I am in some ways responsible for those twenty-three who will swim no more."

Flounder started to open his mouth; by habit Ariel just held up a finger to silence him.

"Two, I think about what *I* would do as ruler of Tirulia. If I were Eric, thrown into this mess now. Human politics and life seem far more dynamic than mer. I've never had to deal with anything like it in my time as queen. Nor has my father. Nor my father's father."

"Oh, but what about the Great Kelp Wars?" Flounder asked with a shiver.

"That was over an eon ago," Ariel pointed out gently. "There have been no wars, no battles, no… large *disagreements* since then. We've lost touch with the Hyperboreans and haven't heard from the Tsangalu in decades. We exchange Great Tide gifts with the Fejhwa but little else. We have had nothing but silence and peace for decades."

"Sounds like a utopia," Jona said. "Especially if no one is grappling over the last tasty morsel."

Ariel smiled. "Yes. Nothing but arts and leisure, beauty and philosophy… but it's all the same, and no one has had a desire to go *find out* what happened to the Hyperboreans or Tsangalu, or acquire anything from them besides presents. Surely their art and philosophy would be interesting, and might invigorate our own… somewhat static culture? The humans, on the other hand, are still exploring their world, every crevice and cranny."

"But…" Flounder made a face. "But we were here to get your father back. Not to get involved in human things."

"Yes, but the two are intertwined," Ariel said, though she was impressed with his desire to stick to the point. The old Flounder would have let her talk indefinitely and hung on her every word. This was better. She *needed* friends like him right now. "I had to find out what the consequences of my actions were, and unfortunately, I have satisfied that. I have a duty to make things right for the Tirulians, in addition to, *after*, saving my father. He can help us defeat Ursula once he's back in his original form and king again.

"Unfortunately, it's also going to be much harder to find him now, because as I said before, she has been alerted to my presence. I made the first move, I had the element of surprise and I blew it."

"Stop beating yourself up, Ariel," Flounder said sternly. "There's no guarantee you would have found him the first time you looked, anyway. Ursula isn't *stupid*. She's not going to leave the king around in a vase labelled *Ariel's Father, Don't Touch*. Just because you made the first move doesn't mean you would have been successful. Games take a long time, and a lot of moves, before someone wins."

"But I don't know how much time we have now. I don't even understand why Ursula kept my father around *this* long. Yes, she likes an audience and probably loves bragging about her triumphs to him… but even she must get bored of that eventually. What if she's keeping him around for some other reason? Which I have… interrupted?"

She squeezed her hands in sudden panic, pulled at her braids since she couldn't run her fingers through her hair.

"Now that you've found him, you're terrified of losing him again," Jona said quietly.

Ariel nodded, too full of emotion to trust her words. That was exactly it. What if she had set something in motion by trying to find him? What if something happened? It would be her fault, all over again. And she would never get him back.

"I have to go back to the castle," she said, fighting down

the childish surge of panic. She stood up and tried to give her friends a reassuring smile. "Even though it's a risk. At least I have a better understanding of the situation now. I'd better disguise my voice, huh? Since up until now everyone has only heard Vanessa using it. *Mebbe I shood tahhk liiike this.*"

She deepened her voice and put her hands on her hips, made a frowny face.

Flounder couldn't help laughing. Jona leapt into the air for a moment, letting out a squawk.

She wrung the water out of her skirts and prepared for the walk back to face a castle full of sea witches and soldiers who were probably waiting to grab her.

"Hey, Ariel," Flounder called shyly. "Before you go… could you… could you sing that lullaby? The one you used to sing to me after I lost my mother?"

Her eyes widened. "Flounder, you haven't asked me that in *years*… even before I lost my voice."

"And I won't ask again! It's just that…" he looked around. Jona politely pretended to watch something out in the sea, over by the far rocks. "We're alone here. No one from Atlantica is going to hear us. I don't know when you're going to have another chance."

And Ariel, who lost her voice for years and had mixed

feelings about singing for others, sang more sweetly than she ever had before, or ever would again. And no one heard but one fish, one seagull, the sand and the water and the evening breeze coming over the waves, and the rising moon.

Sebastian (and Flounder)

"I have been waiting over a week now for an answer!"

A barracuda towered over the throne in a way Sebastian was pretty sure he wouldn't have if Ariel had been sitting there, voice or no. The little crab glanced nervously at the guards: one a mer, one a surprisingly large weever fish with venomous spines. The two exchanged a look that was certainly not respectful, but nevertheless leant in protectively, the tips of their spears coming close enough to touch above his head.

The barracuda scooted backwards, but recovered himself quickly.

Fortunately there weren't many there to observe the scene; it was late in the tide and even the most dogged petitioners had gone home to wait until the next day. Or have dinner.

Or do something civilised, because they are civilised *people, unlike this shiny-scaled bully.*

Threll and Klios, the dolphin amanuensis, floated on the dais, but otherwise the throne area was empty except for a few cleaning sardines and some planktonic jellyfish that couldn't fight against the current enough to leave. Dark water curved overhead in a deep turquoise dome, full and empty as the sea always was before a storm. Despite the guards, Sebastian felt very, very alone.

"My boys took care of the wreck," the barracuda said defensively. "We cleaned up everything real good. Now it's time for you guys to hold up your end of the deal."

"Royalty doesn't 'hold up' 'ends of deals'," Sebastian said haughtily, emboldened by the sharp spears overhead.

"Especially when the vendor is asking for far more than what was originally agreed," the amanuensis muttered, looking over a row of figures on his tablet.

"If Ariel was here, she would deal with me fairly." The barracuda opened his mouth a crack, a move that usually foretold a strike.

"Oh, she would deal with you fairly, all right," Sebastian said menacingly, snapping a claw at the fish. "Be glad it is *me* and not *her* dealing with you. Now go away, and maybe if you're lucky I'll see you another week."

The barracuda gnashed his teeth, and with a last warning flip of his tail, angrily swam off.

The moment he was gone Sebastian collapsed on the armrest, a little *ticktickticktick* pile of exoskeleton and claws and sad eyes.

"What are we going to *do*?" he moaned. "If Ariel doesn't return soon the whole kingdom is going to collapse."

"One annoyed barracuda does not a collapsed kingdom make," Threll said with a sniff.

The amanuensis saluted them and swam off into the depths, done for the evening. The little seahorse followed suit. Sebastian raised a weary claw in goodbye.

"What's with everyone being so mopey-looking?" Flounder asked, scooting in from the side.

"FLOUNDER!" Sebastian leapt up in excitement. He looked behind the fish, back and forth, eagerly scanning the sea. "How is she? *Where* is she? Does she have King Triton?"

Flounder stopped where he was in the water, hovering there. "Uh… no. She hasn't found him yet. And she's not with me. She's… um… made progress, but still has… some work to do…"

Sebastian frowned at the large, brightly coloured fish.

"Flounder. You are lying to me about something."

"Me? No. Nope."

Sebastian clicked slowly, sideways, up to the fish. Hunting.

"Is she… *really* all right? Did you lose her? Has something happened?"

At *has something happened*, Flounder's face began to swell. He felt all the blood rush to his front and swished his tail to try to stay calm. He *wouldn't* betray her. He *wouldn't*.

"I didn't lose her," he said tightly. *That* was true, at least.

"Yet you are not *with* her. You are supposed to be *with* her. If she is not here, *you* should not be here, either. You should be *there*. With her. Protecting her."

"I don't know how much good I could do protecting the Queen of the Sea," Flounder said, a little archly. "She sent me back to give you an update, Sebastian. Scuttle and his, uh, great-grandgull are keeping an eye on her on the land."

"YOU LEFT HER FATE TO A PAIR OF SEAGULLS?"

"Settle down, Sebastian. She's fine. More than fine. And she's not a helpless little mer any more, even you should see that. These things just take time."

"Well, I hope they don't take *too* much more time," came a voice from behind them.

Attina hovered in the water, arms crossed. The look on her face was as spiky as the decorations that stuck out from her thick auburn hair.

"I want Daddy back," she announced grimly. "And failing that, I want someone ruling the kingdom who can actually command a little respect around here."

At this Sebastian looked utterly defeated. Flounder saw his friend shrink into himself and frowned.

"Princess Attina, perhaps what is needed is an actual member of royalty ruling the kingdom in their absence," he suggested coldly.

Sebastian gawked at Flounder. It was so… not… Flounder.

Well, old Flounder, anyway.

The mermaid glared at him.

"Nice try, Flipper," she said with a sniff. "But you know that being queen was part of Ariel's punishment for losing our father. She can't escape it by turning into a human and running away to the Dry World forever."

And for the second time that evening, a tail fin was flipped and someone swam angrily off.

Sebastian and Flounder exchanged weary looks.

"This is all… very *hard*," Sebastian said, without his usual loquaciousness.

"I know," Flounder said with a sigh. "But the moon is waning and we're approaching the neap tide, when the ocean is pulled farthest back from the shores."

"Flounder, I know what a *neap tide* is."

"My point is that the trident's power will also be at its lowest, so she *has* to come back soon! With or without her father. Or she'll suddenly turn into a mermaid, flopping around on the land."

"That would be a sight," Sebastian said thoughtfully. "A very, very bad sight."

And for once, the fish didn't disagree with the crab.

Ariel

The first part, at least, was easy. There was no issue trailing along with the other servant girls and boys as they finished up their errands and returned to the castle; many were already gossiping and flirting, done with work whether or not they were officially done. A couple of young men were definitely looking at her. She tried not to smile.

But then… several girls were looking at her, and whispering to each other. And they didn't look appreciative *or* jealous.

Ariel began to feel uneasy.

She had filled her apron with pretty shells, thinking her

excuse could be that Vanessa wanted them to decorate her bath. She had thought that she fit right in with the other servants carrying piles of wood, bins of rubbish, baskets of eggs… but maybe not?

There were *four* guards flanking the servants' entrance this time. Had they been there previously? She couldn't remember. They definitely looked more alert than when she had snuck in earlier, these scanned each and every person who passed, sometimes directly in the eye. Ariel hesitated.

One of the guards spotted her and frowned.

As casually as she could, Ariel turned round and walked back against the flow, peeling off to the strip of beach right in front of the castle in case she had to make a quick getaway into the waves.

What she saw there stopped her dead in her tracks.

At first glance, it seemed silly, no, *insane*. Royal guards were using long poles to draw things in the sand, over and over again, like children punished by a teacher for spelling something wrong.

Why would Ursula do this to them? Had she gone completely off the deep end? Was it some sort of weird disciplinary thing? But then Ariel stood on her tiptoes and saw *what* they were drawing: *runes*.

Atlantica runes.

Upside-down from her perspective, because they were facing the sea.

THE MOMENT YOU ARE SPOTTED ON THESE GROUNDS

YOUR FATHER DIES

Ariel backed away slowly as the letters burnt themselves into her eyes.

Then she turned and ran…

… and slammed chest first into Carlotta, who grabbed her by the arm and pulled her into the shadow of a pine.

"I saw you try to get in just now. *What are you doing here?*" she hissed. "We're on high alert because of what you've done. I assume it was you who took the necklace? Vanessa is in a murderous mood! Surprised she hasn't locked up poor little Vareet. She's rampaging around, doubling the guards, offering rewards for information… and doing strange witchcraft. Those symbols of hers…"

Ariel shook her head. "That is a message for me. She is threatening to kill my father if I come looking for him… which I have."

The maid blinked at her.

"Oh, yes, I can talk now," the mermaid added.

"Does this have something to do with the…" Carlotta

said, indicating her neck. The nautilus. Or possibly a voice.

Ariel nodded and held up her wrist so the maid could see the leather band, the broken bit of shell attached to the golden bail. "I smashed it, breaking the spell, and now I have my voice back again, and she has none. Or her own, rather."

"That *would* explain the whispering and the muffler and the talk of colds," Carlotta said, a little desperately, as if that one bit of logic were her lifeline.

Ariel felt bad for the woman, who was obviously having a hard time dealing with it all, directly confronted with the truth of magic.

"Everything's clearer now, you know," Carlotta said, falling heavily onto a tree stump. She waved her hand around. "That day. The cake I helped make. The lightning. I may… have even… *seen* you… your tail."

She looked Ariel up and down, as if for the first time. Then her eyes rested on the apron full of shells.

"What in the name of all that is good and holy is *that*? Something for a spell? More magic? More… sea stuff?"

"No, it's part of my disguise," Ariel said. "If anyone asked me what I was doing I would say it was for Vanessa."

"*Shells?*" Carlotta asked, starting to laugh. Ariel recognised that laugh. It was the beginning of hysteria. "From the beach? And *driftwood*?"

"They're beautiful," Ariel protested.

"Oh, oh, I know," Carlotta said, laughing and wheezing. "I'm sure you think so. But nobody wants those. Not a princess, not even a fake one, like Vanessa. There *was* a fad for a bit where fancy girls with nothing better to do would glue lots of tiny shells to boxes or frames like mosaics… hideous, really… but those were *tiny* shells. Dear, you wouldn't have lasted a moment even if you'd made it inside the castle. Oh, what are we to do?"

"I have to find my father," Ariel said firmly. "He is the King of the Sea and Ursula's prisoner. She turned him into a polyp. She has him hidden here somewhere. I need to find him and free him. Then, together, we can defeat the sea witch and free Tirulia from her rule forever."

Carlotta just stared at her as she said all that.

Then the maid shook her head vigorously, as if she could physically thrust away all the crazy things she had just heard.

"Whatever else, you can't set four steps inside that door without someone stopping you. You sound exactly like Vanessa! And believe me, everyone knows what she sounds like. Even if you disguise your voice, you still don't sound like a servant girl. I need to think about what to do. Who could help us? Who could be clever and figure out a plan?

You need someone on the inside, more connected than me. Someone like…"

She looked up, her eyes suddenly set and certain.

"Grimsby."

Carlotta led Ariel by the hand into the castle, screaming nonsense at her and waving a hand in her face at just the right time when people looked too closely, especially the guards. The Queen of the Sea just let herself be dragged along; she was too terrified just being in the castle to do much else. Ursula could always be counted on to make good with her threats; Triton's life was definitely being put in danger by this. And Carlotta had only slightly eased her fears, bragging about the number of secret lovers' trysts she had covered for.

Ariel was also strangely embarrassed, and it wasn't just because she was being pulled along by the housemaid like a girl in trouble. They were going to see *Grimsby*. Although the butler bore no real resemblance to her father (and was, moreover, a servant) he nevertheless possessed an air of ancient patriarchal wisdom. His was the final and correct word in the castle. Sometimes more so than his master's.

The butler was downstairs in his tiny 'office', little more than an upright desk in an oversized cupboard. He was admonishing a footman for some indiscretion. The young man was handsome, olive-cheeked and blushing fiercely. While Grimsby spoke mildly, his eyes were ironic and cold.

But when he saw the look on Carlotta's face he changed his tone, hurrying the whole thing along.

"Yes, well, don't do it again. Am I clear? You're dismissed."

"Yes, Mr Grimsby, thank you. Thank you, Mr Grimsby..."

The youth, overwhelmed at the shortening of the lecture and cancellation of whatever punishment he had assumed he would get, practically fell over himself to get out of the room. In doing so he tangled with Carlotta and caught sight of Ariel, who was hiding behind the maid. She smiled at him. A dazed expression came over his face: one of utter rapture. It was a full moment before he recovered himself and ran down the hallway.

"Carlotta, what is the matter?" Grimsby demanded.

She didn't say a word, just stepped aside to reveal Ariel.

Ariel found herself shy, unqueenly, overcome with the urge to look down at the ground. But she didn't.

Grimsby's eyes, sunk deep behind veils of skin like parchment, widened like a child's. There was recognition, and for the most painful fraction of a moment, *delight*.

Then all too swiftly his face hardened and his eyebrows set like thunderheads over a cliff. The change was like a spear of ice thrust into Ariel's heart. She hadn't realised how much she had looked forward to seeing the old man again.

"Ariel, you look well," he said coldly.

"And you look as dapper as ever," she responded.

The thunderheads shot up, high into the sky of his brow in surprise.

"Yes, I can talk, and please," she stepped forwards and took his hand in both of her own. "I know things are… confusing and they ended poorly, and involved me, but I'm here to try to make it right."

"You have Princess Vanessa's voice," he said, seizing the one thing that he could comment objectively on.

"She's not a princess, she's not Vanessa, and it's *my* voice. That *she* stole. If you allow me, I'll fill in all the details of the story that both of you are probably just remembering."

Grimsby shook his head, obviously unhappy with the untidiness of it all. "Well, come in, shut the door and tell me."

It was more than a little cramped in his tiny space; Carlotta's breathing seemed to take up most of the room. Ariel told her story as quickly and succinctly as she could.

When she was done there was silence but for the forlorn calls of a gull outside somewhere.

I've got to make myself seen through a door or window before they get too worried, she thought, imagining an all-out gull attack on the castle.

"You see?" Carlotta said. "That's why I figured she had to talk to you. It's all... very complicated."

"So, Ariel. You fell in love with Eric and became a human, and this... sea witch also became human, probably to make sure you failed in your quest," he recited the facts in his clipped Bretlandian accent, as calmly as a teacher lecturing history.

"Yes," Ariel said.

"But the sea witch never returned to the sea. She... stayed. And became our princess. And now rules Tirulia. With an iron fist."

"Yes," Ariel said, a little less certainly.

"And you're here to find your father, restore him to his rightful throne and depose the sea witch."

When you couldn't speak, you couldn't say *ummmm* or *errr* or use any space-filling noises to indicate thinking or forestall potential embarrassment. *All of which would be very nice right now. But queens don't do that, either.*

"I came to find my father," she answered as truthfully as she could. "Everything else depends on that. We will do all we can to free you from the sea witch, afterwards."

"Yes… about this 'sea witch'. Do we have proof that she is indeed a… cecaelia?"

"Cecaelia?" Carlotta interrupted.

"Half human, half octopus," Grimsby explained. "Like a mermaid, but with tentacles."

"Half in the form of the *gods*," Ariel corrected gently. "We are not humans who are half fish, the way you people always say. We are children of Neptune and are not like you, even half you, at all."

Both Carlotta and Grimsby looked surprised and a little confused. *All right, maybe not the time to get into ancient prejudices,* Ariel decided. Some day if she stuck around in the Dry World she would set it straight.

"Very well," Grimsby said carefully, clearing his throat. From the new look in his eye it was obvious he was re-evaluating her. She wasn't the playful, simple girl who couldn't speak she had been before. She was someone who had things to say, who had goals, plans, *opinions*.

A woman, perhaps.

"There is little I can do myself, besides, er, keeping an eye out for something that looks like a… polyp in captivity. Which I will absolutely do, of course. But it seems now that spells have been broken, certain truths are becoming apparent and our kingdom is driven even deeper into war with our enemies, well, something else must be done about this whole matter *immediately*. And I do not have the authority to decide that. Neither does Carlotta. Ariel, I think you know what you must do.

"You must go talk to Eric."

Ariel felt her cheeks flame and she looked at the floor, not moving her head, just her eyes. But only for a moment. She quickly regained herself and forced herself to look at the old man. His expression had softened.

"I'm a trifle surprised you didn't seek him out earlier, on your own," he said softly. "I don't know much about magic and undersea kings, but I'm fairly certain the two of you felt something strong for each other. Isn't that *part* of the reason you came back? To see him?"

She opened her mouth to disagree… but stopped. The old human was right.

He put a hand on her shoulder, like he might a soldier's. "You two… began a series of events which wound up involving all of us up in this mess. And I think maybe the two of you can get us out of it. It's fate, or some such. It feels rather right. Rather Greek. Don't you think, Carlotta?"

"It's fated," the maid agreed. "I don't know about the Greeks."

"Anyway, Carlotta was right to bring you to me and I am

right in sending you on. Whatever veil has clouded Eric's thoughts is gone now, and I think he would receive you in the right frame of mind."

"But how can I see him without Ursula finding out? She has guards and soldiers everywhere!" Ariel spoke the words clearly while her head was muzzy with possibility. "I won't endanger my father!"

"Eric goes for a walk after dinner," Grimsby said, straightening himself up. "Along the beach, a long way, north beyond the castle. He walks when he's not... *allowed* to get on a boat."

"I can provide a distraction for the princess," Carlotta said. "There's a hatmaker been *begging* for an audience. Vanessa loves posing and preening. We'll keep her tied up in bows and feathers for at least a watch."

"Excellent. It's a plan," the butler said, clasping his hands together.

"Thank you, Grimsby," Ariel said, kissing him on the cheek. "This is all a little... difficult for me. It must be impossible for you."

"Oh, no, not at all, dear child," he said, blushing a little. "And think, when this is all over, I shall be able to publish my memoirs about how I helped a mermaid!"

Ariel

She stood behind an old wreck, the hull of a fishing vessel that had been lost decades before and was then swept far up the marsh during a particularly stormy high tide. Blasted by sand and wind and sea, it now looked like the bones of a whale, its chest facing the sky.

When Ariel and Grimsby were trying to figure out the best place for her to meet Eric, Carlotta mentioned that the boat was a place where many couples, wishing to… speak in private… betook themselves. The thought should have given the mermaid a smile, but now she was overcome by the mood of the place.

The wind picked up and blew tiny whitecaps across tide pools like minnows jumping. Ariel put her hand up, feeling the breeze in her fingers. Things changed *much faster* up here than they did under the sea.

And yet change came nonetheless; it had been several days now since the height of the spring tide, when the full moon worked with the sun to grant the sea her greatest reach over the land. Now tides were lower and weaker, and would become lower still in the coming week. So too the power of the trident dipped.

Soon she would have to return to the sea.

A movement at the edge of the marsh caught her eye. Eric emerged from behind the stand of trees that blocked the view of the castle, and the view of anyone watching *from* the castle. His stride was sure and he looked around boldly, but it was with just a frisson of confusion; he had not been told whom he was meeting, only that it was important. He wore his old boots and beige trousers, and one of the thick-woven tunics sailors in Tirulia wore on wet and chilly days. A faded blue cap was pulled firmly down on his hair. His ponytail escaped out the back, curling round his left shoulder.

Ariel grasped the bleached wood of the boat at the sight of him. He seemed… so much *realer*. All those times she had dozed off with visions of the young, handsome prince in her head… and here he was actually coming to meet her. Life was far more detailed than dreams. His neck bent into his collar, his hands were shoved deep into his pockets like he was cold. Something unimaginable in a fantasy.

Ariel looked down at the outfit she wore, just a dress and apron. How cold *was* it? For humans? Was she dressed inappropriately?

Eric continued to look around for whomever he was supposed to meet. He put a hand to the back of his head and scratched there, pushing up the edge of his cap.

It was this gesture, this boyish, unprincely, unrehearsed gesture, that made Ariel step out from behind the boat.

"Eric?" she called.

The reaction that overcame him was not the one that she expected: his face fell into a snarl of impatience, exhaustion and disgust.

"*Vanessa*, how many times have I told you that I *need* these walks—"

But when he turned and saw her, *really* saw her, he fell silent.

Ariel smiled. Then she carefully took off her headscarf so he could better see her hair.

"You… It's *you*…" he whispered.

"It's me."

He started to open his mouth, but she interrupted.

"Before you say anything else, this is *my* voice. Vanessa stole it. Which you should know… I hear you wrote an opera about it…"

Eric's hands fell to his sides, useless. His fingers fluttered as if there were something he wanted to do with them, some sign, some gesture, but he couldn't think of what.

That's oddly familiar, Ariel thought.

"It's all true… the opera…" He didn't blink as he stared at her. She could almost feel his gaze on her hair, the braids, her eyes, her dress, her feet, her arms.

He rushed forwards, then stopped. His eyes were as clear and blue as the hot summer sky. His skin was not as peachy-dewy as when they first met; it was tauter, drawn more over his cheekbones, his brow, his nose. It was darker and drier too, but no less handsome. Just different. She lifted a finger, overcome with the urge to feel it.

Eric caught her hand in his before she could finish the motion, and took her other hand in it as well.

"You're a… mermaid?"

"Yes."

"And you can talk now?"

"Yes."

"And you came back for me?"

His eyes shone with open emotion: hope and wonder after a long period of darkness, the beautiful look of a child who, having passed through the gloom of puberty, is suddenly shown that unicorns and fairies are real after all.

Ariel was taken aback. She hadn't expected this, not exactly. She hoped for his joy, she expected his confusion. But this was… too much. She wanted to disappoint him about as much as she wanted to put a spike into her own heart.

"I came back for my father," she made herself say. The Queen of the Sea had little difficulty stating the truth out loud; a younger Ariel would have stuttered. "I received word he might still be alive, as a prisoner of Ursula."

"Oh," Eric blinked. "Your father. Of course."

"That's the main reason I have returned. We had thought he was dead all these years. I'm here to rescue him."

"I just thought… I mean… I had hoped… you came back to take me away from all of this. To go live happily ever after somewhere. Under the sea, maybe."

"You would drown under the sea."

"I'm drowning up here. I've *been* drowning. For years. Under water, it felt like. Now that I'm waking up, of course it makes sense that you would come. And… end it."

Ariel had a brief flash of where some of his thoughts were heading: to sirens who sang their lovers to their deaths, the human men and women still ecstatic even as their lungs filled with salt water.

"Ah, no," she said. "That's a little… morbid. I'm not, it's not like that."

They were both silent for a moment.

Suddenly Eric was touching the back of his head again in awkwardness and embarrassment. But there was a lightness to his movements now, an energy that seemed new. A youthfulness.

"I'm sorry, yes, that was Mad Prince Eric speaking," he said with a laugh. "The Melancholy Prince. It's a bit of a role, I'm afraid. To keep me as sane as I am. This is all very strange. I can't believe it's real. That my opera was real… but I *knew* it was real, somehow. But… was it exactly like I recalled? Did it all really… happen exactly that way?"

"I didn't actually see the performance myself. I heard about it second-hand, from a seagull who saw it."

"A seagull?" Eric asked, startled. "Like, a seagull. Like one of those birds flying around up above us right now? One of those… many… birds…"

He frowned. There were at least a half dozen of them circling silently directly overhead. Eerily.

"They're keeping an eye on me," Ariel explained. "Making sure I'm all right."

"Of course they are," Eric said, nodding absently.

"Protective seagulls. Why not. So… wait." He turned back to her. "Is this the story? Because this is how it goes in my opera: You really are a mermaid. You really did trade your voice to come up on land. And it was because you had… you had fallen in love with me?"

He said the words carefully, trying to sound like an adult while sounding more like a child terrified of being disappointed.

Ariel closed her eyes. When put that way, it sounded really epic, the stuff of legends, or painfully stupid. Not just the folly of youth.

"I… always wanted to go on land, to see what it was like to be human." She reached out and touched the Dry World planks of the wrecked boat, the whispery traces left by human hands on its shape, the nails made of iron forged in fires that glowed without the help of undersea lava. "I collected things that I found, that had fallen to the bottom of the sea from ships. I really… I really had quite the collection. I was fascinated with all these things, some of which I still have no name for, the things you people make. And then, one day, I found you.

"There was a storm, and a ship. I think most of the crew died. But I managed to save you and take you to shore. You were so… handsome and strange."

"Strange?" he asked in surprise.

She laughed softly. "You had two legs, silly. And no fins. *Strange.*"

"Right. Of course. Strange from a mermaid's perspective," he said quickly.

" 'From a mermaid's perspective'. Yes. Anyway, I'll skip the more complicated parts, about my father, and other things that happened. Suffice it to say I made a bargain with Ursula the sea witch that if I couldn't make you fall in love with me in three days, she would keep my voice forever, and me, as her prisoner."

"Three days? That seems rather short. To make someone fall in love with you, I mean."

"I'm a *mermaid*," Ariel reminded him. "For thousands of years you people have been falling in love with us at first sight, immediately and forever upon hearing our songs. I didn't think it would be a problem."

"But you weren't a mermaid. You were a human."

"Yes, and I had no voice, which made things even harder than I imagined," she said bitterly. "But, I suppose, *just as hard* as Ursula hoped. I also suspect she had her hand in little incidents that went wrong along the way."

"So I was looking for the beautiful mermaid who sang me awake," Eric mused, thinking back on the time. "And all the while she was right there before me."

"YES."

Ariel said it a little louder, a little more fiercely than she had meant. Her eyes blazed.

Eric looked at her, surprised.

"You had legs," he pointed out.

"I had the same face and hair, Eric," she said, using his name for the first time.

"But you couldn't sing. You couldn't even talk. I remembered that better than how you looked. It stayed with me. I was coming out of unconsciousness, Ariel. Please have a little pity. I had swallowed copious amounts of seawater, I was coughing it up for the rest of the day, and lay in bed with a fever for three nights. I narrowly avoided pneumonia and there's still a little bit of a twinge in my lungs on certain days if I cough too hard."

"Oh," Ariel said, taken aback. She hadn't thought it was like that at all. From her perspective she had saved him, fought with her dad and returned triumphantly as a human to woo him. She hadn't given a moment's thought to what had happened to *him* in the meantime.

Same old Ariel, she thought with a mental sigh. *Impulsive and a little thoughtless.*

"Would you have stayed? A human?" he asked curiously. "If I *had* fallen in love with you, and you got your voice back, and could stay on land?"

"I… suppose so…?"

It was a question she had thought about many times over the past few years. The answer had changed with time. Back then, she absolutely would have stayed, and lived happily ever after as the human princess married to her true love in the Dry World.

But now… as someone who had been Queen of the Sea… and, perhaps, had more time to think… who knew? There were so many details to the world that she hadn't understood back then, when her vision was coloured in bright primary hues and the borders between truth and fiction were defined in bold black lines. Would she have aged and died as a human? Would it have been worth it? Would she miss her friends, her family? Could she wake up every morning and not choke on the dry air?

"… on the other hand, it's also possible my father, the King of the Sea, would have stormed your castle, drowned all the inhabitants and dragged me back home. He's a bit controlling that way."

"*Drowned?* Everyone?"

"I mean stormed quite literally," Ariel said with a tight smile. It was a power she now controlled, by means of the trident disguised as a beautiful and ostensibly harmless hair comb.

Eric took a moment to digest this.

"I guess falling in love with mermaids is pretty dangerous," he finally said.

"Did you?" Ariel asked in a small voice. "Fall for me? At all?"

Eric gave her a measured look, treating the question seriously as she had his. "I *did* fall for you, just not in the way I expected it would happen. And maybe not in the way you hoped. It wasn't a lightning bolt. As I got to know you, I realised you were the most… energetic, fun, enthusiastic… *alive* girl I had ever met." He smiled at the memory, and Ariel felt her breath catch. "You know, for a boy who's all about sailing and running around with his dog and exploring, you were just about as perfect a companion as he could ever want. *And* beautiful, to boot. I would have been very lucky."

He said this wistfully.

Ariel wasn't sure when she was going to start breathing again.

What if, what ifs…

"So… yes. I think I did," he said, taking her hands and squeezing them. "No, I *know* I did. You were one in a million. Even an idiot like me saw that. But then…Vanessa came along…"

He looked confused.

"She had my voice," Ariel supplied. "And you remembered the song."

"Yes! But . . . it was more than that. Somewhere between *Wait, that's the girl who saved me!* and the next moment, everything went… fuzzy."

"Ah. Well. She cast a spell on you. On all of you, I think, somehow. But primarily you," Ariel said bleakly. "I think she knew her stolen looks and voice wouldn't be enough when coupled with her, um, *very original* personality. So she…"

"Stolen looks?"

"That's not what she looks like. At all. Even as a cecaelia. She's much older. And shaped differently. Her arms are shorter."

"She's… half… octopus?"

"No, she's half god," Ariel said impatiently. "And what's wrong with octopuses? You don't seem to mind girls who are 'half fish', as you say. What's the difference?"

"There *is* a difference," Eric said, looking a little sick. "It might not be logical, at all, but for some reason, there's a difference."

"Well, you're married to a person who is old enough to be your grandmother, at least," Ariel said with a smirk. "With or without tentacles."

He looked sicker.

"Besides," Ariel said. "Octopuses are some of the

smartest creatures in the sea, only dolphins and whales and seals surpass them. And dolphins have frightfully short attention spans. Octopuses are creatures of great wisdom, and ancient secrets."

"All right, all right. Octopuses are great. I'm a bigot with tentacle issues." He leant against the boat for support, resting his head on his arm. "I knew my marriage was a sham, but this… surpasses all of my nightmares. I guess in my clearer moments I just figured she was a pretty and somewhat vicious enchantress."

"She is a witch. She is incredibly vicious. I can't speak to her looks objectively…" Ariel replied crisply.

"Oh, you're much more beautiful than Vanessa."

Eric probably really meant it. But he was still breathing funny and his eyes were turned inwards. *Contemplating marriage and tentacles, no doubt.* He ran a hand through his hair and looked like a wild creature for a moment, trapped and ready to bolt. To go mad and die quietly in the wilderness.

Ariel felt a wave of sympathy for the anguished man. If her life had been hell, at least she had been aware of what was going on. He was just now dealing with truths that were even uglier than he expected, and that had been his life for the past few years.

She put a hand on his shoulder. He immediately took it, like a lifeline. He didn't look at her yet, though, still staring into space.

"*Octopodes,*" he finally said.

"I… beg your pardon?"

"Oc-to-poh-dehs." Eric took a deep breath and finally looked up. "The real plural of octopus. Because it's third declension in Latin, not second. *Pus*, *podis*, podes."

"All right," Ariel said uncertainly.

"There was a thing going around last year. Everyone was, well, all my old university mates were, talking about it. Hard to explain. Latin jokes. *Volo*, *vis*, *vulture*, and so on… oh, never mind."

"*Romanorum linguam scio,*" Ariel said mildly. The look on Eric's face was very, very satisfying. "They were known to us, at least in the very earliest days, before the Republic."

"Of course they were," Eric said, rubbing his brow with his palms. "You know what? This would make a real amazing opera on its own. This marriage of mine. A *horror* opera. A new genre. A man wakes up one day to find he's been spending his whole happily married life with an evil octopus witch."

"Were you happily married?" she asked, curious despite her other concerns. *I sound like Jona.*

"Mother of God, *no*," Eric swore. "Actually, it's like many state marriages, I suppose. It could have been worse. We show up for formal functions together, pose for portraits and spend most of our days and… private time… apart. You know, she runs the kingdom and plans our next military venture, and I write operas everyone loves," he finished disgustedly. He reached into the deep pocket on his jacket, pulled out his ocarina and glared at the instrument like it had been the sole cause of all his problems.

"*You* love music," Ariel pointed out. "It's sort of what brought us together. Almost."

"Ariel, I'm a *prince*. I should be ruling. It's my responsibility. If I had been more… awake over the last few years, or less of an idiot, I could have prevented the mess we're in now. You wouldn't understand," he sighed. "I have *responsibilities*."

Ariel regarded him with steely amusement.

"*Prince Eric*, since my father went missing and presumed dead, I have taken his place as high ruler of Atlantica. I am its queen. Informally known as Queen of the Sea. *All* of the sea. This one, at least. *Queen*."

Eric looked, quite understandably, dumbfounded. She felt his gaze change, felt him searching for, and finding, signs of a queen where his playful little redheaded girl had been. She drew herself up taller and pointed her chin, not quite unconsciously.

"Oh," Eric said. "Oh. Right. Oh. I should be… I should kneel to you then, shouldn't I? Foreign royalty of a higher station?"

Ariel laughed. The second real laugh since getting her voice back, and this one was far more burbling and not brittle at all.

"Oh, Eric, it's a little late for that," she sighed. "But… you do love music. Of all the things that should upset you about this situation, getting to do what you love shouldn't be one of them. *I* love music too. I love singing. Taking that away from me was the cruellest form of torture Ursula could have devised, well, next to making me think I was responsible for my father's death."

Eric smiled bitterly. "She should have taken this away, then," he said, shaking the ocarina. "*That* would have shown me. She should have *kept* me from composing and performing and spending all my time with real musicians, and made me rule. That really would have been torture."

"I don't think she was looking to punish or torture *you*, specifically," Ariel said delicately. "I think you were just a pawn in her plans."

"Great. Not even a threat. That's me," Eric said with

a sigh. "You know, speaking of our joint love of music, remember that song you sang? When you rescued me? I never put it into the opera. I could never get the ending right. I think I must have drifted into unconsciousness before hearing you finish it."

Eric moved the ocarina slowly to his lips, looking at her for permission. She nodded, and he played.

It was just like when he had played it in the boat, when she had watched him, unobserved. And just like then, the melody trailed off into silence.

But this time she could finish it.

Even if it wasn't Eric, even if it was Ursula herself playing the piece, Ariel would have continued the tune. The last note had hung there so invitingly, so *unfinished*, it was a blasphemy against nature to let it drop.

Ariel didn't so much sing as allow the song to come up from her chest, from her heart, from her soul, and let it merely pass through her lips.

Eric grinned in pure delight.

When she came to the end of the refrain she took another Dry World breath, to sing it properly from the beginning. Eric hurriedly put the ocarina back in his mouth and played along. This time he didn't play the tune, out of respect for the original artist, he let her sing that alone. Instead he improvised a harmony that was just a touch minor. The main melody still sounded bold and cheerful, enthusiastically describing the world as young Ariel had seen it. But Eric's part added an element of complexity: things weren't as simple as they seemed; details and nuances convoluted a bold declaration. It was no less beautiful, in fact, probably *more* so. Age and wisdom, life and the outside world, observations hitherto unseen.

They finished almost together, Eric cutting off his last note before she was done.

A nod to his mortality? Ariel wondered.

"That was beautiful," she breathed aloud. Of course she had sung duets with the greatest mer singers, male and female, ones who were hundreds of years older than she with voices trained for as long. Somehow what she had just done with Eric was far more powerful and beautiful. All with no audience except for the sea grass, the water and the wind.

And the one seagull who landed ever so delicately on the boat behind them.

"Sorry to interrupt," Jona said. "The skinny grumpy old man at the castle is acting fidgety and skittish, I think about Eric's absence."

"Thank you, Jona," Ariel said with a sad smile. "Eric, she says that Grimsby is getting nervous about you being out here."

"You can talk to seagulls?" Eric asked, eyes widening.

He looked over her shoulder at Jona. "Seagulls can *talk*?"

"Life outside the human realm of understanding is complicated," Queen Ariel said gently. "For you, seagulls will never talk."

"I disagree," Jona said, a little waspishly. *"HEY, FEED ME SOME OF THAT BREAD."*

Eric jumped at the demandy squawk.

"See?" the gull asked triumphantly.

Ariel laughed. "Excellent point, Jona. She's right, though. I have to go. Maintaining this form is beginning to be a little bit of a strain, I have to return to the sea."

"Oh, you can do that. Turn back and forth," Eric said quickly. "But you couldn't before. But you can do it now. Because you're queen?"

"Something like that," she said, self-consciously pushing a piece of hair back behind the comb that was the trident in disguise.

"Right," Eric said, looking into her eyes like he was memorising her, like he could make her stay.

"I have to get my father back," she whispered quickly before she could say anything else. "And then we can work on… you, and Ursula."

"Of course, of course," Eric said, nodding, looking back at the castle. "Of course. Please, let me help you. I'll find him *for* you. It's the least I can do."

"He would be in a jar," she said, wincing at the words as she said them. They sounded ridiculous. "Or a tank. And would look like a slimy, weird piece of seaweed or a tube worm."

"Just like in my opera," Eric said, nodding, but he looked a little queasy again.

There was a moment of silence between them, each fishing for something to say, to make the moment linger.

"Of course! All right, well, let's make a plan to meet again. Hopefully so I can bring you your father, and if not, at least so I can update you on my progress." Eric said it brightly and seriously, like it was a meeting between him and a shipbuilder, or between her and the tax fish.

"When the tide changes back, and the moon is full," Ariel suggested. "Right back here, by this boat."

"Agreed!"

Eric started to put out his hand to clasp hers, then started to pull it away, then shrugged, then put it back to rest at his side.

Did he want to kiss her, instead?

Ariel wanted to kiss him.

But the mood was wrong, weird. It was upbeat and positive: she had a direction and an ally. He had a quest.

Two members of royalty had agreed to right past wrongs.

None of this was romantic.

None of this fell in line with the smell of the briny wind, or the tumult of the clouds, or the breathy, eternal sound of the waves coming in against solid ground.

She took his hand in hers and squeezed.

"Agreed," she said gently.

Hopefully, there would be time for other things later.

Eric

How epic! He was going to help rescue the King of the Sea!

His heart exploded a little each time his thoughts came close to the idea. All his life he wanted to set sail for adventure, and here it was, *right here*! And it was greater than anything he could dream of, greater than discovering a golden city in the deepest jungles of the lands in the west. The king of the merfolk, cousin to gods, in *Eric's castle*… hidden as a polyp in jar.

All right, that part was a little strange.

But mysterious!

And then of course there was the king's daughter, Ariel.

Who, now that she could speak, said things Eric could not have imagined the old Ariel would have. Yet at the same time she was far more reserved now than she had been on those happy days long ago. She held herself in: proud, stoic, still. There was something both wonderful and sad about that, not unlike the reduced state of the sea king. And…

She was *beautiful*.

Before, she had been pretty and gorgeous, lively and smiley, all red hair and perfect skin and quick movements. Now her eyes were deeper. He could fall into her face forever and happily drown there, pulled into her depths. There were worlds in her mind that were only just forming before.

"What a damn fool I was," he muttered, entering the castle. All of this… *all of this*… could have been averted if he had just gone with his heart instead of his, what? Ears? *Ironic, really, when you think about it.* A good composer could summon human emotions and transform them into music. A true love would have been able to resist the witch's spell somehow. He hadn't listened, to his heart, at all.

"Good evening, My Lord. A perfect night for a walk. One couldn't ask for better. Can I…" A footman approached him, hands out to take the prince's jacket.

Eric pushed past him. The smarmy young man wasn't one of Vanessa's two despicable manservants, but he wasn't one of the original staff, either. The prince had no idea when he had turned up. Depressing, since he used to pride himself on personally knowing all the people who worked for him, how their parents were doing, how many children they had… even if he didn't know their name days, he made sure that *someone* did and passed along a little present or extra silver in their wages.

Grimsby appeared like a shadow at his side.

"Yes, we met, we'll talk later—" Eric began.

"It's not that," Grimsby said, keeping pace and not looking at the prince, as if the two were just speaking casually. "The emissary from Ibria was found while you were out… dead. On the unused balcony on the third floor. Causes unclear."

Eric cursed under his breath.

"Poor fellow. Not the worst sort, for a known spy."

"Absolutely regrettable. But it's a dangerous occupation, sir."

Then the prince considered the situation more deeply, and the possibilities it presented him.

"Er, it's in rather poor taste, I know, but I could use the distraction right now to follow up on something… privately. If you would make sure Princess Vanessa directs the inquiry until I officially take part, that would be extremely helpful."

"Princess *Vanessa* direct…?" Grimsby said, eyes widening.

"I need her attention elsewhere," Eric said, giving him a look.

"Ah. Very good, sir. At once."

Like a well-trained military horse, Grimsby peeled away, intent upon his mission.

Eric felt his shoulders relax. He could depend on the butler with his life. And now he could devote himself to his own task without worry. For tonight, at least.

Now, where would Vanessa hide the King of the Sea?

Eric wondered for a crazy moment if he could somehow get Max to help him, to sniff out the merman. Or if he could convince one of Ariel's seagull friends to help. He glanced out a window, but there were far fewer birds in the sky now that it was dark, and those gliding were utterly uninterested in the castle and its inhabitants. He redoubled his steps to Vanessa's room, urged to speed by the ending of the day.

He did pause for a moment at her doorway, readying himself as if for a plunge into cold water.

Dear God, what a tacky mess.

First he went to her shelf of trinkets, picking up goblets and statues and what looked very much like reliquaries but really couldn't be, *because that would be too much, even for her, right?* In his zeal he forgot to be careful; suddenly he realised in a panic that he hadn't remembered exactly where each thing sat or how it was turned. He was behaving like a reckless idiot.

He made himself stop, took a deep breath and began again. If worst came to worst, he could claim he lost a medal or recognised one of her treasures from a book and wanted to see it close up. It never even occurred to him to blame his mess on a maid.

But he found nothing.

"Trinkets and gimmicks aplenty," he swore. "Devices and doodahs galore, what the heck is she *doing* with all this?"

The shelf of terrifying, unknowable black instruments and dangerous-looking things made *some* sort of sense, at least. She was an enchantress. Or witch. Or something. The rest of her collection could only be explained by a childlike, endless need to find, keep and store any sparkly, or horrifying, thing she saw.

He pushed aside books, clawed through chests, even looked under her bed and pillows. He went through the walk-in wardrobe that led to the baths, shaking out each dress and squatting on the floor to look in the back corners, under petticoats. He tried not to think about the rumours that would result if he were caught doing that. *Mad Prince Eric indeed.*

Exhausted, with maybe only a few minutes before Vanessa returned to dress for the evening, he threw himself disconsolately into the poufy chair in front of her dressing table. The top of the dressing table was covered with strange little bottles and jars and vessels and containers of every unguent known to man. Another ridiculous symptom of her never-ending collecting of rubbish.

He looked at himself in the mirror. When they were first married, and he actually paid some attention to his beautiful, mysterious wife, the prince would watch her apply all these oils and astringents while she talked to herself, posing, primping and making moues for her reflection.

(As time with her passed he chose instead to lie on his own bed in his own room with the pillow over his head, wishing she would shut up so he could sleep and escape his nightmarish existence for a few hours.)

The way she behaved would be pathetic, if she weren't actually evil. She *always* needed an audience. In public she surrounded herself with nobles and hangers-on. In private it was extremely rare that she was without her two slimy servants, or her little maid, Vareet. And when she was utterly alone, her other self was always here, listening to her boasts from the other side of the mirror.

Wait—

Eric frowned.

Was she talking to herself?

Wouldn't a jar labelled as something else be the *perfect* place to hide a polyp? He grabbed one and opened it up. Nothing, just some rose-scented powder.

He picked up another one.

Vanilla oil.

He picked up a third… and it didn't feel right in his hands at all.

It *sloshed*. Despite its very clear label, BRETLANDIAN SMELLING SALTS WITH BRETLAND-GROWN LAVENDER FROM BRETLANDIAN FIELDS MADE AT THE REQUEST OF HIS MAJESTY KING OF BRETLAND, complete with a little Bretlandian flag, the contents flowed back and forth nauseatingly like a half-filled bottle of navy grog.

Eric's first instinct was to shake it, but he caught himself just in time.

The tin had a pry-off cap, but as he looked around for something to wedge it off with, a knife or a make-up spade, suddenly it *changed*. When he tried to focus on the box, however, it was just itself again, silver, red, white and blue.

He pretended to slowly turn away, but kept his eyes fixed on the label.

The outline blurred, as if it knew it wasn't needed any more.

"AHA!"

The prince couldn't help calling out in triumph when he whipped his head back, 'catching' it.

What was once a tin of stupid Bretlandian cosmetics was now a glass bottle with a cork stuck in the top. There was a little gravel in the bottom and it was filled the rest of the way with cloudy seawater. Sucking at the sides was a hideous thing: oozing and pulpy, with what looked like soft claws *and human eyeballs*. Yellow, but sentient. Barely.

It blinked at him forlornly.

Eric resisted the urge to throw the thing away from him.

He looked beyond it, back at the dressing table. As if the spell had given up entirely, at least half of the cosmetic jars were now similar bottles full of similar slimy things. Emptied of beer or rum or wine, full of seawater and sadness. No two were alike: they were all shades of black and green with four, three, or no appendages. Some had suckers; some had horrid tendrils that they couldn't seem to control. All had eyes. Some had heads so heavy even the buoyancy of the salt water they were in wasn't enough to support them, and their faces looked up awkwardly at the prince from their prone positions.

Eric swallowed the bile rising in his stomach.

There were at least a dozen… all prisoners? Transformed merfolk?

It was like her own personal prison. Or a medieval torture chamber.

The prince crouched down to get a better look at the feeble creatures. They turned to follow him with their eyes.

"All right," he said, clearing his throat. Whatever they looked like, whatever they were, now or before, they were prisoners of an evil witch and he was a good prince. There was protocol. "I promise you, each and every one of you, I will help free you. I'm not sure how to go about doing that right now, I admit. I don't suppose I could just put you all back... in the ocean?"

There was a flurry of slow but desperate head shakes that was sickening to watch. Some let off little clouds of what he hoped was like squid ink, darkening the water around them.

"All right, all right. Find the king, set him free, defeat the sea witch, *then* turn you back. Nothing until then," Eric said with a sigh. "So which one of you is King Triton?"

The large eyes looked at him unblinkingly.

"Any of you? Raise a... flap? A fin? Anyone?" Eric asked.

The one he had first picked up shook its head dolefully and made what looked very much like a shrugging motion with its appendages.

Slowly the rest copied it, shrugging and shaking.

"Oh, boy," Eric said with a grimace. "This is going to be harder than I thought."

Ariel

If a person had been watching, she wouldn't have seen the obvious transformation of a human to a mermaid. She wouldn't have been able to believe her eyes, or explain what had happened so quickly in the dusky half light of early evening. It could have been a trick of the light, a curious seal, a strangely shaped piece of driftwood; anything but what it actually was.

Ariel did a couple of rolls and then floated on her back, looking up at the mixed sky of clouds and stars. Everything was quiet. She felt her hair loosen from its braids, yearning to float free in the water as it once did. She took the comb out, and it was a trident once again in her hand, but the braids remained firmly wound.

Half in and half out, she thought, then rolled and submerged herself into the depths. It was slightly slower going this time, what with the burlap sack of apples she dragged along.

Flounder appeared surprisingly quickly; he must have had every undersea eye and electroreceptor keeping watch for her.

"*Ariel!* You're back! Do you have him? Is that him... uh, in the sack?"

"No, I failed. Those are apples. But I am back, for a little while."

Flounder bumped his head against her hand, a safe gesture because no one was around. He didn't need the world to see that he still enjoyed being petted.

But he wasn't young any more, and didn't miss the meaning below her words.

"You're going back with the full moon, aren't you? When the trident is back at its peak power?" he asked, full of disappointment.

"Flounder, I didn't find him. I *need* to go back," she said gently. "But I have a clear path now."

"*Clear path?*" he said with a snort. "I can't *wait* to hear you say that to Sebastian."

Ariel smiled. Flounder was one of the very few people

who could use that tone with her. He was dead right. Now that she could speak again, she was already using words like a trickster. *Clear path.* What did that even mean? She had allies, she had a goal. That was all. It wasn't like a parrotfish had just chomped through a snarled lump of dead coral, revealing a beautiful cave of treasure beyond.

She needed a plan, a *direction*, in case Eric failed.

She ran a hand along the base of Flounder's dorsal fin. "Nothing is easy. I can't go back to the castle at all now, although Eric is looking, for me. And I assume Ursula knows I'm back, and has hidden my father somewhere better."

"All those things sound like the exact opposite of easy."

"I *know.* Also, *why* is she keeping my father around at all? You'd think she'd at least want to use him as leverage for bargaining… like, she would give him to me in return for our never bothering her and Tirulia again."

"Would you take that trade?" Flounder asked curiously. "And abandon Eric?"

"Well… I think I've learnt the hard way that there is no fair bargaining with a sea witch. Also, I wouldn't just be abandoning Eric. I'd be leaving his kingdom to a terrible fate as well. Our worlds should never have collided, and the people of Tirulia are dealing with the results of…" *a rash decision by a lovesick mermaid*, "choices I myself made years ago."

"Fine, but," her friend said with wry smile, "you still have to come down and check in with His Crustaceanness. And explain all of this to him too."

"Fine. Race you?" she asked, darting ahead.

"Hey, wait, no fair!" Flounder squealed, shaking his tail as fast as he could.

"OH, ARIEL, THANK THE THOUSAND SEAS OF THE WORLD YOU ARE BACK. IT HAS BEEN A TERRIBLE NIGHTMARE OF BUREAUCRACY SINCE YOU LEFT!"

Ariel, Sebastian and Flounder were alone in the deserted throne room. Ariel had her audience very much to herself.

She opened her mouth.

"YOU HAVE NO IDEA THE THINGS I HAVE HAD TO BEAR." Sebastian clacked a claw against his foreshell dramatically, turning away from her. His eight walking feet clicked tinnily on the armrest of the throne.

Ariel took a breath and opened her mouth again.

"The constant fighting," Sebastian continued, "the interminable discussion of *rituals*. *Taxes*. The stupid sharks and their stupid sea-grabs. Distributing parts for the Sevarene Rites. And no one knows where the Horn of the Hyperboreans went!"

The little crab collapsed in a heap, more like a moult than a living creature, burying his eyes under his claws.

Ariel and Flounder exchanged an exasperated look.

"Not a moment for *me*. Not a moment for my *music*. Not a moment to compose, or prepare a chorus for the Rites," Sebastian continued feebly. He poked his eyes piteously up through the crack in his claw. "What is a musician to do?"

"Maybe stop whining and be grateful for a chance to serve his kingdom," Ariel suggested dryly.

Sebastian's eyes twitched in a crab version of blinking.

"ARIEL! You can TALK!"

Using quick scooting motions, Sebastian swam sideways to plant himself on her chest, pressing his face against her skin. A crab hug.

"Oh, my dear, dear girl. I am so happy for you. I want to shed!"

"Ugh. Please don't," Flounder said.

Ariel picked the little crab off her and held him, cupped in her hands, before her face.

"But how did this happen?" he asked, looking around. "And where is your father?"

"It's… complicated," Ariel said.

"Ariel!"

Attina was frozen in surprise behind them, staring at her sister. Then with a snap of her tail she was next to and around her, holding her shoulders and looking her all over, as if she would be able to see a physical reason for her change.

"Ariel! I'm so happy for you! How did you…? Where's Daddy? Is everything back to normal now?"

"Not… precisely." Ariel wished she could stay there, basking in her big sister's good humour and attention. But there were truths to be told.

"Oh," Attina said, her face falling. "So… does this mean you're back to assume your responsibilities again? For good this time?"

Ariel thought about the twin meanings of that word: *good*.

"Why don't you listen?" she suggested, making her voice lilting, not quite begging, but the sort of *come on* sound a younger sister would use to wheedle sense out of an older sibling. "I was just about to tell the story."

"I'm all ears." Attina crossed her arms and drifted away from her.

Ariel decided to ignore her sister's tone and just leapt into the tale, starting with Jona and Scuttle's furious attack on the guards and ending with a slightly censored and greatly abbreviated retelling of the conversation she had with Eric.

It was hard to tell that part. Her lips moved as she recounted their official discussion, but her heart wandered away from the conversation. She could still hear echoes of their duet lingering in her mind.

"*Help* from the human prince," Attina drawled. "I'm so surprised."

"All right," Ariel said mildly. "Do you have a better idea to get our father back? Because if you do, *I'm all ears.*"

"Now, girls," Sebastian said, holding up his claws. "It's good that he's searching the castle, but… Ariel… he's the reason you lost your head to begin with."

"I'm not going to lose my head again," the queen said with a steely look. *No, really.* Despite the flutters her heart felt when she thought of him. "I'm older and wiser, and I have a mission. I'm not going to be distracted from rescuing my father by a human boy. Even Eric."

"Even Eric," Attina said with a sigh, throwing her hands up. "There are *millions* of 'human boys' up there. You're the *queen of the merfolk.* Don't you ever think about that? Are *any* of them worth *one* of you?"

For a dizzying moment Ariel saw things from her sister's, and her father's, perspective: countless humans swarming everywhere on the Dry World; only a tiny kingdom of mer below in the World Under the Sea. Losing a daughter to a human wasn't just tragic on a personal level; it also meant the loss of one of the dwindling mer to the ever-growing mass of humans. Triton had already lost a wife to them, and Ariel, a mother.

"Just… forget about Eric for a moment," she finally said. "You'll just have to take my word that my father and my kingdom come first. That's all I have to offer."

"I guess," Attina said uncomfortably. "It's strange to hear you talking like this, now that you can talk. 'Take my word' and everything. Like a queen."

"I was talking like that before I could *speak* again," Ariel reminded her sharply, signing the words as she spoke. "Were you listening?"

"Oh, yeah, of course," Attina said, unsettled and chastised. "I just meant, in general. The last time you could speak, aloud, you were all… 'Guess what I found, Attina!' And 'Listen to this song, Attina'… and all those silly stories about what you saw or thought you saw."

"And then I lost my father, and my voice, and the boy I loved, and then you made me queen. I guess that will change a person."

"Yes, I guess so."

The two sisters regarded each other silently. Ariel had no idea what was going on in Attina's head, and that was strange. Some secret part of her hoped it was jealousy, that Attina was regretting her decision to make her littlest sister the queen, that she felt she should have taken the crown herself. Jealousy would have been simple, though sad, and easily dealt with.

Not so this quiet reassessment, this weighing and evaluating from her oldest and closest sister.

Ariel swished her tail.

I'm going to rest for a bit and then give an update to the council before I have to leave again. Sebastian, Flounder, I hope you join me. Her hands wanted to sign these things.

"I brought you these apples," she said aloud, holding out the bag.

Attina's eyes widened as she peeped inside.

"When did you… how did you…?"

The king's daughter greedily grabbed one in both her hands, holding it before her face like she was afraid it would disappear.

"There's enough for all of you. *Us*," Ariel corrected quickly.

Attina shot her a look, but it softened almost immediately.

"Thanks. This is… thanks."

"I'm going to rest for a bit and then update the Queen's Council on what has happened before I have to leave again. Besides the usual agenda, I plan on opening discussion to possible strategies for rescuing our father, since currently I am at a bit of a loss, maybe heads older and wiser than mine can think of something. Sebastian, Flounder, please work with Klios and Threll to come up with an official announcement about the return of my voice. It's best if everyone else learns it at the same time. Cuts down on gossip and chatter. After it has gone out, join me in the council."

She swam away, trailed by her friends, resisting the urge to look back at her sister.

I guess that will change a person.

Something inside of her tore a little.

But there were sharks to manage and taxes to go over.

Carlotta and Grimsby

Grimsby and Carlotta sat in the butler's private office having tea together. Carlotta was wedged in; it would have been even harder for her to fit if the door hadn't been left open 'for modesty and propriety'. Carlotta had tried not to laugh at that; the dear old Bretlandian gent was never going to change his ways, not at this age.

As chiefs of their respective staffs they often worked late together, revising lists for parties, making sure the right number of footmen were there to serve and coordinating what they needed to order. The chef usually came as well.

But this time it was just the two of them, and instead of beer or soup or tankards of wine, what most of the lower staff drank, they were having tea. Grimsby had invited her *specifically* for tea, prepared the Bretland way: in a proper tiny cup, with no more than two lumps of sugar for ladies.

Carlotta sipped it as slowly as she could, since there was actually very little of the hot beverage in its adorably minuscule vessel. Not her thing, really, but as far as tea went it wasn't bitter and even a little floral. *Delicate*, like the rose-patterned teacup. Funny how formal and fussy the old gent was!

But once the ceremony of pouring and serving was over, they sat in awkward silence.

"A bit… a bit surprising, isn't it," Grimsby eventually ventured.

"With the…" Carlotta moved her hand like a mermaid, back and forth through the water.

"Yes, precisely…"

"And the…" She waved her hand, indicating everything else.

"Yes, quite." Grimsby leant forwards eagerly.

"Yes, it is," Carlotta agreed.

They lapsed into silence again, falling back disappointedly into their seats.

"What do we do about it, Mr Grimsby?" the maid finally asked.

"I really don't have the foggiest idea. It's not our place. I have sworn to protect and serve the royal couple; it is an oath I cannot break..."

"Yes, yes, yes." Carlotta almost used the cup to gesture with, scattering scalding hot tea everywhere. The fine bone china weighed so little in her hand that she had almost forgotten it was there. "But I never signed on to serve an undersea hag, if that's what, you know..."

Grimsby turned white at the term *hag*, as if she had mentioned something as terrible as her own unmentionables.

"No, neither did I," he haltingly allowed. "And she's certainly not acting like a proper princess..."

"Oh, hush on that. There's been plenty of warrior princesses in both of our lands, Mr Grimsby. But she's not even acting like a proper warrior, or *any* sort of normal human being, because she *isn't* one. She's like a rabid dog, er, shark, biting everyone and everywhere. Mr Grimsby, we, all of Tirulia, are in thrall to an evil supernatural being, oaths or no!"

"I think I could forgive whatever she was, if Eric truly loved her."

Carlotta almost dropped her teacup at this heartfelt admission from the old gentleman's gentleman. It was only shocking because the very Bretlandian Grimsby was usually as sealed up as a clam when it came to what he felt or believed.

"You've been with the prince a long time, haven't you?" she said softly.

"Well… you know, our careers don't often give one much time for things like family," the old butler said mildly. "I care for him very deeply. Like a son."

Carlotta looked stern. "Then we should let our hearts and souls dictate our actions, Mr Grimsby, not contracts. There are others who can judge us, maybe, for what we swore and didn't swear. But they aren't on Earth, if you see what I'm saying, Mr Grimsby."

"I don't like talk of mutiny, Miss Carlotta, it's not our place—"

"Oh, heavens forfend, Mr Grimsby. But if you meant what you said about Eric, I believe there is *another*… girl… thing… whom the prince might indeed have feelings for."

"I always thought he did, I always wished that he had…" Grimsby trailed off wistfully, thinking back to earlier times. Then he redirected his attention on the maid. "All right, then. Perhaps if you have something in mind for an… acceptably subtle and appropriate course of action that might benefit our original employer, given the circumstances, well, I might be persuaded to go along."

"First thing we do is find all the downstairs folks we can trust and put them to work looking for the sea king. As for other ideas… I'm sure an opportunity will present itself, Mr Grimsby," Carlotta said, eyes twinkling over her teacup. "It is a very *small* castle, after all."

Eric

In the world of operas, when a hero is searching for something, be it the identity of a woman who rescued him or the letter that will free his daughter from being unjustly imprisoned, the tenor sings heartbreakingly about his quest, wanders around on stage, picks up a few props and looks under them. He finds the thing! Voilà. Done.

Real life was a lot more tense and a lot less satisfying.

And, unlike in opera, Eric's search for the King of the Sea was often interrupted by real-life stuff: sudden appearances of Vanessa or her manservants, meetings, rehearsals for the opera's end-of-summer encore, formal events he had to attend, or princely duties, such as hearing a coroner's report on the death of the Ibrian.

(No foul play discovered, although why such a healthy youngish man had keeled over would remain a mystery for the ages. Vanessa had no trouble getting along with his replacement, who was much more amenable to collusion anyway.)

Often when interrupted Eric would forget which was the last object he had looked at and have to start a room from the beginning.

Then he hit upon a brilliant idea to keep track, inspired by his life as a musician. He would carefully mark the first thing that he looked at in a room, observing its precise placement, and the last thing he looked at before leaving, and then *he would write it all down in his musical notebook.* The altitude of the item was indicated by a note: high G over C, for instance, for the top shelf of a bookcase, middle C for the floor. A portion of a room was a measure of music; each room was a refrain. He filled in the details with what could very easily have been mistaken for lyrics.

Some parts were harder to put into code than others; the library, for instance. He pulled out *every book* because Vanessa was known to spend entire afternoons there, especially in the sections on history, folklore and magic.

An hour going through all the floor-level shelves resulted in a whole page of middle C notes. Very suspicious, even to someone who didn't know much about music. In a burst of inspiration Eric labelled the sheet *Part for Upright Bass, Picked: Anticipating the Coming Storm.* It was a bit more experimental than the sort of music he normally composed, but these were modern times, and the Mad Prince was nothing if not eager to try new things.

Progress was slow but steady. He had no doubt that soon he would find the king.

And then something so unimaginably horrific occurred that Eric couldn't even gather his wits enough to escape it.

Chef Louis said to him:

"Eet has been a long time since the royal couple has dined *en privé*. Maybe a special dinner is required?"

The entire staff was in on this decision, reacting exactly like an extended family scared that Mum and Dad were drifting apart, what could they do to keep them together?

Grimsby and Carlotta, bless them, did their best to quell the whole thing. The maid yelled, the butler made Bretland-accented speeches of disapproval.

It didn't matter. The dinner would be happening.

Part of Eric thought he deserved this. He had been avoiding Vanessa like a coward and not behaving like a true, brave prince. It was only a matter of time before he was forced to face the villain, he just hadn't expected it to be at opposite ends of a long dining table with a white linen tablecloth and golden candelabra; a multicourse feast for two lonely people in a giant empty room that overlooked the sunset sea.

When Vanessa came into the dining room Eric stood up, as was only right. He looked at her, *really* tried to look at her. But whatever spell kept her appearing human was different from whatever hid the polyps. Her form remained. And it was a beautiful form; very curvy in the right places, maybe a little too skinny and waspish in the waist. *Implausible.* Her hair was radiant and her face was symmetrical and prettily composed. But what looked out of her eyes and tugged the corners of her lips wasn't married to the flesh it wore and seemed hampered by its limitations.

Tonight, as befitted the 'romantic' occasion, she wore a blood-red velvet gown and matching bolero to cover her shoulders. A fox was draped round her neck, behind which sparkled the chain of a golden necklace Eric didn't remember seeing before. But besides the fur there was no other nod to the sickness she kept pretending to have. The weather was far too warm for velvet, really, but Vanessa never seemed to get hot or cold. And she never pretended to feel faint like other ladies.

That, at least, Eric could appreciate.

He wore a military-style dress jacket, royal blue, with a sash across the front indicating his brief service in the army that was required of all royal sons.

"Good evening, My Prince," Vanessa whispered. They air-kissed, like cousins. He pulled her seat out for her. "Thank you," she simpered, oozing down into it.

Chef Louis himself came out to present the first course, small golden cups of perfectly clear consommé.

"It should be good for your throat, eh, Princess?" he said before bowing out.

Eric was feeling annoyed and reckless. He gazed at the woman opposite him daintily sipping from a tiny mother-of-pearl spoon.

"I don't think I've ever seen you sick," he observed. "Not the entire time we've been married."

"Oh, it's this ghastly summer weather. Cold one moment, hot the next. Plays havoc with the… nerves… oh, I don't know, whatever it is the silly little things say about the weather," Vanessa finished, too bored to bother completing the thought.

She pulled the fur from her neck and let it drop to the floor. Eric flinched when its taxidermied nose made a soft *clack* against the tiles. There was no reason to disrespect an animal you killed. It wasn't a *thing*; once it had been a living being.

"You haven't been… yourself lately, either," she said, somewhere between a purr and a growl, letting the whispering part of her act die off as well. "It seems like you've been acting different since… well, almost exactly since the time I lost my voice."

"Perhaps so. I *do* feel pretty good these days, actually," Eric responded airily.

They finished their soup in silence, looking into each other's eyes, but not like lovers.

Not at all.

Eventually a serving boy came in and cleared the bowls; they clattered against each other loudly in the vast room.

The next course was a magnificent chilled seafood salad on three tiers of silver dishes mounded with ice. Glittering diamonds of aspic decorated the rims.

Eric picked up a tiny three-pronged golden seafood fork, thinking about the trident in Ariel's hair. She hadn't worn it years ago, when they had first met. Maybe it was a sign of royalty.

"Don't suppose your feeling good has anything to do with a pretty little mermaid, does it?" Vanessa asked casually.

Eric froze.

Vanessa smiled coyly down at her plate.

"Why, yes, as a matter of fact, it does," he said as he speared a tiny pickled minnow and delicately eased it into his mouth.

It was extremely gratifying to see Vanessa's eyes grow huge in childlike surprise.

"Yes, I definitely started feeling good when I managed to get Sarai to hit the high F over C in her final aria, 'The Goodbye.' Like this."

And then the Mad Prince sang in a terrible falsetto.

Vanessa just sat and watched, unblinking. Through all seven minutes. No doubt people in the kitchens were listening in fascinated horror as well.

When he finished, Eric took a few pickled bladderwracks in his fingers and popped their air bladders thoughtfully. "It was a real triumph. Now I just need to get her to do it onstage."

Vanessa narrowed her eyes.

He tried not to grin as he ate the seaweed. The princess slowly pulled out a piece of fish and cut it, thoroughly and assiduously.

A different serving boy came out with a basket of steaming hot bread and, in the Gaulic fashion, little tubs of sweet butter. Eric preferred olive oil, but along with all the other terrible things going on in the castle, Vanessa had embraced Gaulic culture with the tacky enthusiasm of a true nouveau riche.

"I do so love baguettes, my dear, sweet, *Mad* Prince. Don't you?" she said with a sigh, picking up a piece and buttering it carefully. "You know, we don't have them where I come from."

"Really? *Where you come from?* What country on Earth doesn't have some form of bread? Tell me. Please, I'd like to know."

"Well, we don't have a grand tradition of baking, in general," she said, opening her mouth wider and wider. Then, all the while looking directly at Eric, she carefully pushed the entire slice in. She chewed, forcefully, largely and expressively. He could see whole lumps of bread being pushed round her mouth and up against her cheeks.

The prince threw his own baguette back down on the plate in disgust.

She grinned, mouth still working.

"Your appetite is healthy, despite your cold," he growled. "Healthy for a longshoreman. Where *do* you put it all? You never seem to gain a *pound*."

"Running the castle keeps one trim," she answered modestly. "Military planning, offensive strategies, tactics, giving orders, keeping our little kingdom safe, you know. We could be attacked any time. From the land… from the sea…"

"Actually, Tirulia's biggest problems are with those who *leave* the sea and come *here* to live… hey, maybe I should write an opera about that."

He gave her a bright smile.

"You're so very clever," Vanessa said softly. "Such a *clever* little musician. With your *clever* little operas. You're giving everyone a free show at the end of the month, aren't you? One wonders if you would even have time to devote yourself to the kingdom or anything military, even if you had an interest in it."

"No interest whatsoever. I'm just the Mad Prince, that's all. Don't mind me," Eric said, saluting her with the butter knife. "Carry on with your little war games. It does seem to keep you occupied."

"I will, then, thank you," the princess said primly. "By the way, I have orders out to kill Ariel on sight if she shows up on castle grounds again, you know. Not just her father."

Eric choked.

When he recovered Vanessa was smiling at him venomously.

Eric worked his jaw, trying to quell the rage that would have him across the room and throttling her if he didn't stop it.

When the immediate anger subsided he felt a terrible emptiness, a sick, sinking feeling that drained his whole body. He sat back in his chair, feeling defeated.

"Do you really have tentacles?" he asked flatly.

"Yes," she said wistfully, through her full mouth. "Really nice ones too. Long and black. I miss them."

The serving boy came in and pretended not to notice the exasperated, obviously *not* eating prince, and the princess who had to keep chewing ponderously because of the amount of food she still had in her cheek pockets. Off a silver platter the boy took two paper cones, *Bretland* style, of course, filled with perfectly deep-fried baby squid gleaming in a crispy golden batter. After carefully setting one down in front of each of them, the boy immediately withdrew, trying not to look over his shoulder. The mood in the room was palpably icy.

Vanessa looked at the cone with delight, and the moment she swallowed the bread, another large, loud, disgusting gesture that showed the bolus going down her throat in an Adam's apple-y lump, she picked up a squid with her fingers and popped it into her mouth.

"How can you do that?" Eric burst out, unable to contain himself.

"Do what?" Vanessa asked innocently.

"Eat... something that looks like you. Something out of the sea. Can't you *talk* to sea creatures?"

"Well," Vanessa said thoughtfully. "There are seas, and there are *seas*. There are the seas that you know and fish out and dump your rubbish into and generally destroy in your careless human way, and the seas you *don't* know. Seas that hide secret treasures and kingdoms of merfolk and portals to the Old Gods. And there are seas beyond that... between the waves, between the stars... where some of the truly Elder Gods come from. What I'm trying to say is..." she leant forwards and popped another squid into her mouth, "... these are *very* delicious."

"Disgusting," he muttered.

"Like you humans care," she said, rolling her eyes. "Have you ever tasted latium shark?"

"No. Is it good?"

"No idea, because you idiots ate it into extinction. Along with several kinds of sea anemone, such beautiful fronds, sweet-hake and other fish whose names were literally also the names of food. We could have quite a long discussion about tuna and lobster and cod and shrimp if you cared. I don't. But then again, I'm what all of *you* call an evil witch. 'Evil' indeed. Meanwhile you humans scuttle across the sea and land literally devouring everything even remotely edible.

If only you knew, you're not that different from the more apocalyptic Elder Gods. Not really."

Eric slumped, all the fear, anxiety, anger and energy draining out of him.

"What do you want?" he asked wearily.

"What?" Vanessa asked, surprised. A squid was poised halfway to her mouth.

"What. Do you *want*," he repeated. "Why are you still here? If my… memory… and legend has it right, you really are a powerful witch under the sea. What do you want to be *here* for?"

"Hmm," Vanessa said thoughtfully, chewing on the squid. "*Powerful witch under the sea.* My, I *do* like the sound of that. I suppose I was. But… does *legend* have it? Or did a certain little ridiculous mermaid tell you?"

"You got all the revenge on her you wanted!" Eric said, smashing his fist down on the table. "You got rid of the King of the Sea, you stole his daughter's voice, you kept her from getting the prince… me. Why stay here? Why not return to the ocean, where you're a powerful witch? Why do you *linger*? Why stay married to… me?"

His last words sort of trailed off, like a weak wave returning from the shore to a vast sea, disappearing in the limitless water.

Vanessa laughed throatily and deeply. If Eric didn't look directly at her he could easily imagine a much older, much larger woman, voice husky from years of cigars or hard living. But he did look at her, and the dissonance he experienced while viewing the weirdly innocent face was too much like a fever dream.

"Oh, dear, no," she said, moving her face in a way that implied she was wiping tears of laughter, but her hands moved differently, still breaking the legs off baby squid. "I will say you have a certain… charm. And youth is always attractive. But, my love, you're short at least eight tentacles. Maybe six, if I were generous and counted your legs. Also, I like my partners with a bit more… heft to their physiques."

Eric was unsure if he was more horrified or relieved.

"It's always the case, isn't it? Men are pretty much the same the world around, regardless of their race," Vanessa said, exasperated. "They always assume they have the complete, undivided attention of whatever female creature happens to be in the room."

"All right, yes, I get it, this is a marriage of convenience, thank you. But *why*? *Why are you here?* If you don't even like me? What is there keeping you here? You're not even doing magic any more, are you? I haven't seen you conjure any spells or do any magic since we've been together, since the initial one you cast over me and my kingdom."

Vanessa looked up at him sharply.

Huh, Eric thought, noticing her reaction. *She hasn't because she* can't. Maybe in human form she couldn't do magic. He decided to file that thought away for later.

"Well," she said. "You're not quite the dumb, handsome prince you look like. Here's the truth, then, if we are speaking plainly. I find I rather *like* you humans, I didn't expect that at all! You're so venal and short-sighted and power hungry and imaginative and… such a mess of wants and desires. And so short-lived! Hardly any of you has the wisdom that a century or two of living endows one with. Such fun to play with… and there's so many *more* of you than merfolk. The possibilities are endless."

She gave him a winning smile.

Doctor Faustus's Mephistopheles has nothing on Vanessa, Eric thought. *Toying with souls and bodies like it's all a child's game for her.*

"And here's the thing," she said, changing her tone. She stabbed five mussels in a row with her knife and shovelled them into her mouth but continued to talk. Like the hungriest, most brutish old sailor in a pub after months at sea. "True, I was a powerful sea witch. But can anyone really have *enough* power? Even with Triton gone there are seven sisters defending his crown, and a mer army, and countless other soldiers, guardians, priests and allies who would effectively keep me from running the show. Here? I *am* running the show. And all it took was a marriage! Not a drop of blood spilt. Or a person transmogrified."

"Not a drop of blood spilt?" Eric demanded, leaning forwards. "We lost twenty at the Siege of Arlendad and three in the attack north of the Veralean Mountains when you were trying to 'send a message' to Alamber. That's twenty-three young men who will never give their mothers a grandchild, who will never see another spring, who will turn into dirt before they reach twenty!"

"My, you really are quite the poet," Vanessa said, perhaps really impressed. "But those were the result of empire expansion. My ascension to power, in itself, was bloodless. Also, I don't remember you being quite so eloquent on behalf of Tirulia's young male population at the time I first proposed these ventures…"

"I was under your bloody *spell*!" Eric shouted, standing up.

"Dear, the staff," Vanessa said primly. "Let's not let the help know about our marital issues. They're all terrible gossips."

Eric made a strangled cry and pounded his fists on the table.

"Just be a good boy and let mummy Vanessa run things.

Soon Tirulia will be a power among powers, to rival Druvest or Etrulio. Then you'll be grateful for what I've done. And what will *you* have had to do, to get all these new lands and resources? Nothing. It's just me, sweetie. You go and write your plays and operas and let the people love you.

"Actually, we make quite a good team together, when you think about it. You're the spiritual side of the operation. I'm the tactics. And the… *body.*"

Eric looked at her blackly.

And that was when the chef chose to come back in.

"How waz everything?" he asked, clasping his hands together.

Vanessa hurried to pick up her fox and wrap it round her neck. *"Quite good,"* she whispered.

"Oh! Zat is wonderful. I will attend to ze palate cleanser now…"

The idea of spending another half hour, another ten minutes, another *course* with Vanessa, made Eric sick.

As soon as the chef was gone Vanessa gave him a nastily patronising smile. "Don't fret, darling. I really do have Tirulia's best interests at heart."

"I highly doubt that you have Tirulia's *best interests* anywhere near what passes for a heart on you."

"Well, I suppose hearts are a mostly human condition,

aren't they? Especially *yours*. You're so full of *love* and *feeling* for everyone around you. Your country, your little mermaid, your dumb dog, your butler… say, speaking of hearts, his is rather *old*, isn't it?"

Her words chilled Eric to his bones.

"Hate for anything to happen to it. A man at his age probably wouldn't recover from an attack," she said thoughtfully.

"I… I'm not sure how you could arrange that," the prince stuttered. "Since we just established you don't perform your witchery any more."

"Oh, there are other magics, my dear," she said coyly. "And things besides magic when one must make do."

Eric fumed, unable to think of a snappy retort. The dead Ibrian lay like an unspoken nightmare in the middle of their table.

"So while you're keeping everyone's best interests *at heart*," she continued through clenched teeth, "perhaps it's best if you stay out of my way. If I so much as *suspect* you're helping the little redhead, Grimsby will be dead before the day is out. And if anything should suddenly happen to *me*, he is also dead. Along with a few others I have my eye on. Am I clear?"

"As seawater," Eric said, through equally clenched teeth.

And that was how the chef found them, glaring silently at each other, when he came back in with the sorbet. He shifted from foot to foot for a full minute before fleeing back into the kitchens.

Ursula

Of *course* her spells didn't work on land.

Idiot.

She was a *sea witch.*

The cantrip she had cast over the prince remained because she had begun it in the sea, just like the one for her new body. So too the mass hypnosis she had blown across the sleeping citizens of the land like an ill fog, it had been created while she was in the ocean. Flotsam and Jetsam were transformed while they were still in the shallows. Ursula had also disguised her favourite polyps on her last trip down to the bottom of the ocean when she realised her future lay on land. She had waved a cheery goodbye to the prisoners who remained in her 'garden', selected a few to keep Triton company, cast a quick perceptual slanter on the rest and never looked back.

Mostly she viewed her current situation as a minor inconvenience that could be handled, like all things and people. It didn't bother her. Systems where there were prices and balances and choices were the world where she lived, and lived very nicely. It was never a question of what was fair; it was a question of how far you could push the rules.

Of course, then she had found that black-bound book from Carcosa, the one with the complicated circuex that would give her powers she could use on land. While this was still an option, it was a difficult and dangerous undertaking. Only the greatest magics could break the rules of the Dry World and the World Under the Sea.

Only the sacrifice of many, many people would be enough to propitiate the Elder Gods.

And only one very, *very* rare ingredient could complete the spell: blood that contained within it the might and heritage of an Old God.

Like the body she currently wore, she had kept Triton around for just such an unexpected emergency.

She played with the heavy golden chain she wore under her dress, thinking. Things were in fact getting a tiny bit out of hand in Tirulia. Although the stubborn Iase had been taken care of, his otherwise agreeable replacement wasn't taken seriously by the king of Ibria. She was still three warships short of the fleet she had promised potential allies. The number of soldier recruits were down this week, the townspeople were growing uneasy about her military manoeuvres. There was a mermaid amok in Tirulia, and Ursula's power over Eric was effectively gone. All she had left were threats and promises.

Every piece of this mess could easily be cleared up with a bit of magic.

But things would be very different after the circuex. There would probably be a larger mess. There might not be much of Tirulia remaining afterwards. And it would certainly mean an end to her current experiment with humans.

Plus she would lose Triton, whom she so loved to hold over Ariel. Actually, she loved just holding him in general: *I have a king! Ursula the exiled has a* king *for a prisoner!*

Bah. Speaking of Triton, if she was going to keep him around for much longer she would have to throw the dumb little redhead off the trail. Maybe she could kill two polyps with one hook: repair her relationship with the king of Ibria *and* get the King of the Sea somewhere safe, far away from the ocean and meddling princesses. *And maybe have some fun while I'm doing all this…*

"She's here, Princess," Flotsam hissed.

"Do send her in," Ursula said, remembering to whisper at the last moment. She would wait a little longer for the big spell. Preparations had to be made, times and places, and sacrifices, prepared. In the meantime there was a country to lead into war and an empire to carve, for which she needed a voice.

A young woman stepped tentatively into the room. Yet it was obvious that this was a girl utterly unused to being tentative, or shy, or cowed. The strain on her face showed as she tried to wrest her feelings under control: excitement, eagerness, fear, a trace of anger that she felt any fear. All on a proud, beautiful countenance with clear sand-coloured skin, bright brown eyes and dark rosy lips. *Put a few pounds on her,* Ursula thought, *and she'd be a very pretty mouthful indeed.*

"Julia, is it?" she said in a kindly whisper.

"Yes, Princess." The girl dropped an elegant, if last-minute, curtsy. Her dress was tacky, all flounces and far too many underskirts and weird pastel colours that didn't go with her complexion. Her hair was so brushed and oiled and coiled it shone more like eel skin than anything human. She was so *not* noble it was painful.

But her voice…

Ah, her voice. Real potential there. Musical and lilting but with far more substance than the dumb little mermaid's. *Now* that's *a voice I could work with!*

"I have heard so much about you," Ursula whispered, "… in that I have heard anything at all, which is, you understand, unusual for someone in my position. And yours."

"Yes, My Princess," the girl breathed, not even reacting to what was probably an insult, too anxious to hear what was next.

"I hear you like a boy," Ursula purred, giving her a twinkly, knowing look.

Julia gasped.

Ursula tried very hard not to roll her eyes. Even if the girl's father hadn't told her, the sea witch would of course have guessed. Silly girls were the same wherever they lived – the Dry World or the World Under the Sea. It didn't matter. There was always a boy. Or a girl.

"Or, should I say, a *family* of boys," she went on. "Handsome, adventurous, *good* boys from a good family."

"Yes, My Princess," the girl said, eyes wide with shock. "But how—"

Ursula shushed her, tsking. "You think I don't understand? Of course I do. I of *all* people. You think I don't hear the rumours, however faint, about *my* lineage? 'Where did that girl come from' and 'Who is her family' and 'Is she truly a princess?'"

Julia said nothing but began to look thoughtful.

Not stupid, Ursula thought. Sometimes that made things harder, sometimes it made things easier. Intelligent people who knew what they wanted and *thought* they understood the consequences were the most fun. They were also the most impatient: they saw her shiny, barbed hook and often grabbed it voluntarily, swallowing it themselves. No force or trickery needed.

"Look at me," Ursula said, twisting her body, showing off her jewels and the room. "No one dares says those things aloud. I know what it's like, girl. I utterly sympathise."

"I'm sorry?" Julia said, terrified of saying it too loudly, leaning forwards. "I didn't quite hear you… your throat…"

Ursula closed her eyes, beating back fury. Pretended she was *working up her strength.*

"I can help you."

"I-I am grateful," Julia stammered. "Your attention and

hospitality are already more than I could ever imagine. But why…? Why me?"

"But my dear, sweet child, that's what I do! It's what I live for. To help unfortunate mer… uh, *towns*folk like yourself: poor unfortunate souls with no one else to turn to."

Ursula could see hope and doubt fighting one another in the girl's eyes. True, when it came to charity, Vanessa hadn't exactly been the poster queen. Or princess.

"I would be eternally thankful for any advice or aid you would give," Julia said softly. She was as beautiful as a medieval maiden, chaste and penitent, praying on the beach.

Ursula had seen a number of those in her time.

"Of course, my dear," Vanessa whispered. "Of course. But we must keep it our little secret for it to work properly. You need my help, I need a little help from you. Meet me at the Grey Lagoon at midnight and we will discuss matters further. Trust me, and all shall be yours. I *promise*."

And so that night Ursula struck a bargain with the beautiful, desperate girl: her voice in return for a title for her father, invitations to all the right social events, some wardrobe adjustments, three days to win a noble son, etc., etc. The usual terms. Ursula would have a new voice, a new polyp in her little collection and she would go on ruling properly, and live happily ever after in her new kingdom *by* the sea, if not under it.

Only… not quite.

This is what actually happened.

The Grey Lagoon was an artificial folly on the north side of the castle, fed by the tides. Originally it was protected by a cavern wall decorated with shells and fake stalactites in the fashion of Etrulian bathing grottos. Over the years it had fallen out of use and now slowly decayed into that shabby grandeur Bretlandian tourists so liked to sketch. Locals avoided the place because it had become more or less a swamp, overgrown with tall grass, clinging vines and sharp, scrubby trees. It fairly screamed *cholera* and *malaria*. Also *haunted*.

So it was deserted, this weird landscape feature shielded from the castle by drippy, unhealthy trees, and most importantly: *it was fed salt water by the sea*.

Ursula arrived at ten to make preparations, and it was a bit of a pain because taking Flotsam and Jetsam along would have rendered the whole undertaking too obvious. That was the worst thing about the Dry World: how hard it was to lug things around. Things *fell*. Heavy things fell *harder*. Feet *hurt*. Sometimes after a day in the stacked-heel booties she wore it felt like knives were impaling her through her soles, like obscene torture out of some fairy tale.

She had to manhandle a smaller-than-she-liked

cauldron out to the middle of the shallow water all by herself, along with all the other things necessary for the spell: ingredients and mordants that she managed to keep away from prying eyes.

Getting a little sweaty and trying to keep her tentacles under control, they burst free of their own volition upon touching the salt water, Ursula was ankle-deep in muck and agitated when Julia showed up. The girl was like a picture: her hooded, innocent-yet-arrogant face lit by the small lantern she held before her. She stepped carefully round the bracken, not wanting to snag her precious clothes on the sharp twigs.

"You came," Ursula said, accidentally in her own voice.

The girl, already nervous, jumped at that.

"I don't understand what we are doing, My Princess," she admitted, trying to remain calm.

"My dear, we need to just alter a few things about you," Vanessa said with a smile. "Not just your clothes and introductions. Fortunately, I know a little magic…"

"Magic? Like the devil?" Julia stepped back, pulling her cloak tighter.

"Not at all," Vanessa said with a smile. "Like the kind you use to make love philtres and predict who you will marry with the blow of a dandelion."

It probably would have sounded a lot more carefree and girlish in the dumb mermaid's voice...

Julia looked uncertain.

"Just step forwards into the water," Vanessa urged. "Not all the way, just your feet."

"Into the water?"

"Yes, dear, like for... a baptism. Nothing more. A blessing of magic."

Julia looked sceptical.

"And this will turn me into a princess, like you?"

"It will not turn you *immediately* into a princess, but remember, dear, I didn't 'become' a princess until I married Eric. Everyone just went along with my insistence that I was a princess, to keep up appearances and the family line. I'm going to help you get to that point too. Now, into the water, dear."

"And you ask nothing in return?" Julia asked.

Ursula sighed. *Clever girl.* For a moment she regretted that she had neither time nor inclination to take on an apprentice, or daughter, or whatever you called a young version of what you were. Julia had flexible morals and a quick wit that was lacking in so many of the young mer the witch had often dealt with. It was a shame she had to simply eat her up and use her, rather than take her time...

"Yes, child, there is always a price. But it is not for *me*, it is for… the universe. You can't get something without giving something. That would be unnatural, and against the good order of things."

She almost couldn't believe how easily this rubbish came out of her mouth. Once she had a decent voice again, Vanessa would be unstoppable.

"What do you… I mean, the universe… want?"

"Nothing much, really…"

"My immortal soul?"

"No, no, child!" Ursula didn't have to pretend too hard to be shocked. She was continually surprised by humans' single-mindedness when it came to religion. "Nothing so precious. Just your voice."

"My voice?" Julia touched her throat. Such an obvious gesture, so predictable. Once again Ursula had to work not to roll her eyes.

"Yes. But you get it back once you achieve your wishes, in three days."

"Is three days how long I have to seduce and marry one of the lords?"

Damn, this girl catches on fast.

"Yes. And time is wasting… the… ah… clock is about to strike the quarter hour, and we must proceed before… the halfway point…"

Julia looked at Vanessa, standing in the water: the princess with the wet skirts, in the deserted lagoon filled with black flies and the smell of rot.

"I do not like the feel of this, My Princess."

"Don't be silly, dear girl," Vanessa spoke softly, wheedling. "It will be no problem for you. Three days is nothing. You will come to the banquet tomorrow night and sit by me, as my special guest. They *have* to pay attention to you then. Lords will be falling over themselves for you."

"But why does the universe need my *voice*?" Julia demanded. "What am I getting in return that you couldn't give me for free, without magic? The invites and the dresses and the introductions?"

"Oh, all right," Ursula swore, giving up. "The universe doesn't need your voice. *I* do. I want a young pretty voice to match my young pretty body. And if you don't pay up, you will be nothing, nothing at all, for the rest of your life. Just a stupid, worthless, want-to-be member of the nouveau riche, never quite making it into the exclusive club of nobility. So make your decision, girl. Are you going to stay Julia, the gold-digging flirt whose father builds ships with calloused hands, or become Princess Julia?"

"I am going to keep my voice," Julia said, backing away.

"Come *here*!" Ursula ordered, wading through the water towards her.

Julia turned and fled.

Ursula lunged.

She missed entirely, flopping forwards into the fetid, murky water. Slime ran down her borrowed, beautiful hair. Tentacles scrumped and played in the mud, happy to be free for a moment.

Julia didn't even have the decency to drop the lantern and cause a big, gothic fire on the marsh. She just ran on, the lantern bouncing and growing smaller like the glow from a fading anglerfish.

Eric

The King of the Sea remained stubbornly hidden.

So the prince continued to stubbornly look for him.

Sometimes Eric wondered if he was still under a spell or suffering dementia. If the Mad Prince was rummaging around the castle in the middle of the night and stolen hours for imaginary friends and other things he had made up.

Well, if so, it was a pleasant way to devolve into insanity.

"Prince Eric, I'm afraid it's time for the memorial service with the families of the deceased soldiers."

Eric was just jotting down a tune for the knick-knacks and bric-a-brac that decorated the public drawing room when Grimsby caught him. The prince was especially diligent around the orchids and assorted tropical plants in glass jars, they seemed like the perfect sneaky place to camouflage a polyped king.

"O-oh, yes. Of course. Immediately. I'll go change," he stuttered. "I'm just looking for… I just… misplaced… my… composition book. Again." It was hard to lie to his old friend.

"Surely not the one you're holding," the old butler said dryly.

"What? This? Oh, no. This is… uh… *another* composition book… that I need. I'm redoing a bit for the encore performance of *La Sirenetta*. Fixing some things… can't remember which page, you know? 'Mad Prince Eric' and all that. Maybe I've an early form of dementia."

Grimsby sighed.

"Eric, you trust me with your clothes, your thoughts, your ideas, your *Max*… perhaps you would be willing to trust me on other things as well."

The prince looked at him for a long moment, weighing his old friend's words. How much did he really know?

No, he couldn't risk it. Vanessa had been quite clear with her threat.

"Grims, you can't help me here. I won't let you," he finally said, putting a hand on the butler's shoulder. "The best thing you can do right now is *be* there for me. A lot of this mess is my fault, and I don't want anyone in the crossfire while I clean it up."

He winced: terrible metaphor. Embarrassing for a poet. Mixed and meaningless.

"I understand, Eric. But sometimes… helping people isn't about you at all. Or even the help. Sometimes it's about the people who *want* to help."

"Grimsby, I…" Eric wilted. He hated how this hurt his old friend. He hated how he couldn't say what he wanted to say.

What he actually said was, "Just don't ever find yourself alone in the castle. And don't hang out near balconies. And don't eat anything I don't send to your study myself."

"I am currently subsisting on a diet of biscuits directly from the homeland, thank you. In sealed tins. They are a tad dry but nutritionally sufficient. Here." The butler pointedly handed him a folded piece of paper. "A receipt for the postage on a private package to be delivered to Ibria. Very expensive, I believe you stated a desire to approve all unusual expenditures above a certain amount?"

And with that he spun on his heel and clicked out of the room.

Eric sighed. It broke his heart to treat Grimsby this way.

But I would feel even worse if something happened to him.

He opened the paper, wondering why the butler thought it was worth his time. It wasn't even that high an amount, although ludicrous, really, for the shipping of a single package. There were international carriages for that sort of thing now. And all the instructions that were tacked on were absurd:

KEEP IN THE SHADE AT ALL TIMES; DO NOT ALLOW TO GET TOO HOT; ENSURE THE HOLES IN THE BOX AREN'T BLOCKED SO AIR CAN CIRCULATE; HANDLE CAREFULLY, LIQUID AND GLASS WITHIN…

Eric blinked.

He reread the instructions:

TO BE DELIVERED DIRECTLY TO THE HANDS OF KING OVREL III OF IBRIA, AND NOT A SERVANT OR FOOTMAN. ALSO CONDOLENCES ON THE LOSS OF YOUR EMISSARY, FROM PRINCESS VANESSA.

Glass… liquid… holes so air could circulate… *Vanessa was shipping the King of the Sea out of the castle right under Eric's nose!*

Grimsby *knew.* He knew what Eric was looking for, and had found it.

Good old Grimsby!

Eric's first instinct was to call out a princely order to stop the whole thing. He would head to the Office of the Treasurer immediately to do so.

Then he stopped.

Vanessa had the whole castle on alert, spying for her. If he did anything and was caught, a very likely possibility, Vanessa would punish Grimsby. *Or Max.*

What should he do?

Ariel

When the time came she changed in the deep channel between thickets of razor-sharp grass on the northern side of the marsh, farthest from the castle and its guards. The tide was still coming in, so the water hadn't been sitting in the muddy marsh for hours, growing still and stinky.

On cue Jona dropped down from the heavens and settled on the top of a sturdy tuffet.

Moments later Eric came striding on the path through the grass. He looked lost when he didn't see her by the boat as he expected.

"Eric!" she called out quietly.

"Ariel!" His face broke into a wide smile that warmed her from the inside. "I was afraid you wouldn't be here!"

"Have you found him?" she asked eagerly.

The prince took a deep breath and gripped her shoulders.

"I did find some polyps, but not your father. Some other prisoners of Vanessa's. Horrible things, disguised in her cosmetics."

Ariel felt the sea inside her retreat into the depths of her soul.

What a happy ending it *could* have been, Eric bringing her father; freeing Triton right there, on the marshes…

But life was complicated.

Eric saw her wilt and he held her steady.

"I'm so sorry, Ariel," he said. "Also… Vanessa knows I know about her."

Ariel shook her head at the multiplicity of bad news. "But how did that…?"

"Long story. Terrible dinner. Actually, *great* dinner. Just terribly awkward. But there *is* a little bit of good news."

He showed her the receipt.

"I believe Ursula is trying to sneak your father out of the castle right under my nose… and impress a potential ally at the same time. She's giving Triton to the king of Ibria as a specimen for his zoo."

Ariel looked at the paper, the edge of her lip rising in disgust.

"A specimen for his *zoo*?"

"Yes, and according to a little prying I've done on my own, she even told him directly that it was the King of the Sea, transformed. I doubt he believes it, but still. A lovely story for his noble guests."

"Can't you stop this? Grab the, uh, *package* from her?"

"Ah... yes... well... besides knowing that I know who she is, Vanessa also knows I'm helping you. She has threatened to kill Grimsby if she finds evidence of it."

"Grimsby?" Ariel cried. "He's harmless! That *monster...*"

"She knows how much he means to me," Eric said darkly. "*That's* her magic. Not real magic. She's brilliant at finding the thing you love most and threatening to destroy it."

Ariel groaned. "I wish I had that insight before I visited her the first time."

"Age brings wisdom," the prince said with a dry smile. "But look, it's not actually such a bad thing. If I act like normal Eric, like I don't even know what's happening with the gift or the mail at all, that makes it far more unlikely that she will suspect anything, or try to stop us."

"Good point. So what do we do?"

It didn't even cross her mind for a moment to trade

Grimsby for her father. Throwing an innocent under Ursula's chariot for her own gain would make her no better than the sea witch herself.

"Well, when I said 'we', I really meant 'you.' The carriage leaves for Ibria tomorrow. It will stop in the market to pick up other packages for delivery beyond the kingdom at midday and leave from the tavern at one o'clock. You could waylay it with your storm powers and grab your father, and no one would be the wiser! At worst they might think it was the work of a highwayman looking for gold."

"I can't," Ariel said gently, although she was amused by the image: Queen of the Sea and Highway Robber. "My powers don't work on land. Only water. Just like hers."

"Oh." Eric's face fell. His lower lip was stuck out a little. It was a tiny bit childish but terribly endearing. She almost felt bad that her godlike powers had presented this limitation to him.

"Couldn't you… stay in the sea… and direct a single, tiny wave or wind to hit it?"

"It's not that precise. And it's less like shooting out a bolt with my trident than encouraging the powers of nature to do something of their own accord. It's not… neat. But if it's just one or two men in the carriage, I think I can manage, with some help from my friends."

"The seagulls?"

"Also my… mermaid charms." She smiled. *Too bad Sebastian won't be there to hear me, singing like a siren.* "Trust me, we can do it."

"Perfect! By this time tomorrow it will all be over."

"And I will have my father back!" Her heart leapt. There was still going to be a happy ending after all.

"And then we can get rid of Vanessa," Eric said. "The sooner, the better. She's far more dangerous than I ever realised."

"It's a plan," said Ariel. "All we need to do now is carry it through!"

"Absolutely!"

"Great!"

"Good!"

"Excellent!"

A moment passed as they smiled at each other.

Another moment passed, somewhat awkwardly.

And then a third.

"All… right, then! Good luck! Hopefully when we next meet you'll have your father back!" Eric blurted out.

"Yes! That will be great!" Ariel replied enthusiastically.

They shook hands and parted.

I hope Eric feels as stupid as I do, Ariel thought grumpily.

Ariel

She entered the town late the next morning, and kept her headscarf close around her.

The market was different today, different vendors selling entirely different wares. In Atlantica it was always the same people selling the same things to the same people, only a slight variation with the seasons. *It's Red Kelp Festival Day! Oh, it's the Incredibly Rare and Beautiful Blue-Tipped Anemone Spawning Day! Oh! It's that guy who makes those little wood carvings of the gods out of shipwreck material!*

Actually, those were pretty great, Ariel allowed. She owned at least a dozen of them.

Jona flew above her, occasionally landing on a roof when it was convenient. Several dozen gulls circled close by. Ariel hoped they wouldn't be necessary; she didn't want to draw attention to the situation. With any luck she could just distract the coachman, maybe sing a sireny tune or two to mesmerise him, then grab the package. And then she could return to her kingdom triumphantly, her father in hand, and it would all be over.

The carriage pulled up behind the tavern precisely at ten. There was only one driver.

Easy, the Queen of the Sea told herself.

But the driver was staring at her.

Leering at her.

In a strangely familiar way.

Ariel fell back, suddenly realising who it was.

Run! she told herself.

Somehow she didn't.

The door to the carriage creaked open, pushed from inside by the footman, who was the driver's twin.

Out stepped Vanessa.

For just a moment, Ariel saw Ursula. Grinning and sharp-toothed, surrounded by her waving black tentacles. All predator, all evil. Sharks killed to eat. Ursula *enjoyed* the pain she caused.

Then the moment was over and the princess of Tirulia

stood there, 'disguised', wrapped in a long, flowing shift that made her look like an actor playing a foreign priestess in one of those operas Sebastian conducted from time to time. Her eyes were large and doe-like, but her smile was vicious and exactly the same as the sea witch's.

Ariel felt a cold rage settle on her shoulders, and the world narrowed down until it was just the two of them.

"Were you expecting something from the postman, maybe?" Vanessa purred, in Ursula's voice. "A package, perhaps?"

"Very amusing, Ursula. You're so… *funny*," Ariel said, trying not to let her anger show.

"Thank you. Nice legs, by the way."

"Thank you," Ariel said. "I made them myself."

"Oh, yes… you're 'Queen of the Sea' now. With all the powers and privileges thereof. *And the trident.*" Her eyes flicked greedily over Ariel, looking for some sign of the weapon. "Isn't it funny…? Your father could have turned you into a human any time he wanted to. But he didn't. Withholding his abilities so selfishly… trying to keep you locked up at home…"

"He was trying to protect me," Ariel said flatly. "It's not the choice I would have made in his position, but he thought he was doing the right thing."

"But you *are* in his position now," Vanessa said, eyes

wide and innocent. "Are you telling me that if you had a daughter, you would just, let her go?"

"If I had a daughter I would make sure she had every opportunity to do what she wanted to enrich her life. Sometimes being a good parent means knowing *when* to let go."

"Well, well, isn't *that* a thoughtful and mature philosophy," Vanessa said, looking at her nails. "Never really had the inclination for children myself, except as dessert."

Ariel just gave her a look, and it wasn't one of horror. One of the most tiring aspects of Ursula wasn't even her villainy; it was her constant bid for attention, for shock value, for turning the conversation back to herself.

"I believe you took something of mine," Ursula said.

"I believe you took something of *mine*," Ariel retorted.

"I believe I traded that from you fairly, in return for something of *mine*. My magic to help you win your man."

"It wasn't a fair trade. You were preying on my desperation and knew that I would fail."

"I believe you were, as they say, of sound mind and body when we made the deal. No one forced you into it and you knew exactly what you were doing."

"I was a dumb, innocent girl!" Ariel snapped, disappointing herself.

You're a queen now, not *that innocent girl. Do not sink to her level. She is beneath you.*

"And it's been… what? Five or six years since then?" Vanessa asked innocently. "*Nothing* in the span of a mermaid's life. The tiniest fraction of a percentage. But I suppose you're all grown up now?"

"I have grown," Ariel said frostily. "And I am queen. And I suspect that if we were to go back and re-examine those three days from all sides, like a god, we would see that you had cheated somehow. Even before you used my own voice and someone else's body and your magic to steal Eric from me!"

"There was no non-compete clause," Vanessa said, almost reasonably. "I never said I couldn't go after the same lovely human. He *is* lovely, by the way."

Ariel knew the witch was trying to get a rise out of her… and she was succeeding; the mermaid could feel warmth rising to her cheeks.

"*Please.* He has no tail or tentacles. I doubt you find him attractive at all. He's just a pawn in an elaborate game to punish me and my father."

"You got me there," Vanessa sighed dramatically.

"Thank you. Now give me my father."

"He's not in the carriage, sweetest. He's not anywhere

you can get him. I have *other* plans for the King of the Sea, none of which involve you or the zoo of the king of Ibria. Both of you fooled… it's quite delicious, really. The king *is* getting a gift, a lesser member of my pretty polyps. Not that the stupid human could tell the difference."

"Very cleverly done," Ariel said coldly. "I suppose you have to resort to plain trickery since your powers don't work on land."

"Well, perhaps my *magic* doesn't. Not *yet*," Vanessa allowed, but a quick twist of fury that came and went like lightning across her face spoke of something that irked her deeply. *That definitely merits further investigation later.* "But I have other powers, you know. Power over the infinite corruptibility of humans. Power over absolute *sacks* of gold, which you and I couldn't care less about, but these people worship more than their gods. Power over life and death in that castle where your darling prince lives."

"Ursula. I know Father exiled you from the kingdom, and you wanted revenge on him. But why involve me?"

"Well, you were a pawn, dear, of course. Another *lovely* pawn," Vanessa said with a sensual shrug. "The best way to get at Triton was through his favourite daughter."

"I'm not—"

"Please," Vanessa interrupted sharply. "The *youngest.*

The *prettiest.* The one with the *beautiful voice.* The one who looked the most like his own dead wife. Everybody knows it. Humans do the same thing, have children who are their favourites, but *they* constantly rail against the habit in their religions and laws. They try so hard to defeat their own base natures. It's one of many things I find rather attractive about them."

Ariel didn't answer immediately, processing this. She almost wished she still had no voice so she could stall for time while coming up with the right signs.

"Is that why you're still here, causing trouble?" she finally asked. "Because you like the humans you live among?"

"Well, yes." Vanessa put a finger to her lips, seriously considering the idea. "They are so rash and easily manipulated and full of *feelings* and quick to agree to anything, more like a race of children than a real race, if you ask me. You know, I almost understand your fascination with them now. Before, I thought it was because you were just a dumb bored teenager looking for a way to shock your father."

Ariel opened her mouth to respond but Vanessa cut her off, coming near. She lowered her head and hunched her shoulders, like Ursula preparing to attack, and Ariel was pretty sure that if there had been shadows in the alley, the one behind her would have shown tentacles waving high, poised to strike.

"You will never, *ever* get your father back. You, the merfolk, everyone under the sea, you have all lost the great King Triton *forever.* And you will lose so much more… That is what you get for exiling Ursula. *That* is what happens to everyone who crosses her!"

Ariel said nothing, she just raised an eyebrow, as if to say, *Are you done now?*

"And you can just forget about ever getting Eric back too," the sea witch added snidely. "Whether or not he remains devoted to *me*, he is oddly devoted to his people."

"It's not odd," Ariel responded, a little sadly. "A good ruler, a successful ruler, loves her people and governs at their will. She doesn't use them up for her own selfish purposes. Some day you might actually learn that, even if you triumph against me now. The humans will not put up with you forever."

Vanessa's face dissolved into another Ursula-style snarl.

"If I catch Eric helping you in any way, Grimsby will die."

Ariel *almost* said, *I know this already*, but stopped herself just in time.

She wasn't a great actress and couldn't feign last-minute

surprise. So she spoke the truth.

"You're a monster."

Vanessa crossed her arms. "You're up to something. I can tell. You're trying to cheat, somehow."

"How does that feel?" Ariel asked innocently.

"If you're going to play a game of knives, you had better prepare to *win*," Vanessa growled. "All you have ever done so far is lose. Lose your voice, lose your prince, lose your father. Don't for a moment think you have gained the upper hand just because you have a crown now. Content yourself with ruling the merfolk; they are about all you can handle.

"Go back to the sea, little mermaid. Go back and leave the human world forever. Leave them… to me."

Ursula

She made a suitably dramatic exit, stepping languidly up into her carriage and having Jetsam slam the door and Flotsam whip the horses to move off.

It was a *little* bit uncomfortable in the carriage, it being a mail coach and not made for the transporting of royal princesses. Also, there was indeed a large wooden crate for eventual delivery to Ibria, random and delicate polyp within.

But at least it was dark and cool inside. She pulled down the shade, which cut the glare further and also amused her: its translucent material was made from the swim bladders of fish. As she ran a finger down its textured surface she grinned at the number of lives given just so she could avoid a headache.

The coach slowly began to roll off and Ursula's smile faded. She had come out on top in their verbal sparring… she should have been exultant. She should have celebrated the fact that the stupid mermaid princess, *excuse me*, queen, had appeared just as she predicted. And did the sea witch ever show *her*! She had all the cards, all the leverage and the mermaid had none. Ursula was at the top of her game. There was *nothing* Ariel could do but swim back to her little home under the waves forever.

"Stupid minnow," she said aloud.

"Ridiculous *hussy*," she added a moment later.

But she was uneasy.

It wasn't a feeling she liked.

She looked out the window at the passing scenes: gigantic ancient trees with their hard stems and their weeping branches, a group of soldiers sharing a flask, a school of little brats chasing each other around in the dirt. *Almost* in the way of the carriage. Tempting.

Being among the humans for all these years had been fun. There was a learning curve, of course, but that was fine: up till then it had been literally decades since the witch had been forced to learn anything new. Her mind had relished the opportunity and the chance to start again. In the Dry World she had remade herself into a ruler. In the Dry World she had no magic powers, yet, but something almost better: power over people. In the Dry World, blood flowed down, in a stream, to the ground and pooled and dried there.

But… that stupid little mermaid. Just when Ursula was about to launch her wars and move up the ladder to queen, or empress, Ariel came back. *To take it all away.* Just like Triton had taken it all away from Ursula: the kingdom, her title, her entourage, her *life*.

What was wrong with the two of them? Why couldn't they just leave her alone?

Ursula twisted in her seat, really thinking about the sea for the first time in years. The place where she once had power, and where the stupid mermaid should have stayed. All of Atlantica just sat there, smugly, under the water, not caring if the sea witch was exiled to a nearby cave or the Dry World or the moon. She didn't matter to any of the merfolk at all any more, except for Ariel and her father. It was like her revenge counted for nothing.

She began to drum her fingers on the ledge of the window. Thoughts ponderously swirled in her mind, like the slow circling current that foretold an eventual whirlpool.

Real revenge would be wiping the mer off the face of the planet. All of them.

Even if the humans never found out or understood what she had done, *she* would know. Anyone who survived would know. The fish would know. They would all know about an ancient, mysterious civilisation that had just… vaporised one day, leaving relics and mysteries behind them.

And… if Ariel were on land when it happened, trying to find her father, and escaped the destruction of her people… she would also know. And so would her father. They would have to live with that for the rest of their lives.

And merfolk, even as polyps, lived for a very, very long time.

But if Ariel were in the sea and died with her people, well, that would mean a tidy end to all of Ursula's problems. She would be free to play with her humans, unimpeded, until the end of time. Or until she grew bored. And bonus: Triton would be extra miserable.

A hideous grin began to spread across Vanessa's features, far wider than should have been possible with the lips she had.

How perfect! No matter what happened, she won! Those were the sea witch's favourite odds. And no messy spells involving the Elder Gods were needed.

"Flotsam!" she shouted, knocking on the window. "We're making one stop before the castle. Take me to… the shipyards."

Flotsam touched his hat.

Ursula began to laugh, feeling like her old self again.

Ariel

She lay in the warm sand, exhausted and not a little stunned. Clean, fresh seawater lapped at her feet.

Flounder turned sad circles just off the shore. Jona stood close by Ariel's head, obviously resisting the urge to comfort-groom her.

"What now?" Flounder eventually asked.

"I thought this would be it this time, I really did," Ariel said, a little hollowly. "Once again, I thought I would rescue Dad and he would forgive me and we would return home and everyone would be happy. Am I *stupid*?"

"No, you're not stupid, Ariel!" Flounder said, worried at her tone.

"I believe your sea witch has been practising evil and trickery for centuries," Jona pointed out reasonably. "You haven't even practised evil once. She's much better at it than you."

Ariel smiled tiredly. "Thanks, Jona."

She sat up and hugged her knees, looking at her toes, the sand, the water beyond.

Ursula isn't sitting around gloating, or maybe she is, but she's also *planning her next move.* Get up, *girl! No time for self-pity.*

She stretched the kinks out of her body and stood, ready to make the sad walk back into the sea.

"What about Eric?" Flounder asked. "Are you going to let him know what happened? So he can go back to searching?"

Oops. Of course she had to let Eric know what had happened. She was so consumed with her own failure she had entirely forgotten the prince, who had a whole kingdom resting on the fate of Ursula. *Thoughtless, Ariel.*

"Oh, yes… but I don't know *how* to let him know. I can't get near the castle."

"I can," Jona volunteered.

"That's right, you can! Hmm…" She took off the leather strap she had been wearing on her wrist, the one with the little golden bail that once held the nautilus. Then she tossed it into the air and touched her comb, using the power of the trident to summon and affix something to the end.

"Here." She threw the necklace to Jona. "Give this to him. He'll understand. And now… I have to return to Atlantica and face everyone."

"You won't do it alone," Flounder promised, patting her with a fin.

Eric

He paced the castle anxiously, waiting for… *something*. Some kind of word. Everything, the last few years of his tortured life, could be resolved in the next few hours if she succeeded! And if not…

… *well, if not, we'll deal with it.*

He was so deep in his thoughts he slammed, head-on, into Carlotta.

"Egads! Sorry!" Eric extricated himself from the folds of cloth and aprons and clothes she was carrying.

"It's all right," Carlotta said, patting herself down as best she could with one hand and fixing her little hat. "I was just coming to do the princess's linens."

"*You?* Isn't that one of the younger maids' jobs? Maria, or Lalia, or one of those younger girls?"

"Well..." Carlotta bit her lip, "... it takes a special touch to, er, tuck in the edges properly and... *poke around a bit*, you know..."

Eric gave her a severe look. "Carlotta, is the entire downstairs staff in league together or something?"

"No," she answered primly, refolding a pillowcase expertly over her arm. "That's why *I'm* the one fussing about the princess's room, and not someone as can't be trusted."

The prince sighed. "I don't know whether to be relieved or annoyed that you're involved. I suppose I'll tell you as straight as I can: Grimsby will get into serious trouble if he's caught helping out, er, *foreign* powers. So far I've heard nothing about you."

Carlotta growled and put her hands on her hips, pushing her chest into the prince's. "Why, that low-down, dirty... *so-and-so*! She threatened Mr Grimsby? How much more can she get away with? Prince Eric, it's not my place, but Tirulia is a *modern country*. We will not be subject to the policies and habits of such arcane despots! *You must reveal her to the public as the beast she is!*"

"Er..." He looked side to side desperately for an escape.

She had him pressed practically against the wall.

"And also *that she is a murderer,"* Carlotta whispered, raising her eyebrows suggestively.

"Carlotta, hush, you're talking about Princess Vanessa. That's treason. And besides, she couldn't have done it. Her powers don't work… uh, I mean, the Ibrian just seemed to have *died.*"

"She's a clever little sea princess," the maid said. "Do you think she might not be working on ways round her… limitations? That she hasn't found some? Perhaps, Your Highness, you haven't been following her latest hobbies." She gestured with her chin out the window. "Although many noble ladies do garden, I suppose, there's nothing unusual in that. And now, I really must make the lady's bed before the lady threatens *me* with something or other." And with that she flounced off.

Eric looked out the window she had indicated, at the neat rows of flowers before the willow grove. Everything looked normal, if a little dull since his grandmother had grown too frail to keep taking a personal hand in her seaside garden.

Then, squinting, he saw a patch that looked different from the rest. Freshly turned, and irregularly planted.

He leapt downstairs as fast as he could and ran outside.

The fact that there was an entirely new, if tiny, garden on castle grounds that Eric hadn't heard anything about was… disheartening. It was just one more detail that cemented Eric's flailing, ignorant and useless place in his own castle. His grandmother would have known about it immediately. Would have been told the moment the gardeners started spending their time on anything besides her heirloom roses and exotic perennials.

The plants growing in this new patch were not roses, though they did more or less fall into the category of *exotic perennial*. Eric studied the leaves and little identifying tags.

Artemisia. Okay, that was like wormwood, what they made absinthe out of. His grandmother had always liked their pretty woolly silver leaves.

Belladonna. Clary sage, henbane. Old-fashioned herbs.

Mandrake.

He recognised the last because a sailor had once shown him a particularly fine specimen of the root; it looked like a little person. "There's folks in Bretland will pay a king's ransom for this. I just have to tell them it screamed when the farmer pulled it out of the soil."

Eric shook his head in wonder. Even to someone more skilled in the arts of the sea and music than farming, it was obvious Vanessa was trying her hand at a witch's garden.

Her magic didn't work on land. So she was trying to learn new magic. *Land* magic.

Was that… a thing?

Was witchcraft real?

If it was, could Vanessa harness its powers? Would she be able to summon undead armies to do her bidding, call down storms and plagues on countries they were at war with?

Would she be able to cast new charms? Would Eric once again find himself foggy and forgetting, hypnotised and half-awake? Would he do everything his terrible wife said?

He swallowed, trying to control the panic that was coming on.

Boneset. Some said it was good for aches and pains. Modern doctors disagreed.

Wolfsbane.

Foxglove. A pretty flower, and dangerous to animals. It was also known as *digitalis* and contained a substance that destroyed the heart, literally. Eric remembered his father telling him not to let Max anywhere near it if they found some in the woods.

Whether or not witchcraft was real, poison certainly was.

No one really believed the Ibrian had died of natural

causes. And here, more or less, was the proof: holes in the ground where some of the flowers had been pulled out. *Used.* The plant could be put into anything: tea, soup, tobacco mix for a pipe… Vanessa could make good on her threat at any time. Grimsby would keel over from a heart attack and no one would suspect anything, it would be sad, but an entirely natural, predictable death.

Nothing Eric could ever do would convince the butler to abandon his post, short of tying him up and putting him on a boat to the lands in the west against his will. Eric ran his hands through his hair, frustrated and at wit's end.

A large bird landed on a statue behind him, casting a cold black shadow. The prince turned, fully expecting a crow or raven, as befitted the mood of the garden.

But it was a seagull. With something stringy and brown in its mouth.

"Hello," Eric said politely. "Did Ariel send you?"

The bird answered by dropping the thing it held onto the ground. It squawked.

"Thank you…?" He picked up the leather cord; it was the one Ariel wore round her wrist. Now, letting it flow through his fingers, he realised it was the strap from the necklace that Vanessa used to wear, the one with the nautilus on it.

(Now the princess wore a gold chain that dipped down under her bodice. He had no idea what sort of pendant was on it, probably something unsettling and hideous.)

A white scroll was tied to one end of the strap; it unfurled of its own accord into his hand. On it, sketched in gold, was a carriage with a half-octopus, half-woman thing emerging through the door. There was also a drawing of a crown with what looked like a slash or a tear through it.

Eric swore when he realised what it meant. "It was a trap. The king wasn't even there!" The little scroll faded into glitter, disappearing entirely even as he tried to grasp at the bits.

But if Ariel had cast this pretty little spell, he realised, it meant that she had to be in the water. Which meant she was safe. Just… disappointed and probably grieving. His heart went out to the poor queen of the merfolk. They had both been so sure their respective ordeals were almost over.

"Is it back to searching the castle again, then?" Eric asked aloud, partially to the seagull. "Well, if that's what we have to do, that's what we *will* do. Guess I'd better expand the search to the rest of the grounds too, huh? I wish *you* could help. I could use another set of eyes. Ones that aren't easily fooled by magic. I wish I had an animal friend who could watch Grimsby for me. I'm afraid Max isn't much up to the task."

The bird squawked again and shook its tail. Almost like it was saying, *Yes, but what can you do?* Then it settled down to preen itself.

Eric laughed and reached out to scratch it on its neck, like he would have Max. The bird seemed to enjoy it immensely.

Ariel

I deserve this, Ariel thought as she delivered the news of her failure again and again and again. Of course the general populace was disappointed. She expected the frowns and the occasional dramatic tears.

Telling her sisters was extremely unpleasant. They wept *real* tears and swished their tails back and forth in dismay. And then they swam off, all but Attina, who gave her a quick hug before leaving.

The Queen's Council was also disappointed, though not terribly surprised, and quick to talk about the future, and Ariel's loyalty to her people, and how maybe further rescue attempts should be turned over to those who weren't the acting queen.

"We should send an army of merfolk, with legs, up through the castle, and seize it," the captain of the merguards suggested. Her eyes shone and her partner, a giant bluefish, nodded eagerly. "It will be like battles of old, sword against sword! We will retrieve the king triumphantly and remind humans of our might!"

"And while you are waving your shiny swords, the humans will be shooting at you with their guns," Ariel said wearily. "That's why I wanted to do this alone, and stealthily. To limit the loss of life."

"Forget the army. Use the power of the sea," a merman senator suggested. "Use your trident and teach the humans a lesson!"

"Yes," Ariel said, leaning back on her throne. "I've actually thought of that. I could destroy the castle and everyone in it with one mighty wave. The advantage of killing Ursula this way is that my father and *all* of her prisoners would be transformed immediately upon her death and released directly into the sea."

Flounder and Sebastian exchanged surprised, and shocked, looks. Had she really considered this?

Ariel turned her eyes to the glowing dome of the surface to avoid seeing their faces. Yes, she *had* thought about it.

If her goal was truly just to get her father back and wreak revenge on Ursula, it was probably the most direct and efficient route. A giant tsunami wiping out a kingdom's castle and all within… some would call it a natural disaster, but others would suspect the truth and tell stories. Maybe people would start respecting the sea again, properly. Maybe they would stop fishing it out and dumping their rubbish into it.

And, from an artistic perspective, how utterly apocalyptic and perfect: destroying her enemy and possibly her lover at the same time. *Very* Old God. They'd be singing about her for centuries.

One side of her mouth tugged into a wry smile. The old Ariel wouldn't have even had these thoughts; she would have dismissed them immediately as horrific and unthinkable.

Now she could think them. She just couldn't *do* them.

"No, guys," she said aloud. "I'm not actually killing everyone in the castle in a tidal wave of utter destruction."

Sebastian and Flounder looked chagrined that she had read their minds, but also relieved.

"Your Majesty, I must attend the Planktonic Life Interior Committee meeting," Klios the dolphin said apologetically, with a bow. "I will continue to ponder our problem of rescuing the king. But for now, other duties call."

"Yes, go. We could all use a break anyway," Ariel said,

rubbing her head for the second time that week. "We'll reconvene on the next tide to discuss further."

As most of the council swam off, Sebastian approached her, sideways and slowly. "Well, then, while we are taking a break thinking about all *this*… maybe we can talk about something *else*? My next masterpiece, maybe? A celebration of the tides. A celebration of the sea. A celebration celebrating the return of your voice, starring…"

Ariel narrowed her eyes at him.

"… well, your voice?" He gave her a winning crabby grin.

"Queens. Do not. *Sing*. Sebastian."

"But Ariel, now that you *can* sing again…"

"My father did not put on pantomimes or act in farces. My mother did not perform burlesque. My station does not allow for such gross frippery. No one would take me seriously again."

"Your mother's voice was terrible."

"Sebastian!"

"Sorry, but it's the truth. And you are not your father…"

"No, but would you suggest this if I were a *prince*? Somehow I think not."

"But Ariel! Think of your people! They have lived without hearing your voice for so long! Don't they deserve to hear your singing?"

"My singing is *my singing*," she said, bending down to put her eyes on level with the little crab. "My voice is *my* voice. I gave it away myself and I got it back again myself. It is not for anyone else's enjoyment or amusement. If I want to sing, I will sing. Right now I use my voice to give orders and run a kingdom. Some day, if our situation changes, perhaps I will consider your idea. Until that time, however, I ask that you not speak to me of it again."

Sebastian clicked his claws together in the crab equivalent of fists and ground his mandibles, trying to keep from saying anything. Flounder put a steadying fin on his back.

"Let it go," he whispered, pulling the little crab away.

As the two left together, Sebastian might have been heard to mutter something about her being *exactly like her father…*

Ariel gloomily looked over the piles of paperwork that were her 'reward' after the meeting.

She sighed and tapped on her desk with a pen, a sharp-tipped whelk, and rested her chin on her hand.

It was no use. She couldn't concentrate. All she could think about was her father… and losing her temper at Sebastian.

She would have to make it up to the little crab somehow. Maybe she would commission him to write and prepare a celebratory chorus for *something*. Maybe that would assuage his wounded ego.

She thought about her duet with Eric. It was almost uncanny how the boy she had fallen in love with once had managed to enrapture her again as his current older self. He was sadder, captive to a strange fate, but still possessed the heart of the old prince and his love for music. After all this, even if they were confined to their own worlds forever, she would love the chance to sing with him once last time.

… nope. Actually, she didn't want that. She was going to be honest; that's what queens did.

She wanted to kiss him.

She wanted to embrace him. She wanted to try spending time with him somewhere, his world or hers, it didn't matter. One more duet was meaningless. She wanted to own his heart.

That hadn't changed.

"Working hard?"

Ariel jumped. Attina had swum up in her usual sneaky, silent way.

"I just… there's so much here. Got lost for a second."

"Is life down here getting boring?"

"Attina, just… all right," Ariel said, throwing her pen down. It bounced slowly in the water, raising up a little bit of settled coral dust on the edge of her perfect marble desk before eventually skittering off the side and over to the sea floor. The two mermaids watched it in surprise.

"A little defensive, aren't we?"

"You're picking at me. Please just admit it."

"Settle down, little sister. I know that you're upset about not getting our father back, *again*." But before Ariel could open her mouth to yell at her, Attina continued, louder. "*And I know you are taking it much harder than the rest of us*. Please."

She added, more softly:

"I know how hard you're trying. But you may, at some point, have to admit to yourself that it might not be enough. That it's too hard a task even for the great Ariel, Queen of the Sea and Walker on Land."

Ariel opened her mouth to say something, but couldn't find the right words, overcome with what her sister had said. It was so understanding, so deep, so…

"*Also,* you are completely bored under the sea. It's totally obvious."

Ariel snapped her mouth shut. Attina was looking at knick-knacks on her desk, specifically not at *her*, but there was a twinkle in her eye.

The Queen of the Sea managed a little smile.

"Well… to be honest, it *is* boring. But I have a thousand other, more important things on my mind! Why *has* Ursula continued to let our father live despite my repeated rescue attempts, and yet refused to use him as a bargaining chip? It's unsettling, and it's probably for very bad reasons. Where is he right now? What is she doing to him?

"I'm worried about the fate of two kingdoms and one old butler. I'm worried about time passing… and meanwhile, I have to go over some bizarre ancient contract specifying which member of the lineage of Kravi gets to perform which Rite of Proserpine in the Equinocturnal Celebrations. Like it matters?"

Attina looked over her shoulder at the paper. "Give the lead to Sumurasa. Her brother would just muck it up."

"I mean, I know, but he was born first. There's no way around that."

"Well… find something else for him to do that sounds good but doesn't have any real responsibilities. A nice title he can brag about."

Ariel raised an eyebrow in surprise.

"That's not a bad idea. Maybe you should start coming to the council meetings too…"

"Nahh, not really my thing. Boring, like you said." But Attina again avoided her gaze, drifting over to a golden bowl of bright sea leaves. She examined them closely: exotic oranges, reds and yellows, a single slender purple… and finally just plucked out the biggest one and began to munch on it. "Bah, not like an apple. How's your little, uh, human toy doing up there?"

"Hopefully he's looking for Father. Since *I* failed to find him."

"You still love him?"

"Irrelevant to the matters at hand," Ariel said primly.

"You are *so strange*," Attina whispered with something like awe.

"I'm not—"

"You *are*. Don't you get that? You always have been. As a girl you never liked *anything* the rest of us liked. We looked for shells, you looked for ship rubbish. We swooned over mermen, you lusted after statues of creepy two-legged Dry Worlders. You had this beautiful voice that everyone envied, and you *gave it away*. You don't like being queen, but you do it willingly and honestly as some sort of penance for what happened to our father. You've never tried to abdicate, though it's *pretty obvious* you hate it.

"You don't want to be here. You *never* wanted to be here."

Ariel raised an eyebrow at her thoughtfully. "Mostly true. Nice use of the word 'abdicate', by the way."

"What I'm trying to say is… your stupid desires and wishes got us into this terrible mess and got our father taken away, and I'm still mad at you for that. But if you do get our father back, you should… you know… go after that dumb mortal."

The Queen of the Sea looked at her sister in shock.

"We'll miss you if you go, of course. But I'd understand. Well, I mean, I don't understand," she added, twitching her tail. "Humans are ugly and dumb and evil and short-lived. But all that aside, there's something a little Old God about you, Ariel. There's something epic about loving a mortal and wanting to leave your eternal, paradisiacal world. Something the rest of us will never understand, but people write sagas about. Even your failure and sadness are the stuff of poetry."

"Um. Thanks?"

Attina sighed. "You know, in your own way, you were once a super girly, carefree, bubbly, beautiful little girl. I still don't understand how you got to be so strange underneath it all."

Ariel was about to answer that very older-sister, not-really-a-compliment remark when Threll appeared.

"My Queen, Princess-Doyenne Farishal and her consort are waiting to speak to you about their children's official Coming of Age?"

"Oh, joy," Ariel said grimly. "Excuse me, sister; duty calls."

"Of course it does," Attina said with a sigh, still chewing on a leaf. "*Hey!* If you *do* see Eric again, have him grab us some more apples, will you?"

Ursula and Eric

"But when will my ships be done and ready *to launch*?"

It was getting harder and harder to pretend that the summer cold that had taken her voice was still hanging on, especially since she didn't act like the rest of the ridiculous, simpering ladies of the court did when they had ague or anxieties or chills or whatever else they complained of. Ursula continued to stomp up and down the castle corridors, and she ate like a champion.

But right then she didn't even care about her voice; she slammed her fists down on the table and bared her teeth at the broad-chested older man standing before her.

The fleet admiral regarded her with icy black eyes.

"We have employed every qualified shipwright in the kingdom, My Princess, and quite a few unskilled manual labourers. The shipyards are at capacity. If we had scaled this up properly, we would have built a second shipyard beforehand. You're asking for a battle-ready fleet to be amassed in almost no time, out of thin air. Give us more space and another month and you will have one of the finest armadas on the continent."

"In a *week*, if I wanted to, I could… set certain *things* in motion that would allow me to no longer require a month, or your pesky ships, or even *you*," Ursula growled. "A month is too late. For your own health, if nothing else, get those ships on the sea and loaded with explosives, *now*."

Anyone else would have looked uncomfortable at the order, but rarely did any emotion pass over the dark skin stretched tightly over the bones in the admiral's face.

"I don't care if you're actually a witch," he finally said. "I don't care if you believe the moon gives you special powers or if you can control the seas. But neither spiritualism nor cetaceamancy nor threats to my person will make these ships ready any faster, unless you have the power to conjure a hundred more men and another dock. If all goes well we will launch and begin our assault on the Verdant Coast by the end of the summer."

"Who said anything about attacking the *coast*?" Ursula

demanded. "Forget about the stupid forts and towns for now. You have new orders, drawn out here. And you will get those ships done in two weeks, because I am your princess and that is your job."

"Then it is *not* my job any longer," the admiral said crisply, undoing the medal at his chest. He neatly, not viciously, threw it on her desk, where it landed with a *thwap*. Then he took off his blue tricorn hat and put it under his arm. "Good luck, Princess."

He spun on his heel and marched off, every inch the military man.

Bother.

She had been really looking forward to wiping out the mer as soon as possible. It was like the best treat ever. It would still happen, of course, just later than she wanted. But she hated waiting around for things. Was it time to try the circuex?

No… things weren't that bad. Yet. Just mildly annoying.

But ah, there is that other *idea I had for getting to Ariel. It's not as grand, but would keep me amused for a while, and give those pesky townsfolk something to think about besides their own worthless opinions on my military expeditions.*

Eric came striding into the room a moment later. "Why is Admiral Tarbish in such a huff? I've never seen him like that!"

"He quit," Vanessa said mildly, picking up the medal and examining it. The admiral's move was unexpected, but not necessarily unwelcome. It was a definite opportunity, and surprisingly, conveniently done.

"QUIT?" Eric exploded. "Our fleet admiral just *quit*?"

"Yes, I'm afraid he lacks the confidence to amass our *fleet* of ships in a timely fashion. Never mind, I have the perfect replacement. Lord Savho very much likes the sea and has been looking for some way of… contributing… to our current military endeavours."

"Savho has never captained a ship, much less led an invasion! Or an exploration! Or a trading mission! I doubt he's ever been beyond the bay!" Eric swore, taking his cap off and throwing it on the ground in the most unprincely display of humours Ursula had seen yet. It was almost amusing.

"But he does have a lot of money, and he would be extremely loyal," Vanessa said with a shrug. "I'm sure the first mate or whatever can bring him up to speed."

Eric felt his anger collapse under exhaustion and the weight of it all. How did you get rid of a woman who, with no magic powers to speak of, managed to manipulate and twist the whole world round her finger?

Or tentacle, really.

"Listen to me," he said wearily. "I don't like you. I don't love you. But I'm married to you, and you are, currently, the princess of Tirulia. And you are tearing Tirulia apart. I'm not going to let that happen. For now we are still Prince Eric and Princess Vanessa, and you have to stop communicating with my generals and admirals without me. Starting now."

"Careful, *Prince Eric*," she said, trying to sound calm, but a quaver crept into her voice. "What might have been yours at one time is now shared by us. Should anything happen to you—"

"Should anything happen to me?" Eric laughed dismissively. "I'm not Grimsby. I'm hearty as a horse and everyone loves me. There are many who do not love you. Including my parents, who are king and queen, or had you forgotten that? You've been lucky so far: they don't like to get involved in the territories their children control. They believe we should be able to rule independently. But if something 'unusual' happened to me, you would be out in less than a day, possibly tarred and feathered and my sister Divinia would take the castle. She never liked you anyway."

Vanessa turned pale.

Interesting, Eric thought. *Had she not considered the possibilities before?*

. . . or no, she just hadn't thought *Eric* would think of the possibility. She was counting on his still being hazy from her spell and perhaps not that clever to begin with. The princess was a haughty egotist who thought that everyone around her was dumber and less capable than she. *Just all-around generally unpleasant, besides being a tentacled sea witch,* Eric thought. How did any of the nobles and commoners she manipulated put up with it? Couldn't they see through to her hateful, egomaniacal self?

Well, maybe humans were, as a race, just fallible... Everybody wanted something. Maybe it was as banal and 'evil' as gold, but maybe it was as sweet and basic as true love. Maybe it was a baby you couldn't have, or some way to keep your family from starving. Maybe you needed a friend. Maybe you just *wanted* to believe that all these things could be received as gifts, from the universe or God or the spirits.

And here is an evil, comely witch who promises it all. It would be so easy to overlook her shortcomings with your wish so close to being granted. Maybe only luck saved humans from having to deal with terrible creatures like Vanessa on a regular basis, who make people sign away their... oh! Wait a moment...!

"Vanessa, you *cannot* hurt me," Eric said aloud, feeling a very Mad Prince smile forming on his lips. He loomed over her.

"You... signed... a *contract.*"

"I didn't! I never!"

"A *marriage* contract."

The shocked look on her face was infinitely pleasing.

"Princess Vanessa, you signed a *legally binding* document in which you promised to have and to hold, to support, to act as a partner in, our royal marriage."

She looked sick. Actually sick. Green and yellow, mouth hanging open like a dog's. She swallowed dryly once or twice. Her eyes glazed over as she stared at something that wasn't there, between the floor and his face.

Maybe she was remembering their wedding day. It all happened very fast, thanks to her overwhelming need to win against Ariel. There was a thrown-together cake, a hastily fitted white dress and a piece of parchment quickly scrawled out by the one counsel who stayed in the seaside palace of Tirulia.

(Who, it's only fair to say, never thought he would have to do anything so crucial and important; his job was mostly a sinecure, reading through various real estate documents and decrees while lounging by the beach.)

He had pleaded with Eric not to marry at least until the king and queen had been informed and Vanessa's family had been checked out. Under the spell, Eric had shaken his head and shoved the paper under the poor man's pen.

Still, even under pressure, the lawyer had managed to turn out a fairly solid little marriage contract that referred to previous contracts with a lot of *ibids*, *see-above*s and *refer-to*s.

With a flourish and a smirk, Vanessa had deftly signed her name, adding what looked like a cute little octopus as a heraldic crest. The sun set, they kissed and it was over for Ariel and her father.

Eric smiled indulgently. "As I understand you immortal creatures, and I do, because I'm a Mad Prince, and also because I'm married to one immortal creature and friends with another, contracts are even more important to you people than they are to us. You have signed with your soul."

"Not legal. Not binding," Vanessa wheezed, trying to catch her breath and stave off what looked like a panic attack. "Signed… as Vanessa… not me…"

"Well, the thing is, you kind of look exactly like Vanessa," Eric said, cocking his head and pretending to look her over. "I think even someone as unschooled in legalese as I could probably make the case that as long as you look like Vanessa, live on land like Vanessa, and have no tentacles, like Vanessa, well, you are pretty much one hundred percent Vanessa. Although Vanessa, it's true, might actually be a girl prone to fits of dementia who believes herself to be a half-octopus undersea witch. Oh, and by the way: there's always a line in royal marriage contracts that deals with demented spouses, especially wives. I don't think you'll like what it spells out."

Although she still wasn't looking at him, Ursula's eyes widened as she realised the implications of what he was saying.

"And speaking of *wives*, I should also add that there are other, *nastier* little clauses in typical royal contracts. Ancient stuff, like what happens if you fail to produce a male heir, most of which would be dismissible in court today. But even in our modern era of astronomy and steam engines, well, I'm afraid Tirulia is still a bit backwards. Anything you own is technically mine, any inheritance you receive is mine, any property you manage is mine, any decision involving purchases or transference of goods, schooling of children, firing or hiring of domestic help… it's all. Ultimately. Mine."

He took a step closer with each final word and grinned down at her.

Vanessa's eyes finally cleared; she looked at him with raw hate. Eric repulsed the look with a sunny smile.

"You see," he added almost apologetically, "you immortal creatures have your powers, your promises, your wish fulfillments and your contracts, it's true.

"But we humans have *lawyers*."

Vanessa's face stretched into a rictus of a smile. She slowly straightened herself up and adjusted her dress.

"You're not quite the dummy everyone thinks you are," she finally said.

"Just you," Eric pointed out. "Everyone else thinks I'm distracted and creative. Only you think I'm actually stupid."

"Fair enough," Vanessa conceded. "I always knew playing with humans would be fun. You're all a lot more, *fun*, than I imagined. It's really astounding, the propensity for evil the least of you have. Here I was thinking that *I* was the master of tricky and binding agreements. Apparently I have a lot to learn. What's that saying? 'The devil is in the details'? You make me think that humans *invented* the devil."

Eric said nothing. He wasn't, as she said, stupid. And he was a little wiser than the first time around. There was no celebrating his victory over her yet. Something as horrible and ancient as Ursula no doubt had another shoe to drop, possibly seven shoes.

She shook her shoulders and settled back into a proper Vanessa pose, prim and pretty.

"All right, then, Prince Eric, a *partnership*. 'For Tirulia'. At least until one of us figures out how to… *dissolve* it."

"All I care about is my country," Eric said with feeling. *Don't think of her. Don't think of Ariel. Don't think of how you're continuing to help her, looking for her father.* While he was unsure if the witch could read minds, it was clear that Vanessa could read faces and would. "And its people. As long as they are safe and happy and prosperous, I don't care what mad little witcheries or whatever it is you do on the side."

"What a generous offer. *Thank you*, My Prince," she said, giving a very ornate bow, not a curtsy. "*Mad little witcheries*, indeed. Time was I would turn you into a barnacle for such language."

"Those times are over, Princess," Eric said with a thin smile. "Welcome to the human race."

The Good Folk of Tirulia/Rumours

AT THE ABSINTHE HOUSE:

"I don't know, Lord Francese. Do we even wish the good prince to return to his senses? At this stage? It seems that all is going along rather splendidly… I've already received several nice… shall we say… *returns* on my investment in the clearing of the Devil's Pass. A pair of vineyards, in fact. Let the lad write his songs and the lady lead us into wealth!"

"I don't object to the general idea of expansion, Lord Savho. And I've made quite a bit myself on the shipment of munitions from Druvest. But I think it's rather ridiculous to consider us Druvest's *equal*, or Gaulica's. The world is changing, and I am not convinced Tirulia is ready to be the world power our dear princess wishes it were."

"Oh, I agree, darling. And I feel nothing but empathy for that lovely prince of ours. He's so haunted, such a handsome young man."

"He is indeed, Lady Francese. I was just having tea with the princess, and upon leaving I saw him cutting such a lovely, gothic figure kneeling in an overgrown garden."

"Whatever was he doing there, Emelita? Practising his poetry?"

"Honestly… it rather looked like he was talking to a seagull…"

AT THE MARKET:

"Mad he might be, but I don't think he wants us to be all over the place starting wars with which and who. And I agree."

"Don't you say that! Florin came back from the assault in the mountains with a necklace for me. There's opportunities in the army for the youngest son of seven that don't exist elsewhere."

"He could get a place on a ship like everyone else, Lalia."

"Yes, and come back with stinky fish. Not necklaces."

"Well, *I* don't like it. None of you are old enough to

remember the troubles of Thirty-Five—"

"When none of the boys in your village came back alive, yes, yes, we've heard it before. This is different. Vanessa is clever! She has all these modern weapons, *explosives* and tactics… our boys don't even need to risk themselves."

"Really? Dead times twenty isn't a *risk*?"

"I may hire on to a fishing boat myself. There's enough work to go around, though not enough boats…"

"Plus there's that contest! A chest of treasure for finding a magic fish! That could buy you a *thousand* necklaces, Lalia…"

AT THE DOCKS:

"I think our prince has taken for the worse, have you heard? He's started talking to seagulls!"

"So? He's an artist. That last opera of his was supposed to be mighty fine. I can't wait to finally see it when they put it on again. But maybe all this music work took something out of him, something vital."

"You ask me about taking something vital out of him, I'd say you're looking in the wrong place. It's that princess of his…"

"Keep your voice down, Julio! Or we'll be next to the front lines, feeding crows with our bones and not seagulls with our fish."

Eric

After Ursula made her (predictably) dramatic exit from her study, Eric stayed, pulling out his composition book and turning to the piece called 'Interlude for a Villain's Lair'. Since the sending Triton to Ibria thing had all been a ruse, Vanessa was probably still keeping the king as close to her as possible. If she had just killed him, she wouldn't have hidden the fact; she would have bragged about it. The sea witch wasn't terribly complicated once you got to know her. Almost predictable in her less dangerous habits.

He carefully checked off everything that was the same as the last time he searched the room: creepy, evil dagger? *Check.*

Teapot and tea accessories? *Check.* It all looked pretty much the same. In fact, the only really new item was an untidy pile of maps and charts on the table. Eric riffled through them. Some were immediately obvious and discouraging: troop numbers, approximate locations of enemy forts and towers, friendly towns. There were atlases with arrows drawn on them in pencil, where future land grabs might be made. There was a list of world leaders, mostly minor, with notes next to each name: *Friendly! Neutral. Mad? Aggressive.*

Her plans were like a little girl's fantasy, all sketched out in a book titled something like *Princess Vanessa's Plan to Conquer the Known World*, in curlicue letters, with hearts dotting the Is.

Eric shook his head and pushed the papers aside. Beneath were the plans for the new warships and marine cartographic charts, with coasts, depths and dangerous reefs sketched in, channels described, destinations plotted…

He frowned at the coordinates.

She wasn't sending the fleet up the Verdant Coast to harass and intimidate their neighbours like she had threatened, and as would be logical, were one beginning to conquer the continent.

It looked like…

It looks like she's sending them out to sea? Deep *sea?*

Along with the charts was a map, mostly blank and unlabelled. There was no key, no compass rose, no marks round the outside to indicate latitude or size. The background was plain as if it were just open sea or field, but with no decorative patterns to indicate either. On this was drawn what appeared to be islands, sketched by an unskilled hand, but ringed as if the topography were known. One large bean-shaped mass had a few details to differentiate it from the others: a scalloped edge on one side, and what looked like a tiny crown in the middle of the right half of the bean.

Eric stared at it, puzzled. It didn't look like any part of the world he knew, or even illustrations of New South Wharen. He looked around on her desk to see if there was anything else that might give a hint as to what it was, but only found different versions of the strange map, smaller and even more crudely drawn. First drafts. Some of these had arrows on them in the same way the war maps did, but they floated over the open spaces and had no troop numbers or anything indicating enemy defences.

Mysterious. Was it a map to invisible sources of power? Were the arrows ley lines, flows of magic or power that were all the rage among modern seers and bored gentlefolk?

He took the smallest, crudest map and folded it into his pocket.

Maybe Ariel would know. They would meet again at the next tide, in nine hours. In the meantime, he would go through atlases and research it as best he could until that time. Her father might have to wait a bit while he did.

On his way to the library he passed through the drawing room, where serious visitors were entertained with brandy and harpsichord music and interesting books and globes. Vareet was sitting at the fancy mahogany desk, drawing.

Eric walked by her and then stopped.

He had *never* seen the little maid entertaining herself with her own pursuits in public. He rarely saw her smiling. Once in a great while he saw her skipping through the halls, overcome by some fancy, or grinning as she exited the kitchen, special gifted treat in her hands. But whatever she did when she was given her, *precious little*, time off, she did it on her own, somewhere hidden.

"What are you doing, pretty lass?" he asked, kneeling down. It was a little awkward. He had no trouble throwing balls to children who were chasing each other outside, or getting into mock fencing bouts with young footmen. But he had no clue how to approach a quiet little girl.

Vareet's face was carefully neutral. She showed him her pictures: standard five-legged horses, unrecognisable human-monster things, squiggly grass, all the sorts of figures children normally drew.

What she was drawing *on* was remarkable, however: strange vellum, whose tactile surface was almost unpleasant to touch. As Eric looked at the pictures and tried to figure out what to say, Vareet impatiently turned them over so he could see the back.

On that side were runes, but not by a child's hand, as outlandish as they were. It was definitely some sort of written language.

"Oh… are these Vanessa's?" Eric whispered. "Are you trying to tell me something?"

The little girl said nothing, just quickly gathered up the rest of her drawings and prepared to go.

"I'm just going to hold on to this for a while," the prince said of the one he still held. He would show it to Ariel, to see if she could make head or tail of the writing. "I really like the way you made the horse's neck. It almost looks like it's… really… moving."

"It's a *bunny*," Vareet snapped. Then she skipped off, exasperated.

The prince gave a wry laugh. Mad Prince Eric, indeed, who had secret friends in butlers and maids, but also in seagulls and little girls, and who could understand neither.

Ariel

As the tide turned she surfaced on the north side of town, on an isolated beach. Sheltered from the sea by grass and the mainland by sand dunes fringed with scrub, it wasn't only perfectly hidden from the castle and its spies; it was *also* the perfect place to raise baby seagulls, and to tend to older ones.

She hadn't seen Scuttle in a while.

But as soon as the mermaid emerged from the water she saw something strange was up. The gulls were screeching even more loudly than usual, wheeling and crying and diving so furiously she couldn't understand what they were saying. She shaded her eyes against the sky and scanned the bright edge of the dune for her friend.

"Scuttle?" she called.

"*Ariel!* Look, everyone, it's my friend Ariel!"

An inelegant but enthusiastic tumbling mess of a bird thrust his body over the edge of the dune, letting gravity drag him towards her, opening and closing his wings in more of a controlled fall than an actual flight. The sand was soft and Scuttle wasn't going that fast; Ariel wasn't too concerned. When he finally came to a stop, she knelt down to stroke his head, pulling her hand back at the last moment when she saw several fish tails sticking out of his beak.

"Sorry," he said, smacking them back in and down his gullet. "Sorry, Ariel. But they were already dead. But I don't like you seeing that."

"Uh, thanks."

"Jona, she's a first-rate great-grandgull, that one. She's been bringing me a *feast*. Everyone else was just stuffing their own gullets. Not her. She thought of her great-grandfather first." He preened his chest feathers and wings to remove any lingering fishy oil. "What's up? You got a lead you need me to check out, or something?"

"No, I just came here to see how you were doing." She scratched him under his chin, but was distracted by his words.

"Awww, that's great, Ariel. That's really nice. I appreciate that."

"Scuttle, what 'feast'? What are the gulls 'stuffing their gullets' *with*? What's going on?"

"Oh, you don't know? All the fishing humans are going *crazy*! Worse than us, if you can believe it! At least that's what they say. Piles of fish for the taking."

Ariel took this in, trying to figure out what it meant. *Piles* of dead fish? That seemed unusual, even for humans. Surely with everything else going on with Ursula, it wasn't a coincidence.

"What are they, I mean, the humans, doing with the piles?"

"I dunno. Not guarding them very well, I gotta say. You getting any closer to finding your dad? Jona told me all about the carriage and Ursula and everything."

"Nothing yet," Ariel said slowly. "I think I want to go see what's going on before I meet Eric. Where *is* Jona? I'd like to get her help."

Scuttle turned over his shoulder and squawked. Someone else squawked back.

"My boy here says he saw her out over the water, away from the docks. I'll bet she was looking for you."

"All right, if I miss her and she comes back here, tell her to meet me back in town."

"Will do, Ariel," Scuttle said, giving her a salute. She turned to go. "And… Ariel? Thanks for… thanks for just coming to visit. Not just 'cause you're the Queen of the Sea and all important and everything. I *missed* you, Ariel. It was hard… those years… when you didn't come to the surface any more. I mean, I completely understand why. You had every reason. But… I still missed you."

"Oh, Scuttle, I'm so sorry…" She nuzzled his beak with her nose, closing her eyes. "As soon as I get my father back on his throne, I'll have way more time to visit."

Scuttle looked delighted and a little surprised. "So you're just gonna… come up now? To the Dry World? To stay? Or visit a lot? I mean, after whatever happens with your dad?"

Ariel paused. Once it was all over, of *course* she would go back to hanging out with her friends, old and new, in the world beyond the sea. But… how would she do it without the trident? Would her father help her? Even if she successfully rescued him, his views on the matter certainly wouldn't have improved by years of imprisonment. What if he refused? What if he didn't let her go?

I'll just have to find a way on my own.

But… another part of her pointed out, *that was how this whole thing started in the first place.* Her father had refused to let her go, so she found another way and it led to him being captured and her losing her voice and Tirulia gaining a tyrant. She squinched her face up at the conflicting thoughts.

Deal with it later, Ariel, she ordered all the voices, wrapping her headscarf tightly round her face and neck once again. She would get the job done first, find her father, defeat Ursula, set everything right. *Then* she could work on the happily ever afters.

She had just reached the edge of town when Jona wheeled down out of the sky to perch on a rock nearby.

"I was looking for you," the gull said. "Be careful. There are a lot of shiny buttons walking around. I think you're a *persona non grata* here."

She tried not to look proud of the words she used, but failed badly.

"Shiny button… oh. *Soldiers.* Yes. That's why I… wait, how did *you* recognise me?"

She had to push the headscarf fully out of her face to see the gull clearly at all.

"I can spot half a sardine carcass sticking out of a flower pot a quarter mile away," Jona answered. "I'm a *gull.*"

Ariel smiled.

She carefully clambered up the rock next to the bird.

Climbing things was still a tricky proposition; you *hurt* if you fell in this world, where everything was heavy and hard and inclined to falling. A very light breeze tickled her forehead as she stood on her tiptoes to get a good view of the town…

… which brought with it one of the most revolting odours she had ever smelt. Bodies, rotting flesh. Death and decay in staggering amounts.

She almost fell off the rock.

"Are you all right?" Jona asked politely.

"What is that… horrible… stink…?"

"You mean the gigantic piles of dead fish the humans are leaving on the wharf."

She had, at least, the good taste to avoid smacking her beak as she spoke.

"Scuttle said… I didn't think… why aren't they being…" she tried to swallow her nausea; she had to know, "*eaten* by the humans?"

"Don't know," Jona said with a wingy shrug. "But it's been a very popular development among us and the rats and cats."

Ariel couldn't see anything from her higher position, and the wind was terrible, so she slipped back down from the rock, stomach still a little rocky itself. *You're a queen.* She pulled herself upright as best she could.

"I'm… going to go look into this," she said, trying not to breathe through her nose. Eric, even her father could wait. She had to find out what was going on to leave her subjects dead and rotting in piles. Jona nodded and launched herself into the air above her.

As she approached the main street Ariel noticed that even the humans who regularly ate fish were covering their faces and noses with cloth; she didn't stand out in the crowd wearing her headscarf. The stench was overwhelming. Some people looked sour and complained bitterly. Others looked excited and rushed to and fro, mending nets, grabbing friends, chatting and shrieking in glee.

And there, on the docks, just as the gulls had said, *every kind of fish* was rotting in piles. From the species that humans loved to hunt and eat to the ones that were deadly poisonous. Squid, octopodes, eels, sharks, sea bass, rays, hake, oarfish, at least one small dolphin… they were all represented among the dead, baking and decaying in the sun.

The Queen of the Sea just stood there staring, overwhelmed by horror and sadness.

Finally she began to do the only thing she could for all of them now: she whispered a prayer. Again and again, willing their spirits to find the eternal ocean of heroes, where they could be happy and free forever.

Ariel had repeated it twelve times, with no intention of stopping, when she was interrupted by a familiar voice.

"I'm so sorry, my lady."

Ariel looked up. Argent the Inker stood there, a disgusted look on her face. She put a hand on the mermaid's shoulder.

"I wanted to see you again to thank you for the extra coins and gems you gave me, but this isn't the way I'd hoped we would meet."

"What goes on here?" Ariel demanded.

The old woman made a face, the divots and wrinkles in her skin pulling into a rictus of contempt. "The castle is offering a reward for the capture of a 'magical fish'. A chest of gold and an estate and a title to whichever fisherman brings it in."

"Magical fish?" Ariel repeated slowly, hoping she had heard it wrong.

"Princess Vanessa has finally lost her mind, at least, that's what some people are saying," the woman said with a snort. "Maybe she never had one to begin with. Maybe she kept that hidden until now. But people don't care, who would? A chest of gold and a title for one fish. Whether it's actually magical or not. But I assume, with you here, of course, there's a chance it actually is..."

"What is this magical fish supposed to do? What does it look like?"

"No idea what it's *supposed* to do. I guess that if it grants wishes, it's probably not going to get turned over to the princess, if you know what I mean. They say it doesn't look like the normal fish we catch around here. It's slow-moving, and fat, with yellow and blue stripes."

For the second time that day Ariel felt a wave of nausea pass over her.

Of course. Of course. She should have guessed.

Flounder.

Ursula had set a reward out for the capture of her best friend.

Something changed in Ariel.

Over the span of a single breath, the nausea subsided, along with the sadness and sickness and helplessness. Something far more solid, and terrible, took its place.

"I would suggest you and whomever you love stay off the ocean for the next tide," she said as calmly as she could.

"What...?"

Argent searched Ariel's eyes, huge and aquamarine, clear as the seas in Hyperborea. She must have found something there. Blue anger? Or perhaps it was just Ariel's confidence: the calm assumption that she could back up insane statements with an even more insane reality.

The eyes of a queen.

"Yes, thank you. Of course, I'll tell them," the old woman said quickly. "Thank you, my lady." She practically bowed. Her earrings jingled as she ran away on her long, rangy legs.

Ariel spun around and regarded the piles of fish, the laughing and angry men and women, the boats out at sea, one last time.

Not caring who saw, she took off down the dock and dove into the water, her tail beating the water into foam before she was even submerged.

Ariel surfaced just beyond the bay. She was consumed by fury over so many things: the piles of dead fish, Ursula tricking her with the carriage, her own inability to find her father, the loss of her voice, the loss of who she was when she first had a voice.

A wave formed, swelling around Ariel's body. It lifted her up higher and higher, or maybe she herself was growing; it was hard to tell. She held the trident aloft. Storm clouds raced to her from all directions like a lost school of cichlid babies flicking to their father's mouth for protection. Lightning coursed through the sky and danced between the trident's tines.

Ariel sang a song of rage.

Notes rose and fell discordantly, her voice screeching at times like a banshee from the far north.

She sang, and the wind sang with her. It whipped her hair out of its braids and pulled tresses into tentacles that billowed around her head. She sang of the unfairness of Eric's fate and her own, of her father's torture as a polyp, even of Scuttle's mortal life, slowly but visibly slipping away.

Mostly she sang about Ursula.

She sang about everyone whose lives had been touched and destroyed by evil like coral being killed and bleached, like dead spots in the ocean from algae blooms, like scale rot. She sang about what she would do to *anyone* who threatened those she loved and protected.

And then, with her final note, she made a quick thrust as if to throw the trident towards the boats in the bay, pulling it back at the last moment.

A clap louder than thunder echoed across the ocean. A wave even larger than the one she rode roared up from the depths of the open sea. It smashed through and around her, leaving her hair and body white with foam. She grinned fiercely at the power of the moment. The tsunami continued on, making straight for Tirulia.

But… despite her rage… underneath it all the queen was still Ariel. Her momentary urge to destroy everything came and went like a single flash of summer lightning.

She pulled the trident back.

As the wave travelled through the bay it grew weaker.

Not so weak, however, that it didn't smash Vanessa's anchored fleet with a satisfying, wood-cracking explosion against the wharves.

The other boats, the fishing vessels that were out in open water, were tossed like toys or bits of flotsam and jetsam.

The ocean rose and flooded the docks, taking the dead fish back to their home, allowing the few living ones left to escape.

Eventually the water calmed. The wave Ariel rode slowly diminished, and she returned to the relatively tranquil surface of the sea. Dark clouds lingered but lightened their load by letting out a soft rain. The storm was over.

Ariel dove into the depths, exhausted. Hopefully Eric would have the sense to realise their meeting would be delayed for at least a tide.

She would send some dolphins up to rescue the drowning.

Ursula

She stood in the hall, one hand on Vareet's head, a distant look on her face. Someone passing by might have taken the scene for that of a distracted member of royalty lecturing the lesser staff with a patronising if affectionate air. But she was thinking about her three destroyed warships. She had been close… so close… to absolute victory over Atlantica.

And now the explosive cannonballs from Druvest lay somewhere on the bottom of the bay, undetonated, *useless.*

In a month, if she was *lucky,* she would have three new ships, but three was not enough. She wanted to make sure she had enough cannon and firepower to defeat whatever the mer tried to throw at her, and enough munitions to obliterate everything down there. Not to mention her failing alliance with Ibria. Once again she would be short three ships…

As for the cannonballs and explosives themselves, well, it was hard enough wheedling them out of Druvest, and getting Eric to pay for another batch seemed unlikely.

Ariel had ruined her whole plan.

Again.

Vareet squirmed under her touch as Vanessa's nails dug deep into the roots of her hair and twisted them in anger. But the little maid had sense not to cry out. Or try to escape.

Ursula wished it was Ariel's hair she had her tentacles sunk into. Pulling and tearing those stupid red locks, ripping them from her flesh. Oh, how she would love to drag the mermaid through the water as she struggled and screamed, forced to watch as everyone she loved died…

Unable to hold back any longer, Vareet let out a single whimper.

Ursula looked at her maid with vague surprise, as if she had forgotten the little girl was even there. Vareet paled, plainly expecting punishment.

But something else was occurring to the sea witch. A

calm detachment settled over her like a warm current from a sea vent. Her rage dissipated as her next, her *only* action became clear.

If Ariel would wield the power of the gods in this battle, then so would she.

All she needed now was a time and place.

Eric strode by, stuffing his hat on his head and buttoning his cloak.

"Going off on your… post-prandial constitutional?" she asked hollowly.

"Oh, yes, yes, walking does wonders for the stomach," Eric said, patting his and trying to keep moving.

"Tell me… are you still planning the big performance? The free one, for everyone in town? That everyone will come to?"

"Of *La Sirenetta*? Yes, of course. Why?" He looked unsettled, nervous.

"I was just wondering. You heard the news about the fleet." It was more a statement than a question.

"Er, yes. Terrible," Eric said. "I'm very glad no one was hurt."

"I think there's something you should know," she said, finally turning and looking at him directly.

"Yes? What?" the prince asked impatiently.

"As a result of this… incident… with the fleet, I find I have time now to devote to another project of mine." She spoke almost light-heartedly. "Something big. Something terrible. Something your puny little human mind could not possibly comprehend. Far beyond my usual *mad little witcheries.* And when I am done, Ariel will wish she had taken my advice and fled back to the sea, far, far away from me."

She enjoyed seeing Eric's face go pale. It was the only fun she had all day.

"Pass the info on, if you happen to see the mermaid," she added, walking away, pulling Vareet with her.

The girl, resigned to her fate, didn't even look back at Eric.

Ariel and Eric

Eric was already at their meeting place, looking nervous and fidgety in the moonlight. He tapped his lips with a piece of paper clutched in his hands. His eyes looked positively ghostly in the moonlight.

"Eric?" She spoke softly. Despite being less deft on her feet than anyone naturally born to the Dry World, she moved silently, as all magical creatures did. And from the way he jumped, it was obvious he hadn't heard her at all.

"Ariel!"

He put out his arms, then stopped.

"What did you do to my ships? To *all* of our ships?" he cried.

Her eyes widened. *Not* what she expected him to say.

"Sorry, sorry." Eric ran a hand through his hair. "No one was killed. A couple people were hurt. Weirdly, those at risk of drowning were rescued by a couple of friendly dolphins, and, if I am to believe what the cabin boy said, one particularly old and giant terrapin."

"Eric," Ariel firmly interrupted. "I am the Queen of the Sea. I protect my people. There are rules in place to allow us and you to live side by side. But if something threatens my realm beyond the scope of those rules, I will respond with all the force in my power. We must put up with your fishing to some degree. But if I hear *anything* else about some sort of reward for the capture of my friend Flounder the 'magical fish' and it involves killing hundreds of other perfectly innocent fish for no reason, I will destroy every boat within my demesne, as well as the towns they launched from. Understood?"

"Oh, the devil," Eric swore. "I thought I caught wind of some foolishness like that. Now it all makes sense. Fishermen pulling in great piles of fish, looking for something… I heard the stink was unbelievable. Flounder is… a… friend of yours?"

"Since he was a fry."

"I'll put a stop to it at once," Eric promised. "For now and forever. Believe it or not, things like this have happened before. There was a rumour once that the Narvani, to the east, believed that the poisonous spine of the chimaera fish would help with… uh… let's just say it would help them have babies. It's a deepwater fish, ocean floor, but that didn't stop every idiot from just netting up every fish around and picking through them like an old woman through spoilt lentils."

"The greed of Dry Worlders continues to shock me," Ariel admitted.

"Yes, well, the greed of some tentacled sea-dwellers continues to shock me too."

"Good point. I don't know where the mer fall in that. I think their sin is complacency, not greed."

Eric sighed. "I wish I could see them. It sounds like a paradise. *My* kind of paradise. Here, on earth, in the sea. Maybe… some day… you could take me there?"

He asked so innocently, so plainly, she was taken aback. He sounded like a little boy.

Or a little mergirl, dreaming of the warm sand.

"I'd love to," she whispered.

He took her hand and squeezed it. She held her breath, waiting for whatever was going to come next. He started to open his mouth…

"But speaking of tentacled sea-dwellers…" the prince said reluctantly, instead of kissing her. "Vanessa has threatened something… well, large and unspeakable and terrible. Magic, I think. She seemed quite serious. She said you'll wish you had taken her advice and returned to the sea. And she told me to pass it along to you."

Ariel swore and tried to lash her tail. Instead, she made a funny kick-kick move, which was far less satisfying.

"*Everything*. Everything she does. Every time I think I have her beat, or at least in a corner, she figures out something to do! I get my voice back; she keeps me from going back to the castle by threatening my father. You help me; she threatens Grimsby. I think she's sending my father away, and it turns out it's all a trick, a trap. Now she threatens something vague and terrible. Is it true? Isn't it? Who knows? She knows my weaknesses and yours. So we all wind up just like we're children rearranging pieces on the board of a game of koralli."

"I guess that's like chess?" Eric asked.

"I guess."

They fell into a sombre silence. The air felt chill and alive against her skin. The sky was almost starless because of the moisture in the air; not quite clouds, and not quite clear, the ether was veiled. The moon had set. Tendrils of breeze picked up the edge of her skirt. She sighed again and hugged herself, something she would never have done while she was underwater, queen. She constantly felt if she did anything that was even a little less than regal, she would be ignored even more than she already was when she was mute.

"I'm sorry," Eric said again. "I wish I had better news to bring you, but I'm still having no luck finding your father. Believe me, I'm trying. But I *did* find these things. This first drawing was among the military papers she still tries to keep away from me. The places on it make no sense to me at all, they are of nowhere I know. It's where she was intending to send the fleet before you destroyed it. It's not of any of our neighbouring countries. Maybe somewhere near the western lands? Some uncharted islands off Vespucci? Or hidden in Arawakania? Or nearby, in the Ruskal Sea? Do you recognise them?"

Ariel took the paper and carefully unrolled it. There were indeed blobs that could have been islands, surrounded by multiple outlines, like mountains that had been cut into slices and redrawn. She turned the map this way and that, trying to make sense of it.

And then it suddenly clicked into place, like when the water is foggy with plankton and a current comes and sweeps it clear so you can see the reef on the other side, or when the sand stirred up by a blenny finally settles.

"This isn't a map of Dry World islands," she said slowly. "This is a map of my home.

"Ursula means to destroy Atlantica."

Ariel and Eric

"Atlantica?" Eric asked. "You mean… your kingdom?"

"Yes, look." Ariel tapped at the parchment. "This is the Canyon of Dendros. This is the Field of Akeyareh, where ancient mer warriors fell in the battles against the Titans. Their bodies drifted to the sea floor and their bones turned the sand white. This is the Cleft of Neptune's… uh… 'Back', a valley with hot geysers and occasional magma flows. This is the Mound of Sartops, where our priests and artisans tend to live; it looks out into the great depths of the ocean, some say to infinity. I know this map like the ribs in my tail fin."

If she *had* her tail right now, it would be tipping and

thwapping the water in consternation. Kicking her foot didn't seem the same somehow.

"The munitions Ursula ordered..." Eric said, thinking. "They're not to wage war on our neighbours, or even Ibria, as I thought she might eventually do. It all makes perfect sense now! Tarbish's reluctance, all the explosives, the dynamite. She's going to drop depth charges, they'll detonate gunpowder-filled mines down on your city."

Death from above.

Ariel looked at the map. She had no idea what those extra words meant. She understood *explosive* and *your city*. Ursula could direct her ships exactly where she wanted them, and then, thanks to the cursed gravity that made life so hard for Ariel on land, the witch could simply *drop the weapons* on Atlantica and obliterate it. Eric talked about *gunpowder* and *die-namite* with the same trepidation he did her own powers.

"By destroying her fleet you might have saved your kingdom," Eric said softly.

Ariel was seized by a strange fit of panic. What if she *hadn't*? What if she hadn't lost her temper and impulsively done that?

"*Why?*" she finally asked, voice cracking. "She's got my dad, she's got your kingdom, she's got me beat no matter what I do! What more does she want? Why does she need to destroy *everything*?"

"She's not a rational being, Ariel. She's like… a walking mouth that's hungry all the time. She sees something and she wants it. So she does everything she can to get it. She wanted revenge on your father and you. She *thought* she got it, and was content, and moved on to the next thing – ruling Tirulia. But then you showed up again. To stop her. You're like an annoying gnat she can't slap away."

"I don't know what a 'gnat' is."

"Um… kind of like a remora? Tiny thing that bites you and sucks your blood and irritates you?"

"I'm a parasitic fish that has latched on to her and won't let go," Ariel said flatly, trying not to imagine what the words looked like.

"No, that's not, look, forget the gnat. And the remora. She *hates* you, maybe just because you remind her of your dad. Weirdly, I don't think she's just jealous of your beauty or youth, which is how it would go in a traditional fairy tale," he added, looking thoughtful. "That's sort of how I made it in my opera, and it's a motive that most people understand. Audiences *love* that kind of thing; jealousy is simple, it makes sense. But I don't think that's all of what's going on here."

Ariel mentally replayed the scene of going to talk to Ursula about giving her legs, but from a different perspective – Ursula's. There she was, a pretty, talented mermaid princess with a voice people would kill for, not a care in the world and a future paved in pearls. And she had basically told the sea witch she was utterly discontented with her lot and wanted to be someone, and somewhere, else entirely.

And there was Ursula, perhaps *rightfully* exiled from the kingdom, but exiled nonetheless. Aged. Forced to deal with her fate alone. Bitter and resentful. In swims this pretty mermaid…

"Oh, my *cod*," Ariel said, putting a hand to her head. "What an *idiot* I was. I didn't even stop to think… she's a *witch*. 'Hello, could you give me a pair of legs? For close to free? Even though you don't like my father?' "

"Exactly. Then she wins the bet, you lose your voice, she gets your dad, she becomes princess, you swim sadly back down to the bottom of the sea. But then you resurface in her life, and you're *Queen of the Sea*. You manage to get your voice back. You control storms and the heart of the man *she* is married to…"

"I do?" Ariel asked with delight.

"*I'm just telling a story here.* But yes, obviously. You've become a queen, a woman with a complicated personality. You have hidden depths and a wisdom and intelligence that all went unnoticed before by an idiot prince whose heart couldn't listen to anything his ears couldn't hear."

Ariel felt a little giddy. "I control storms and the heart of a prince. I like that." If she were in the sea she would have been swooning, thrashing her tail and spinning in circles until she was dizzy.

Well, as a girl. Not as queen, not where anyone could have seen her.

Eric smiled. "I think my character would have a song about how he's been caught by a siren and is under her spell."

Ariel made a face. "I'm not a siren. Trust me. I have cousins… distant cousins… we don't get along. But what were you saying? About Ursula?"

"Just that everything she did to you and your father didn't keep you down. You popped up, older, stronger, more powerful than ever. She realises she didn't beat you *enough* last time. Now she wants complete victory, which involves wiping out your home."

"If she wants complete victory, why not kill my father outright?"

"Well, that's the thousand-gold-piece question, isn't it?" Eric said with a frown. "Why bother pretending to ship him off to Ibria? Why bother keeping him here at all?"

"She's up to something," Ariel agreed. "Something involving him. I feel like I started some sort of chain of events in her mind when I reminded her of my existence."

"Well, maybe this has something to do with it," the

prince said, pulling out the piece of vellum Vareet had drawn on.

"Oh," Ariel said, taking it. "What a cute… um… walrus."

"It's a *bunny*," Eric corrected with great dignity. "You've never seen one. Anyway, it's what's on the back that's important. Ursula's maid risked a lot by letting me 'discover' this…"

Ursula's maid again. Ariel's heart broke a little when she thought of the girl, remaining silent so the mermaid could sneak out with the necklace unseen. Despite her life being in danger now, she still chose to help Ariel.

The pictures on the back of the strange-feeling vellum were far more disturbing than the weird Dry World creature on the front. There were lines and shapes that looked like they could be runes but shuddered when she tried to look at them too closely. Curves somehow didn't bend properly on the paper, and constellations of dots made her sick when she studied them, suggesting terrible things.

Ariel shook her head at the blasphemous sigils. "I don't know what these say for certain. They aren't mer runes; they're like a twisted, upside-down version of them. If I had to guess I would say they're black runes of the Deep Ones. Forbidden, evil… the whole deal."

"Can you read them at all?"

"This is just a noise, I think," she said, pointing. "Like *äi äi*. No idea what 'phtaqn' means. This here I think refers to a circuex, a powerful spell that is capable of disrupting, or joining, worlds. This looks like the mer word for 'blood', and that looks like a determinative for 'god'. Or possibly 'great' or 'lots'."

"So..."

"So she needs blood, the blood of a god." Ariel bit her lip, seeing where it was all leading. "Ancient blood flows through my father's veins. That would explain why she's keeping him around. She needs him for something, something involving magic. But for what exactly I can't tell."

Ariel felt sick as she said the words. She pushed the paper back at him.

"Here, please take this. I don't enjoy the feel of dead human skin."

"Dead...? Human...?" Eric took it back, aghast.

Ariel closed her eyes and rubbed her knuckles into her forehead. "This is all... so... *frustrating*! We do one thing, and she does another to block it. We think we know what her plans are; it turns out she has something even bigger and sicker in mind. She always has an answer, always has a countermove. And she *knows* what my weaknesses are, and yours too. If I didn't care about my father, if you didn't care about Grimsby or your people, this would all be over in a flash."

"Back to your old 'children playing a game of koralli'," Eric said with a wry smile. "But if we were human kids playing chess, at least, an adult could come over and put an end to everything eventually."

An interesting point, but how relevant? If it were her and Eric against Ursula, who was the adult in the scenario? Her father? An Elder God? Or…

Something was just at the edge of her mind, like a playful eel nosing in and out of the sunlight at the edge of the shore. Slippery, sparkling and just out of her grasp.

"I think if adults, if *everyone* just knew what she was really like," she said slowly, "who she really was, they would do something. But how do we convince anyone she's an evil tentacled sea witch?"

"I don't know. Even if you just managed to show one person… there's no way to prove it to anyone else, much less *everyone* else. Enough people to do something about it," Eric said.

Ariel thought of poor terrified Vareet, who had seen her mistress change in the tub. She was the only one in the entire castle who knew the truth of the matter, very viscerally, besides Grimsby and Carlotta.

"But don't worry, we'll figure it out," he added, seeing the look on her face. He took her hand and squeezed it. "We have to, and soon. So she doesn't have a chance to do that ritual or whatever."

But Ariel didn't feel as much faith in them as Eric did. Somehow, despite being a rapidly ageing human, he had managed to keep some of his youthful optimism, while she had lost some of hers. It was kind of adorable.

She leant forwards and kissed him on the cheek.

He smiled in surprise. He put his hand up to touch her face, perhaps brush away a stray hair… before his fingers did what they really wanted and pulled her chin closer to him.

He kissed her on the lips.

It was brief, but in the moment their skin touched she closed her eyes and consumed him: his smell, his warmth, the movement of his mouth against hers.

It was like…

A goodnight kiss.

Over too quickly, but every moment of it meant a universe.

All those years before, and all those years in between… she had dreamt so many different scenarios of this moment! Ariel as a human, Ariel as a mer. *Eric* as a mer! Eric opening his eyes right when she rescued him and kissing her, falling in love with her on the spot. Eric kissing her in the boat, when she really, *really* thought he was going to and the night was so romantic. Kissing her on any of the three mornings, or realising at the last minute Vanessa was a fake and kissing Ariel instead, and the wedding would have been for them…

And here it finally was. She was a human, temporarily, and he was a human, and it was night, and they were getting ready to leave, and it was cold, and she had barnacle-bumps on her skin, and her feet hurt, and…

She found herself laughing, albeit a little breathlessly.

"That wasn't the way I imagined it would be…"

"'Imagined it would be'?" Eric asked with a smile. "You've been thinking about me? Does that mean I have indeed caught the heart of a mermaid?"

"You did years ago when she was an idiot minnow, and look where it got us," she said, pushing his chest. "Where it got *me*."

"I know, I was just—" He sighed. "I know."

She kissed him again on the cheek.

"Let's… just… see how it goes," she said, heading off to the water.

He watched her walk straight into the waves, no hesitation, no floating, until it was up to her neck.

"Hey, aren't you going to ruin your clothes?" he called.

She rolled her eyes and dove, letting her tail hit the surface like a whale's, slapping a spray in his direction.

Eric

He watched Ariel's head disappear under the waves and a fin appear in its place. He couldn't help smiling.

He had just witnessed the transformation of a girl into a mermaid. Back *into a mermaid,* he corrected himself. Despite the terrible things they had endured, and probably more before it was all over, despite the years he had lost in a haze to Vanessa's spell, he felt like a delirious little kid who had seen his first firefly, or bioluminescent jellyfish, or shooting star. Everything was beautiful and anything was possible: the world was an amazing place just waiting to be explored.

He laughed and picked up a handful of sand and pebbles, throwing it into the ocean.

Though her whole walking straight into the water without floating or swimming thing *was* more than a little creepy. Almost like a lead soldier.

Eric took off his shoes to walk his way back home barefoot; despite how cold it was he wanted to feel the sand on his feet. It was part of the sea, part of her home.

When he entered the castle with his hair askew and trailing beach detritus, no one was much shocked. It was just Mad Prince Eric, out on one of his walks again.

He thought about Ursula. Sometimes winning wasn't just about playing fair, but knowing the rules so well that you could exploit discrepancies. That was the sea witch's whole method of operation.

He puzzled over ways to expose her true identity to the people who fawned on her and protected her. But as a musician and a prince his ideas were mostly dramatic, elaborate and complicated. Like throwing a magnificent masked ball, for instance, and installing a hall of mirrors like at Versailles, and then having a bathtub full of salt water there somehow as a prop for Ursula to fall into, causing her to revert to her cecaelian state. Then her image would be reflected a thousand times, and everyone would see…

He scribbled that down as an idea for a later opera. Rather unwieldy in real life.

The prince felt bad about the opera he was *supposed* to be working on, he hadn't been to a rehearsal in days. Still, kings of the sea, mermaids and evil sea hags came first. The real ones, that was.

(Eric did, however, make time to occasionally visit the poor polyps still trapped on Vanessa's dressing table. He gave them little updates on things and told them to buck up. He had no idea if they understood, but it seemed like the right thing to do.)

He found it easiest to think logically when he worked at the puzzle the way an artist or musician would: by sketching out a stage direction plot, with Ursula in the middle and, around her, all the people she had vowed to kill if she was ever threatened in any way. He almost felt like his old self, sitting at his desk under the window and scribbling away, but this time clear-headed and glamour-free.

"Prince Eric," Grimsby greeted him, a trifle coldly, bringing in hot tea. It was served the traditional Tirulian way, with lots of sugar and cinnamon and cardamom.

Eric sighed. The other man had still been distant and, well, grim, since the prince had ordered him to stop helping.

"Grimsby old boy, *some day* you're going to have to

forgive me for trying to protect your life. It's what princes do. Well, good ones, anyway."

"Of course, sir," Grimsby said crisply. He put down a napkin and the saucer and eyed Eric's drawing. "Oh, you're still working on the opera. I daresay you have a lot else on your mind right now…"

"No kidding. And no, this isn't for the opera. I should really just put that on hold for a while, until other things… clear up."

"I wouldn't necessarily do that, Your Highness. Everyone is looking forward to the show. Now may not be the best time to ostracize your subjects. And it's a convenient way to keep certain people thinking you're, well, thinking about *other* things. Distracted, you know, when your keen mind is focused elsewhere…"

"That's not a bad point, Grims. All right, then! The show must go on!"

"Good for you, sir. You know… I must really get the carpenters and seamstresses to redo the royal box at the amphitheatre. Apparently, it's been quite… decorated by seagulls and the like. We don't want to upset the… er… *refined* sensibilities of Princess Vanessa. You know how she likes everything around her to look perfect when she's the centre of attention. Probably have to add some gold flourishes or something too…"

"Yes, she… wait… w*hat?*" Eric suddenly looked up at his butler. "What did you just say? What did you *really* just say? About Vanessa?"

"The princess enjoys flaunting her questionable taste and wealth?" Grimsby stammered.

"Grimsby, old man, you're a *genius*!" Eric kissed the confused butler on both cheeks, the Tirulian way, and ran out of the room.

"Thank you?" the Bretlandian said, dabbing at his cheek with the napkin.

"Woof?" Max asked, watching the prince go.

"No idea," Grimsby said with a sigh.

Flotsam and Jetsam

"Sssso, which one did she wind up choosing to send to Ibria, in Triton's place?"

The two eels-become-men were walking side by side, shoulders touching, making their rounds of the castle. Paying out the spies, threatening servants who wouldn't snitch, stealing bits in the kitchen in front of everyone and snickering about it… the usual afternoon's work.

"Garahiel," Jetsam answered, thin lips pulled back over a toothy grin. Neither one of them opened their mouths very far when they spoke; they were all teeth and tongue.

Flotsam laughed a long, hissing strain of laughter.

"Excellent choice! I always hated him. Of course, I always hated all of them."

"Oh, but he was a pretty one. He is so fit to be in the zoo of a king!"

"Well, he *was* a pretty one," Flotsam amended. "And lucky fellow too, escaping what Ursula has planned."

"He'll be the only one!"

They both laughed and laughed, and when a maid looked at them in disgust, they couldn't *quite* hold back from snapping their necks and jaws at her like the predators they were.

Transformations only went so far…

Ariel

It was a puzzle.

Not unlike the puzzle of finding the right member of the Kravi to sing the story of Proserpine in the Equinocturnal Celebrations, but far more important.

(She decided, as Attina had suggested, to have the younger sister sing it, and make the older brother Director of the Celebrations. It was an honour in name only. Everyone already knew what to do and where to stand; they had been performing the Rites for thousands of years.)

How could they expose Ursula's true nature to as many humans as possible?

She signed bills, listened to complaints, chose chariots, finally worked out an equitable payment plan with the pesky barracuda and considered the possibilities.

Ursula could... review all the troops. She could give a speech about the prowess of Tirulia as a military force while striding up and down in front of the rank and file of soldiers. But... by the sea! And then a giant wave could come and splash her... and her tentacles and true form would be revealed!

Ursula could... have a new warship built and take it out to christen it! Didn't humans do that silly thing where they wasted a bottle of wine, breaking it over the prow of the ship? And while Vanessa was there, surrounded by her crew, a wave could lap over the side and...

What if Ursula had a birthday party, and the chef baked a giant three-tiered cake, and Ariel was hiding inside, and when the sea witch went to taste it, the mermaid burst out with a bucket of salt water, utterly dousing the birthday girl?

Ariel laughed quietly to herself. It was a pleasant and deeply satisfying fantasy.

"What's with you, giggle-puss?"

Attina had been slinking around the public work rooms of the palace more and more often lately. A less forgiving sister might have thought she was hoping for apples, like a semi-feral seahorse, or that she found she liked the taste of power after all.

But maybe she just wanted to hang out and be near her little sister, offering what little support she could.

Whatever the truth of the matter was, Ariel was relieved at this new development and always happy to see her.

"You're all smiley-faced and, well, not broody," Attina pressed. "What's going on?"

It was true, since Ariel got back she had been more light-hearted, smiling and flipping her tail more. But when Flounder and Sebastian asked her why, she felt like she had to keep it a secret.

Isn't that what sisters are for?

She put down her whelk pen, deliberating. Attina looked like she was going to explode.

Finally the queen spoke.

"I kissed a boy."

"WHAT?"

With two quick lashes of her tail, the auburn-haired older mermaid was over by Ariel, eyes wide.

"Eric. I kissed Eric. We kissed. Eric and I kissed each other."

"When? How? What? Why? I mean, what took so

long?" she added, trying to sound casual.

"Didn't seem appropriate before," Ariel said, shrugging. "There were too many other things to talk about, to plan..."

"You are so weird!" Attina practically shrieked. "And so is he. Who ever heard of a human *waiting* to kiss a mer? He must be weird too. What was it like?"

"Not the stuff of a teen's fantasy," Ariel said with a rueful smile. "But it was genuine, and it was... nice."

"Well. The sea be praised," Attina muttered. "*Something* is moving ahead. What's going on with our father?"

"I'm working on that. I think we're going to have to get the Tirulians... uh, humans, to take care of Ursula for us. It's tricky. Maybe you can help come up with an idea, like you did with the Celebrations?"

"Sure. Just tell the humans she tastes like candy," Attina said dryly. "Or that a mouthful of her flesh can cure their diseases."

"*Thanks.* I'll give your suggestion the thoughtful consideration it's due."

"Any time, little sister."

Sebastian scuttled on the floor towards them, seeming very pleased with himself. Threll swam above, looking likewise.

"Don't talk about this!" Ariel whispered.

"Talk about what?" Attina asked innocently.

Ariel made a desperate *hush* motion with her finger to her lips, minutely tipping her chin at her friends.

"What are you doing? I don't think I learnt that sign..." Attina said, looking very puzzled.

Ariel glowered at her.

"Oh! But wait, don't you think your *friends* should know as well?" her sister pressed.

"Know what?" Sebastian asked curiously when he reached them.

Ariel floated upright off her stool, fists clenched at her sides, wishing she could pummel her sister like in the old days.

"Oh, that this whole thing with the Equinocturnal Celebrations and the Rites of Proserpine is over. She figured it out," Attina said with a sweet smile, batting her lashes at the queen.

"But we already know that," Sebastian said, confused. "You have the sister singing it. What other news is there? Oh... ARE YOU GOING TO SING?" His eyes twitched in the crab equivalent of widening; he tiptoed forwards, claws delicately tapping each other's tips, as if afraid to scare away the idea.

Attina guffawed silently and swam off.

Ariel looked at the little crab and felt bad. She had felt bad ever since the stern talking-to she had given him about how she would never, ever sing while she was queen. She hadn't changed her mind about that. But how could she make it up to him?

She thought about the other musician in her life, Eric. In his own way he loved an audience as much as the little crab did; he relished the goodwill of the townspeople and was very much looking forward to the encore of *La Sirenetta*, performed for all who had missed it the first time. Composing was one thing, but both of them felt the most fulfilled when they could directly gauge the reactions of their listeners.

That's an idea…

"Sebastian, I was serious. I will never sing for an audience while I am queen. However, *that being said*," she continued quickly as the crab looked like he was about to explode, "two things. One, I want you to devote a portion of your spare time to writing me an aria, a really amazing aria, that I will sing, triumphantly, when my father is returned as king and I can go back to being a mostly private citizen. It should be a celebration of his return. This has to be epic, Sebastian. Things like the capture and return of the King of the Sea do not happen but maybe once in a thousand years."

Sebastian was torn, she could tell. His little black crabby eyes twitched desperately. Everything about this idea appealed to every part of him, from the artist given a truly special challenge all the way to the egomaniac whose work would be performed and remembered forever.

But it still wasn't the same thing as having her sing *now.*

He was trying very, *very* hard not to say that. She could see it in the way his antennules clicked silently against each other.

"And for the Equinocturnal Celebrations, I plan to give a speech to all the participants about my promise not to sing until Father is returned, and what we are doing to facilitate his return." *Did I just say "facilitate his return"? Next I'm going to start saying things like "leveraging the synergy..."* "And then I will talk about the Return Aria and turn the floor over to you, so you may talk about your composition and your vision."

"That sounds highly acceptable," Threll said with an eyecrest raised at Ariel – the closest thing he had to a wink.

"Don't think I don't know what you're trying to do, young lady," Sebastian growled. But then his voice got dreamy. "Still... I can just see it now... 'The Return'! Everyone is seated in the Grand Amphitheatre... no! We will do something unique! We'll build an *all new* amphitheatre!"

"Uh, Sebastian, I didn't say anything about approving funds for—"

"We'll have an *upside-down* amphitheatre! Starting at

the top very big, then rows and rows getting smaller down until it's just you, on the sea floor... n*o!* On the Mound of Sartops, so everyone will be looking at us... I mean, you... and then I will raise my claw, so, and I will give a little speech of thanks for this opportunity and Triton's triumphant return..."

Ariel blinked.

"Everyone will be there because it's a performance," she said slowly. "And they will all be looking at you..."

"Yes, of course, yes," Sebastian said impatiently. "But also you. And then I will raise my claw, *so*..."

It hit the Queen of the Sea like an orca slamming into a plate of ice.

"I have it!" she cried. "I know what to do! Somebody, go find me Jona... Sebastian, you have the helm. I'm surfacing, but just for tonight!"

"But my aria..." Sebastian called out sadly.

She was already gone.

Ariel and Eric

Eric had trouble falling asleep. He had the beginnings of a brilliant idea for a plan, and no way to contact Ariel!

It was late when his dreams finally overcame him, and it seemed like only a few moments later when he was woken up by Max.

"Mmm, what's up, boy…?" Eric murmured, turning over.

Then his eyes shot open.

The old dog slept a lot now, and always through the night. He *never* begged for walkies when it was dark.

The prince pushed himself up on his elbows. Max had

risen on his hind legs with one front paw on the wall for balance. He was staring out the window, gesturing at it with his lolling tongue and interested muzzle. Outside was a gull, its white wings flapping as delicately as a moth as it hovered there.

"You?" Eric whispered. "From… Ariel?"

The seagull bobbed as best it could. Then it peeled away from the castle. Eric watched it descend and then look back at him and give a quiet cry.

It wanted the prince to follow it.

Eric didn't bother putting on shoes; he hastily pulled on a pair of trousers and tiptoed out of the room and down the stairs. His bare feet made no noise on the floor and for a moment he revelled in that; it was like being a young prince again, sneaking out to see the full moon.

Outside, the gull, glowing a pale unlikely white in the night, waited patiently drifting through the air.

He followed it south, past the castle beach and into the stony area with the basalt cliffs. When sand gave way he had to clamber on the rocks; the waves broke over seaweed-covered boulders and got deep very quickly.

Holding on to one of those boulders was Ariel, strangely placid in the turbulent water. Her tail snaked sinuously out behind her, keeping her level and on the surface of the water like a kraken.

"This is *amazing*!" he said, as delighted as a child. "This is how you really are."

"This is how I really am," she agreed, touched that he had phrased it that way. She was no longer a human girl who became a mermaid to him; she was a mermaid first and foremost, and a human occasionally by choice. "But listen, we need to talk."

"I know, I know!" Eric said excitedly. "I had an idea!"

"So did I! I was thinking of some sort of performance, which Ursula would attend, giving a speech or something pompous that would put her in front of a huge crowd."

"Exactly! Something where, for a moment at least, she is the absolute centre of attention—"

"Something that really tickles her vanity, so she absolutely agrees to go—"

"Like the encore performance of *La Sirenetta*," Eric finished.

"Your opera!" Ariel said with a gasp. "It's perfect!"

"It's *so perfect*. Everyone will be watching. The only problem is that I just don't know how to turn her back. Maybe the altos can bring in a giant tub of salt water on their heads and splash it on her? I don't know, though, some of them are surprisingly dainty and delicate. Maybe they could each carry a *small* tub of salt water on their heads…"

"Or… since it's a concert for the people, you could

have it outside in the town square, right next to Neptune's Fountain. And we could just knock her in," Ariel suggested lightly. Sebastian and Eric were more similar than she had even guessed. Always leaping to the most complex and fussy ideas when a simple one would do.

"Oh, right." Eric grinned sheepishly. "I hadn't thought of that. You're sure it will work?"

"Absolutely, and it's foolproof, because the water comes straight from the sea. So you need to make that fountain part of your opera, or at least stage it around it."

"Easily done. This is *great*." He laughed and punched the air. "I can practically *feel* the happily ever afters coming for us!"

"Slow down there," Ariel said cautiously. "This is Ursula. Nothing is over until it's actually over."

"I know, I know, but it seems so… perfect! Artistically too," he added thoughtfully. "You know, ending it with an opera that's actually about the two of you, and there's singing, so it's all about your voice, and that's what does her in…"

"Yes, yes, very clever and semiotic. But I should go, I don't know if this counts as 'castle grounds' or not, but you are definitely helping me. It would be stupid to risk Grimsby when we're so close."

"Agreed. And I should get back and… I don't know,

walk around the beach talking to myself and Jona or something. Maybe sing. Keep up the whole Mad Prince thing a bit longer."

"Oh, I hope you don't ever give it up entirely! I rather like it."

"For you, it will come out of the closet occasionally." He leant over into the water. Ariel kicked her tail and rose up just long enough for a quick kiss, cold, wet, salty and slapped by the sea at just the wrong moment.

Heaven.

Eric good-naturedly laughed at himself as he brushed the foam and seawater out of his now-limp fringe.

"You have to make sure she attends," Ariel warned.

"Oh, leave that to me," Eric promised. "I know exactly what to say. I'll also work hard to keep the original performance date, on St. Madalberta's feast day. Two weeks from now."

"I hope that's soon enough, that it's before the circuex or whatever she's planning."

"Nothing in the castle has seemed out of the ordinary so far. No weird things ordered, no giant cauldrons procured, in fact, Vanessa has been rather quieter than usual since her big threat. I wouldn't worry too much yet. You'll be there, right?"

"I wouldn't miss it for the world," the mermaid said dryly, and dove back down into the depths.

Eric wandered back to the castle, zigzagging to pick up shells and a stray feather, sticking the latter in his cap. Just in case anyone caught him.

He saluted the gull above him and could have sworn it did a victory roll in response.

Ursula

"Come again?"

She was seated on her poufy chair, Vareet perched uncomfortably on a stool at her feet. Sometimes Ursula ran her fingers through the girl's hair, which, while certainly not as pleasant as stroking an eel, was at least a *little* satisfactory.

The prince stood before her with a strange look on his face, somewhere between timid, ironically amused and chagrined. It was impossible to predict what was going to come out of his mouth, and what finally did was mind-boggling.

"I am here to offer a détente, and a bit of an apology for our… argument in your study."

She raised a very sceptical eyebrow.

Eric sighed.

"It was *very* rude of me to point out the technicalities of our marriage contract the way I did. *While it is all still true,* it was very bully-ish of me and highly unmanly. Threatening a woman is the basest of sins." He bowed, but the edge of his mouth twitched in a smile.

"Please leave gender out of this," Ursula said without thinking. *But really.* Even if he meant it as a joke. "Also, apology formally accepted, although I don't believe it for a moment."

"Believe what you will, I have no power over that. The fact is I am genuinely embarrassed by the way I acted. At the very least we can be civil while we're together."

"Hmm," she sniffed. She couldn't detect any obvious falsehood, but since he was turning out to be smarter than she thought, nothing he said or did could be taken at face value any more.

"Here is part one of my peace offering," he said, and gave her the brooch he had been holding.

Ursula looked at it with surprise. She knew about his secret meeting with the head of the metalworkers guild, and had assumed it was to re-explain what she had already said, the way men boorishly did, or to outright contradict her. But apparently *this* was the true purpose of the meeting: a tiny metal octopus, its tentacles all akimbo and curled, detailed down to its little suckers. The eyes looked suspicious and were rubies. It was made from…

"Bronze," she said with a chuckle. Eric gave a little bow.

It was really quite delightful. Normally she didn't care about jewellery beyond what was considered trendy and appropriate for princesses to wear, but this… this was an adorable little trinket. No one had given her anything like it… any gift at all, really… in years…

She fastened it onto her collar and tried not to admire it there, sparkling temptingly.

"Part two is that the encore, and farewell, performance of *La Sirenetta*, I am dedicating to you."

"Why?" She didn't even pretend to be touched. There was a reason behind this that had nothing to do with kindness, she could *feel* it.

"We need to present a united front. As is obvious from that horrible dinner, the staff and probably the townspeople think we're, on the rocks, as it were."

"I don't see why what they think is important. *Riff-raff.*"

"Then apparently you don't understand humans as much as you claim to. At some point one of your friends or enemies is going to use our inimical relationship to drive a wedge through the kingdom. Many countries are already getting rid of their kings and queens and princes and princesses, or at least taking away their power while letting them keep their pretty crowns. Royalty that actually rules is a dying breed. Do we really want to give anyone the opportunity to speed it along here in Tirulia?"

Ursula had never thought of it that way before. It was true, a lot of nasty populist places were having revolutions and becoming republics and democracies, patting their royalty on the head and pushing them on their way.

(If the royalty was lucky, that was *all* that happened to their heads.)

The fact that Eric was concerned about this was a novelty; she had always thought he was just a happy-go-lucky, entitled prince who, yes, cared for his people, but in his own privileged way. She never thought that he actually valued his *princehood*, or keeping it.

"You may have a point," she allowed.

"Thank you. Thus, ostensibly I am dedicating the opera to you as a promise to spend more time on our… ah… marriage, and to me being a good prince. We have moved the venue to the town square so everyone can come and we're constructing a raised dais just for you. I'm having this chair made, sort of muse-of-the-arts-y…"

He unfurled a scroll of paper and showed her the plans: where the performers would stand, where the orchestra would sit and where there was a beautiful velvet-canopied pavilion with an ornate chair that was basically a throne.

She would look like a real queen sitting there.

Not some dumb princess.

The royal purple fabric… the gilt chair… the way it was angled so both the audience and the performers could both see her. She would be queen in all but name.

All would be watching her as she brought down destruction on them, like a true Old God tyrant.

"I… don't… trust you," she said.

"I don't expect you to. I don't trust you, either. But once in a while we may need to actually work together for survival. And as I said, I am, if nothing else, genuinely regretful for the way I spoke to you."

He's a regular Prince Charming, Ursula snorted to herself. If nothing else, it was amusing to see him spend all this effort trying to get her to go to a performance she never had any intention of missing. If he had a trick or two up his sleeve, well, it was nothing compared to what *she* had planned.

Performing the opera outside, in the square, was better than she could have ever dreamt. *All* the people of the little seaside town would be there. A thousand victims to sacrifice, a thousand hearts bleeding together with the King of the Sea.

Thanks to Eric and his *generous* apology dedication of the performance, there was no way the spell could fail. The powers released by all that death would grant her true magical mastery over the Dry World and the World Under the Sea. She would be unstoppable. Atlantica would fall. All would bow to her or fall to her wrath.

Ursula realised she was absently stroking the little bronze octopus and stopped it immediately.

Ariel

When the day of the opera came she wished she had better clothes; it seemed a shame to attend Eric's opera in the rags of a maid. But she changed into what she had, slipped the trident into her hair and looked for Scuttle.

"Right here, Ariel! Just a moment!" the old gull called. He was standing at the shoreline gazing into a very calm tide pool at his feet, adjusting his chest feathers and preening his wings. "All set!" he finally declared and glided haphazardly over to her. "Wanted to look my spiffiest for everyone's big day."

Ariel smiled warmly and stroked him on his head. There

was a bit of slick black seaweed round his neck, arranged to look a little like a cravat.

"Got me a nooserton," he said proudly. "Just like the fancy human birds."

"You look wonderful." She kissed him on the beak, then offered her arm. "Care for a ride? Just so you don't get tired too early."

"It would be my honour to escort you, my lady," he said with a bow, then hopped lightly up.

Well, not that lightly. Ariel had to grind her teeth to stop from reacting. She had forgotten how heavy things were in the Dry World, even supposedly light things, like birds.

They probably made for a very odd sight, strolling from the beach into town: a robed and mostly hooded maid with a seagull balanced on her arm. But there was no one around to see. The houses, churches, markets and shops were mostly abandoned; everyone had gone early to get a good place to sit or stand for the free show. Ariel walked between the empty buildings, regarding them with mixed feelings.

If they failed, there was a chance she would be dead, or at the very least, a polyp, and never again free to go where she wished, either land *or* sea.

There was also a chance, if they *succeeded*, that her

father, once returned to full power, would never allow her to come onto land again. He could make it so that *no one* could become human. Of course, she could always search for another way. But last time that had led to Ursula, and…

Her thoughts spun. There were objects in the window of a shop that she couldn't quite fathom: possibly candy, possibly gems and crystals. There were so many alien things about this world she still didn't know. There were so many more things in the *rest* of the world, both above and below the sea, that were yet to be discovered…

"You okay, Ariel? You seem a little, I dunno, worried or spacey or something," Scuttle said.

"I just… I was just thinking about past choices and future possibilities."

"Huh. Deep stuff. Well, the world's your oyster after today. I can't wait to see Triton again! You think he'll give me a medal or something? For helping? For starting this whole thing?"

"I'm sure he will," she said with a smile. It wasn't quite a lie. Despite her father's distaste for all air breathers, she would make sure her friends were properly rewarded.

They caught up with a few stragglers: families gathering small children onto their shoulders, limping soldiers, farmers from holds farther out. Scuttle took off. Ariel hoped he would find and stay close to Jona, who was, somewhat ironically, keeping an eye on Eric and developments at the castle end of things. And to think she was originally supposed to protect the Queen of the Sea!

"My lady!"

Ariel turned to see Argent hurrying down the avenue to catch up with her. Despite her old age it was easy with her long legs. She swung a heavy walking stick in the air enthusiastically, with little need for it, apparently.

"You're here to see the show?" the apple seller asked with a smile.

"Oh, yes. I promise you, it will be a… *show* that everyone will remember for years to come."

"I sense there's something beneath those words."

"Today it will be revealed who your princess really is," Ariel said, feeling mysterious and queenly. "You shall be witness to something amazing. Watch closely, and be ready to tell the story of what you saw."

"Oh, I can do better than that," the woman said with a wink. "I'll *ink* it, if asked."

"Yes, I think you'll find it very inspirational," Ariel said, thinking about the other sea-themed pictures on the woman's arms. She was pretty sure there wasn't an octopus… not yet, anyway.

"Well, I'd better get a front-row seat," the old woman declared, striding forwards. *"EXCUSE ME!* Old lady coming through! *Make way for a grannie."* She handily pushed people aside, forcing her way to the front.

No frail biddy, she.

Ariel also wanted a close view, though not so close that Ursula could pick her out of the crowd. She smiled and slipped sideways and murmured apologies and, yes, flashed a beautiful mermaid smile at large in-the-way boys when she needed to. She succeeded in getting halfway into the main square, about a third of the way back from the stage. A low platform had been erected behind Neptune's Fountain for the singers to stand on, and stand only. It would be a far less dramatic performance than in the amphitheatre, not much moving around. Ariel felt a little disappointed despite knowing just how ridiculous she was being. But from the way Jona had described the original show, it had sounded like a lot of fun, and she was curious to see how Eric and the humans had recreated her ancient underwater world.

The orchestra was grouped against the wall of the indoor market; their music would echo off its stones and back to the audience. *There's a pun in there somewhere about songs and dolphins and their singing-sight…* but she was too excited to think it through.

On the side of the fountain closest to her and the audience, raised just a *smidge* higher than the impromptu stage, was a jewel of a box seat, canopied in cloth of gold and purple velvet. A banner even flew from the top. Ariel's eyes narrowed when she saw the sigil of the black octopus on it.

The sky was blue, the crowd was happy, the air was crisp and fresh. Everything was bright and pretty and happy, and she was caught up in the mood despite the dire reasons for her being there.

It was like attending the markets and fairs when she was a child, when it was all new and everything seemed exciting. Back then she darted everywhere and begged for treats and admired strange merfolk she didn't know. She missed that and it was nice to recapture it again.

The royal carriage pulled up, the crowd breaking into cheers when Eric stepped out. Ariel hoped they would react poorly when Vanessa emerged, but she was disappointed. The false princess looked stunning. She wore a very modern, highly corseted ocean-blue dress with a half dozen underskirts, and she had jewels and shells intertwined with her hair that looked… almost… tentacle-y. She flashed a sly, toothy smile and the crowd ate it up. No one believed the truth of the opera, but they all loved the *idea* of a villain modelled on their princess. An antihero.

Flotsam and Jetsam oozed to the sides of the box seat, flanking it.

Vareet was right behind them. She wore a simple, pretty frock and her hair was arranged like her mistress's, her naturally curly tresses tightly wound round her head with ocean-blue ribbons. But she was very pale. The little girl could tell something was up, or she knew something was about to happen.

Grimsby made his way to the royal seats from a different carriage, gradually and strangely carefully, and then Ariel saw that he was leading Max, who was nearly blind but still wagged his tail, excited to be there.

She thought her heart would break. He had been there when it all started, and Eric obviously wanted to make sure his friend was there when it all ended, no matter how it ended. She felt tears bead up and her heart continued to flutter.

And flutter.

A *lot.* Scratchily.

Panicked, Ariel put her hand to her chest.

"HEY, WATCH THE FINGERS!" a voice snapped as she touched a strange, hard lump below her clavicle.

"Sebastian?"

The little crab scuttled up so his eyestalks popped up above her neckline. It itched and tickled mightily but the queen restrained herself.

"What… what are you… w*hat…?*"

"I couldn't let you do this all alone," Sebastian said matter-of-factly. "I have done nothing all this time but rule the sea in your place and worry. I had to do *something*."

She carefully reached down her front and unhooked him from the rough wool, then held him up to her face.

"Sebastian…" she said, trying not to smile. Trying to look frowny and fierce.

The crab put a claw over his antennule. "Can't talk. No oxygen out of the water. I have less than a day before I need to go back. Have to conserve."

"Well, thank the sea for *something*," she said, then kissed him on his carapace and carefully placed him on her shoulder. *First a seagull, then I'm hosting a crab. Am I the Queen of the Sea or of random sea creatures?*

Back on the dais, Eric was gracefully making sure Vanessa was on his right side, closer to the saltwater fountain. They stood together, every inch a mighty power couple.

"Good people of Tirulia," he cried. "Thank you for joining me this afternoon. That I could give you this performance fills my heart with no end of gladness… I only wish I could do more for the greatest people in the world!"

The crowd went wild, stamping and hollering.

"No artist can create without an inspiration; no man can work so without a muse. So it is with your prince.

Everything I've ever done, every piece you've ever heard, every tune I've ever scribbled in the wee hours as a Mad Prince does, they are all because of one woman, who owns me heart and soul."

This was met with *awwws* and cries about the power of love.

Eric looked out at the crowd, but his eyes didn't find hers. It didn't matter. Ariel knew he was speaking to her, and she felt her eyes moisten.

He let the moment drag out and then turned dramatically to Vanessa, making a very distinct break between what he had said before and now, but only to those who knew.

"I hereby dedicate *La Sirenetta* to the most unforgettable princess in the world. For Vanessa, and for Tirulia!"

He took out his ocarina, toasted her with it and then hurled it into the crowd.

There was a little bit of a scuffle, but it wound up in the chubby hands of a toddler on someone's shoulder. Everyone cheered madly when she raised it above her head in triumph.

Eric laughed. He bowed and kissed the princess's hand.

Ariel felt her stomach turn. Despite his vow of silence, Sebastian muttered and clicked angrily.

Vanessa curtsied low, then sashayed forwards.

Flotsam and Jetsam were suddenly behind her. They held a chest between them.

"Thank you, Prince Eric," Vanessa said sweetly, or as sweetly as she could, shouting in Ursula's voice. More than a few people looked confused. "And thank you, good citizens of Tirulia. Bear with me while I hack and cough through this… the summer cold I had destroyed my lungs."

Did anyone really buy that?

Sneaking a glance at the people around her, Ariel saw a mix of reactions: surprise, scepticism, and horribly enough, *pity*.

"Could a princess be any luckier to have found such a prince? Truly, I am honoured to be the… *inspiration* for his art. I have just a couple of words to say before we begin."

Ariel tensed, the sea witch had to be pushed into the fountain *soon*. But Vanessa was sort of in front of Eric now, moving diagonally away from where she needed to be. With Flotsam and Jetsam up on the stage with her, it might become even more difficult. Could Eric handle them if they saw their mistress was in trouble?

"First, I would like to thank Lord and Lady Savho, who have generously loaned the government of Tirulia two of their heaviest cargo vessels to fill in while we rebuild our fleet. They are on manoeuvres right now, even as we speak, heading towards the open waters… testing powerful new munitions we plan to use against enemies of the state."

Ariel felt her heart stop. Ursula's eyes glittered and she

looked carefully out over the crowd, hoping to see a reaction, hoping to catch out the mermaid, hoping to gloat.

"What does she mean? So what? I don't…" Sebastian whispered.

"She means to blow up Atlantica. She means to do it *now*, while everyone is at the opera, including me!"

The Queen of the Sea thought quickly. If she ran, she could dive into the water, summon a storm and possibly stop them in time. But the moon wasn't in the best phase; it was already taking most of her effort to remain human.

And this might be the only chance they ever had to stop the sea witch. Ariel needed to be there in case something went wrong. Vanessa said *heading* to open waters. They still had a little time.

Her heart pounding, she decided to stay. For at least a few more minutes.

"Secondly," Ursula said, looking disappointed as she failed to spot Ariel, "I wish to announce the winners of our special fishing contest, to find the magic blue-and-yellow fish. Unfortunately, and somewhat embarrassingly, the prize goes to my own servants, *Flotsam and Jetsam*."

They knelt forwards and threw open the top of the chest they held, sickly grins on their faces.

Flounder tried to leap out.

"But that's—" Sebastian started to cry.

Ariel squeezed his mouth shut with her hand and tried not to cry out herself.

Eric's eyes practically popped out of his skull. He shook his head desperately, looking for Ariel in the crowd. He had managed to stop the contest, but not Ursula.

The crowd booed. Cries of *"Cheaters!"* and *"It was rigged!"* were hurled at the dais. Vanessa deflected them with a cool grin.

"Of course this looks bad. My servants are highly skilled hunters, I mean, fishers. Fishermen. Best of their people."

As she said this she came forwards and seized Flounder violently but securely round his waist. He threw himself back and forth, but behind Vanessa's weak and skinny little arms was the might of the cecaelia, and she didn't even flinch.

He screamed silently, his words killed by the atmosphere of the Dry World.

"Flounder," Ariel whispered. She put her hand to her hair, feeling the trident. If only…

The moment dragged out. The crowd grew impatient and grumbly, but not prone to violence, yet. And Vanessa just stood there calmly, not so much gazing at them as *scanning* them. Looking for the mermaid.

She was doing all of this just to lure Ariel out into the open.

As much as she hated it, Ariel had to resist her instinct

to jump up and rescue him. She would wait.

"My servants are a generous pair of boys," Vanessa finally continued, sashaying closer to the fountain. With a nonchalance that disgusted Ariel to her core, the sea witch tossed the fish into the fountain, then clapped her hands to clean them of water and scales. Flounder dove deep for a breath then leapt out of the water a few times like an upset goldfish, confused and terrified and trying to figure out where he was.

Ariel breathed a deep sigh of relief. Ursula was keeping him alive for now, probably to use as leverage later.

The crowd was still agitating. The sea witch seemed to gauge them for a moment before coming to a decision.

"My servants have decided to give up the prize to the good people of Tirulia!" she cried.

With skeletal leers, the two eel brothers reached into the bottom of the chest that had held Flounder and pulled up dripping handfuls of gold coins. They flung them into the crowd.

There were immediate cheers, and a few shrieks as the heavy coins struck some in the head and face.

Ariel frowned. That was an unexpected move. The sea witch never cared about the feelings of the commoners, even when she was under the sea. She generally referred to them as *riff-raff.* Her goal had always been to rise far above the masses, as princess, queen, or god. Why did she care what they thought of her now? Why was she trying to buy them off?

Unless it was just to keep the crowd calm and happy for some *other* reason…

Eric moved towards Vanessa, slipping in between her manservants while she was distracted, enjoying the cheers.

Flotsam and Jetsam were *not* distracted; they immediately pulled out daggers with their free hands, crossing them in front of the prince.

Most of the crowd didn't notice this; they were too busy looking for missed coins, arguing with their neighbours, cheering, or watching Vanessa.

Grimsby noticed.

"Prince Eric!" he cried, his thin voice barely carrying over the crowd. He thrust Max's lead into Vareet's hands and tried to push his way to the stage. Max howled and barked and lunged forwards, also trying to get to the prince.

Ariel put a hand up to cover and protect Sebastian and also started to move forwards.

A gull called from overhead. Suddenly, Jona dove like a porpoise right into Flotsam's face. (Or maybe it was Jetsam. Honestly, Ariel could never tell them apart.) She stabbed her beak into his face like she was spearing an especially truculent fish.

Flotsam (or Jetsam) eerily did *not* scream, he merely put one hand up to protect his face and very methodically tried to pick the bird off with the other.

Scuttle followed close behind, ripping at Jetsam's (or Flotsam's) nose. That eel also didn't scream; he just knocked the old gull aside with the back of his hand.

Eric threw himself forwards, trying to push through.

One of the eels sucker-punched him in the stomach.

The prince doubled over, falling to the floor.

"No!" Ariel cried.

Vanessa was watching all this… and laughing… and then…

Slowly, like a giant ship sinking, she fell over into the fountain.

The splash was enormous.

There were shouts of confusion from the crowd.

"What happened? What happened?" Sebastian demanded from underneath Ariel's hand.

The mermaid stood on the tips of her toes, trying to get a look.

There, standing at the edge of the platform, panting and exhausted, was Max. Also Vareet, with the empty lead in her hand and a look of triumph on her face.

The dog growled once at the princess he had knocked into the fountain, then wagged his tail and barked happily back at Eric, who was just getting to his knees.

"By the sea," Ariel whispered, grinning.

"He did it!" Sebastian cried, thrusting a claw into the air. "That little girl and the terrible shaggy dogfish *did* it!"

Someone screamed.

The crowd grew silent. The Tirulians watched in horror as Ursula emerged from underneath the water, pulling herself up over the side of the fountain with slick black tentacles that glittered in the sun.

Eric

"Max!" he gasped. *"Good boy."*

Breathing was hard. Jetsam had got him good, up and under his rib. Moving was also hard. The prince gritted his teeth and forced himself upright anyway, leaning hard on his left leg with both his arms. The despicable henchmen had abandoned him to aid their mistress.

Eric gestured Vareet over and used her shoulder to help him the rest of the way up.

He took a deep, painful breath and addressed the crowd.

"Look!" he shouted. "Look at what your *princess* truly is. Lord Francese, do you see? Savho? Señor Aron? Do you *see* the creature before you? The one you gave promises to, and gold, and your loyalty? *Look, people of Tirulia.* Behold not Vanessa, but *Ursula,* witch of the sea!"

"It's real?"

"She's really the sea witch?"

"The opera, it's all true?"

The opera singers and orchestra members drew back in horror. The crowd closest to the stage pushed and shuffled, some surging forwards to see and others trying to get away. But except for confused murmurs, everyone was silent, as silent as a beach before a tsunami.

And yet… Ursula didn't seem bothered. She sort of floated in the water, her forearms resting on the marble rim of the fountain like a child at a pool. Her tentacles danced in a ring around her, splashing in the water as if they had minds of their own and were deliriously happy. She smiled and grimaced and leered at the people as Eric spoke. Vanessa's jacket hung in rags around her shoulders.

"Kill it!" someone in the crowd shouted in disgust.

"She's the spawn of the devil!"

"She *is* the devil!"

"Oh, you humans. *So predictable,*" Ursula purred loudly. Her voice resonated across the square in a way it never had in her tenure as a princess. "You know, not *everything* is about you and your Dry World gods."

Her tentacles grabbed at the sides of the fountain harder, and looking neither fully octopus nor fully human, she pulled herself over the side, flowing like foul black ichor onto the dais.

Flotsam and Jetsam, bloody but uncowed, grinned to see their mistress in her original form. They immediately put themselves between her and Eric, giving him venomous, threatening glares.

The castle guards and soldiers looked unsure of themselves. They kept their muskets trained on the crowd, which was roiling and growing unpredictable. There, at least, was a threat they understood and could stop. Yet some of them separated from their comrades, turning weapons on, well, it was hard to tell whom. Surely it wasn't the other soldiers? Or the prince himself?

Ursula cleared her throat. "Tell me, is there a… is there a *mermaid* in the audience? I have something to say to her. Come forwards, darling."

Ariel looked around nervously. Everyone else looked around as well, confused. For a brief moment there was a space between the bodies and her eyes met those of the apple seller. Argent shook her head: *don't do it.*

"Well, no matter, I know you're shy," Ursula continued,

drawling. "Sometimes it seems like you're so timid you can't speak at *all*. Heh-heh. All that is required from you is to *watch*. And *listen*. And do *nothing* as your entire world is destroyed."

"Silence, Vanessa!" Eric cried. "It's over. Give up. I'll try to keep the guards and the people from killing you."

"Very generous," she said, laughing throatily. "Here, let me make myself a little more comfortable, before we get around to all that..."

With a sneer that was pure evil, she ripped off what remained of Vanessa's jacket. On top of her black camisole she wore a heavy golden chain. And hanging from that chain was...

Triton.

Ariel

Father!

She began to cry the word aloud, but pushed a fist into her mouth at the last second. The people she was standing next to looked at her in confusion, but it hardly mattered.

The large pendant Ursula wore was a glass ampoule with a bronze and wax top. Inside this floated a sad, disgusting little polyp whose tendrils still resembled the beard and moustache of the ancient sea king.

"Oh, come *on*." Ursula swore in disgust, looking out over the crowd. Her hands were on her hips. "I've got your *father*, dear! I *know* you're out there *somewhere*! I know you two were planning something big for me today. Although," she added, looking at Eric, "I rather expected something more than *being pushed into a fountain*. Disappointing."

Ariel took a tentative step forwards.

Sebastian pinched her hard, on her shoulder.

"Don't you dare, young lady," he hissed. "You're jumping in too early, like you always did with your solos. For once in your life stop being so impulsive and *think*!"

Ariel winced from the pain of his words. Was he right? But… that was her *father*! The whole reason she was there! He was maybe a goby's leap from her!

"Guards, seize the creature who pretended to be Vanessa," Eric commanded. "She is a dangerous enemy of the state."

The captain of the guards and his top men jerked into action, finally with a clear path: their prince had given an order.

Yet still, some of them did not.

"Guards, stand down." Ursula waved at them, almost lazily. "Or my boys will kill your prince."

In a wink Flotsam and Jetsam had their daggers pressed against Eric's neck.

Once again the captain faltered, as did the men closest to him.

"All right, I was hoping to draw out the little mermaid queen, but I guess the show must go on without her," Ursula said with a sigh. "In case she *is* here, somewhere, hiding, let me make this very clear to her. And to all of you. My reign as Princess Vanessa of Tirulia is over."

"No kidding," Eric growled.

"It's been fun, and I have so loved ruling you all," she said, blowing a kiss to the crowd. "I'm going to miss you terribly. Well, probably not. But it was a nice growth experience. Just understand that what is about to happen is all *because of* 'la sirenetta.'

"I was perfectly happy being your princess, and then *she* showed up. So I told her to go away. Very clearly. To leave *us all* alone. She ignored me, and came back, infiltrating the castle with her spies and henchmen."

She paused and added, sotto voce:

"I have that dumb broad Carlotta strung up in the basement, and I am *not* feeding her. She could stand to lose some… *attitude*…"

Ariel choked. *Carlotta too?* Was *no one* safe?

"And then, just as a side project, to shut up the dumb mermaid and her idiot people forever, I had planned to destroy her kingdom. Oh, yes, there's an underwater kingdom of peaceful happy mermaids out there, but the point is, it had nothing to do with *you* all. Tirulians. I would have wiped the mer off the face of the planet and none of you would have been the wiser."

The crowd began to mutter, puzzled by this. *Ursula really doesn't understand humans at all if she thinks they wouldn't care.* In one sentence the sea witch had admitted to the existence of a kingdom of mythical creatures, and how she now wanted to exterminate them.

"But she foiled that plan by destroying my fleet… and a number of your own fishing vessels as well. Remember that great storm? Yes, that was her. Every time I've tried to take care of her quietly, she comes back, ruining everything. If she had just *stayed away* none of this would have happened."

It's my *fault that Ursula has my father? I* made *her try to bomb Atlantica?* Ursula was twisting everything around so much, did she even believe her own rhetoric? Or did she just say whatever made her look good, knowing even while she said it that it was false information?

"Some of you who actually saw the opera might already know a bit of my past," Ursula continued casually, regarding the tips of some of her tentacles. "I was a… *powerful witch under the sea.* But really, how much power is enough? So I became a powerful ruler on the land. And that was fun. But then I thought… *why choose?*"

Time stopped for Ariel. Blood filled her ears as the strangely banal question rang loud and ominous.

What did she mean?

"So," Ursula sighed, taking the necklace off and holding the glass ampoule in her hands, "I won't. Thanks to the ancient blood running in this little guy here, and… well, a lot *more* blood, your blood, in fact, I will soon be what you little folk would refer to as a *god* of both the Dry World *and* the World Under the Sea.

"Hold still now, won't you? This won't hurt a bit…"

Ursula

Iä! Iä! Egrsi phtaqn! Bh'n'e vh ssrbykl Y'ryel varrotel phtaqn!

The ancient words flowed like black music through her body. No one had recited them in over three thousand years, and the culture that had spawned that priestess had disappeared into a howling vortex of chaos and agony.

Soon these Elder Gods would come and take the people of Tirulia as her offering and feed upon the soul of Triton. In return they would grant Ursula the unthinkable: power over two demesnes, two worlds that had always been separated under ancient, inviolate law. She would be the mightiest creature Gaia had ever seen, or bowed down to.

Hideous shrieks from beyond the stars rent the atmosphere, preparing the way for their singers to come through.

The crowd went deliciously mad. Like a mermaid's song turned inside out, the verses ripped into their skulls through their ears. People screamed, trying to block out the sound with their hands. They sank down to the ground, and Ursula saw precious, bright-red drops of blood start to seep between their fingers.

Well, all right, she conceded. *It* might *hurt. A little…*

Ariel

"No!"

She cried out before she had a plan.

Sebastian didn't even chastise her, too busy staring in horror at the groaning and screaming people around them.

Ursula looked up. It was easy to find Ariel now; she was the only one still standing. The terrible chant in the forbidden language didn't affect her the same way it did the humans, perhaps because she understood some of its foul purpose and its origin. It wasn't meant for her, only the poor humans.

Ariel pushed her way to the front. *Think like it's a game of koralli,* she told herself. *What do I have that Ursula doesn't expect? What is Ursula's weakness?*

"*URSULA!*" she cried again. "*Stop this!* I surrender!"

A slow, ugly smile grew from one side of the sea witch's mouth to the other. Something like relief and pleasure mixed disgustingly on her face: she really had been afraid Ariel wouldn't show. That she wouldn't witness Ursula's triumph.

The hideous wailing from the blackness beyond the stars wavered and slowly died off.

The groans of the Tirulians could be heard now as they recovered, weeping and bleeding.

"And why do I need you to surrender?" the cecaelia asked languidly. "I have everything I want now. Land, sea, power, a bit of a show, *blood*… *w*hat could I possibly want *you* for?"

"Please," Ariel begged. "I know you want revenge on me and my father. But leave the humans out of it. They have never done anything to you."

"*La sirenetta?*" someone whispered in wonder.

"Is she a mermaid?" another Tirulian asked, slowly straightening herself out, wiping the blood off her face.

"Wait, is the octopus-woman a mermaid too?"

"Is that the mermaid from the opera?"

"She's beautiful…"

"Ursula, I know this isn't what you really want," Ariel guessed. "What you *really* want is to rule Atlantica, to show all the merfolk what you do to those who treat you badly. You want to to reign over and enslave the people who know who you really are. These humans have no idea!" She waved her arms at the crowd. "They have no concept of what happened to you a hundred years ago. Your triumph over the Dry World is meaningless, because they don't even know who Ursula is. Everyone under the sea *does*."

"*Don't tell me what I want!*" Ursula snapped.

But she looked uncertain.

"Don't tell me you actually like it here," Ariel pressed. "It's so *dry* and everything is so *heavy* and things *fall* and people live such short, ugly lives..."

"My feet were killing me," Ursula admitted.

"*Think* about what you're doing. Think about the forces you are calling on. Do you really want to summon the Elder Gods if you don't have to? You know as well as I do that they don't always follow mortal rules or deals," Ariel said.

The sea witch was definitely looking unsure now. Ariel had to reel her in and finish it quickly.

"All right, so maybe *just* ruling Atlantica isn't really what you wanted," she said while she still had the moment. "But here."

She took the comb out of her hair. It sparkled in the sunlight, far more clear and detailed than something that small should have appeared. It shimmered and melted and transformed into a mighty golden trident, flashing brilliantly.

The crowd gasped; even Eric caught his breath at the magic and beauty.

Ursula's eyes grew big at the sight, utterly entranced.

"Just… let the people of Tirulia go. You can have Atlantica, and me…"

"And your father?" Ursula demanded.

Ariel swallowed.

The whole reason for her being here… her one constant desire for the last five years…

Would she trade his ancient life for a town of humans? Some of whom killed her fish… and one of whom loved her?

Ariel nodded. Once.

"Ariel, *no*!" Sebastian howled.

Ursula cackled with glee.

"All right, then! I can always try the circuex another time. I'll still have Triton! Come on down, pretty little mermaid! You've got yourself a deal!"

The Tirulians stumbled out of Ariel's way as she approached the dais and climbed up onto it.

"Ariel," Eric whispered. "Thank you. For my people. I am… so sorry."

She didn't say anything.

Flounder leapt up onto the rim of the fountain.

"Goodbye, old friend," she murmured, going over to give him a kiss.

"Ariel, don't," he begged.

"I'm sorry, Flounder." She stroked his fin. "But one thing you learn as a queen is… *to never trust the word of a sea witch*!"

And with that she let her hand fall into the salty water of the fountain…

… and with her other hand, she shot a bolt at Ursula's heart.

Eric

It took a moment for him to grasp what happened.

Just a moment before, the love of his life had surrendered herself, her kingdom and her father to the evil sea witch to save *his* people, and was saying a sad goodbye to her fish friend.

Then, suddenly, her eyes were blazing as she hurled bolts of magic at Ursula.

The sea witch reacted surprisingly quickly; her tentacles shot up all around her torso, protecting it. Ariel's aim might not have been perfect, but it was enough to singe the side of Ursula's face and char a streak across two of her appendages.

"*Ha!* Ariel!" Eric shouted in joy. Was there *anything* she couldn't do?

Flotsam and Jetsam watched, dumfounded, for only a second before leaping to defend their mistress, throwing themselves in front of her. Eric grabbed one of them by the arm as he passed, yanking him back round and then smashing him in the face with his fist.

It felt really, really good.

"Father!" he heard Ariel cry.

The little mermaid threw herself at Ursula, grabbing at the ampoule.

The other manservant backhanded her away, a terrible, fleshy-sounding blow that sent Ariel reeling.

Eric launched himself at him, with no real plan besides wanting to feel the thug's neck being squeezed in his hands. Jetsam (or Flotsam) brought his dagger up to stop him and Eric smashed it aside with his forearm.

Shots rang out from somewhere behind him. Were the guards firing at the crowd? Above the crowd? Were they warning shots? Was there another threat he couldn't see?

Someone was firing back. *Who?*

Eric delivered a good blow, considering it was his left hand, into his opponent's side, but the man was strangely slippery, wiggling and twisting despite his apparent pain, away from Eric's reach. Out of the corner of his eye the prince could see Flotsam slowly pulling himself up, crawling over to help his brother.

Ariel was rushing the sea witch, trying to grab her father.

"I'll kill you all!" Ursula screamed. *"ALL OF YOU.* Humans, mer…"

She smashed the mermaid aside with some of her tentacles.

Others snaked themselves round Eric's throat.

He flailed his arms, trying to grasp at her face, her neck, anything he could reach, but his arms were too short.

He started to get dizzy as the air was cut off, and the world began to go dark.

Ariel

She fell to her knees, invisible bells ringing and tolling around her. She had never felt such pain, except when her voice was ripped from her body and when it was returned. No one had ever dealt a physical blow to her before. She could hear nothing outside the beats of her own heart.

But her father needed her.

Staggering back to her feet, she refused to let the world swim away from her. Chaos was on all sides: people with mouths open like they were screaming, Flounder with his mouth open like he was suffocating. Eric was struggling. Ursula was wounded and looking around anxiously, trying to decide what to do or where to flee. She didn't move very well in the Dry World, on her own tentacles.

One of which waved slowly in the air and still held her father.

With a scream she could only feel, not hear, Ariel threw herself at Ursula. The ampoule slipped surprisingly easily into the mermaid's hands, suckers didn't work very well on dry land. Ariel tumbled to the ground, rolling, her father cradled in her arms.

More shots were fired over her head. Max whimpered and growled; her hearing was slowly returning.

People screamed. Some tried to run away, some huddled, some rushed the soldiers, some rushed the dais. In the back of her distracted mind Ariel noticed that there were some soldiers who didn't side with the palace guards, they were challenging them and trying to get to Ursula's side.

"*The sea witch!*" a familiar old woman's voice roared. "*Get her!* She's got Prince Eric!"

A mad scramble ensued as people rushed the dais. Some soldiers seemed to align themselves *against* the would-be saviours, aiming their muskets at them. Ariel curled up on the ground, protecting the delicate housing her father was in, like a shell wrapped round a nautilus. *Spirals and spirals…*

Max and Varect came to her side and tried to defend

her against the chaotic stampede.

"I'm fine! Go help Eric!" Ariel begged. "Where is… *oh*!"

The prince was struggling, Ursula's tentacles round his neck. Flotsam was sneaking up behind him, dagger raised.

Suddenly, with a final bit of strength, Eric hurled himself to the side, trying to smash Ursula's head into the base of the fountain.

Flotsam threw himself into the melee, dagger still at the ready.

"*Don't let her touch the water!*" Ariel screamed.

But it was too late. Grabbing the stone basin with her tentacles, Ursula dragged all three of them into the water, where they sank to the bottom.

Ariel leapt up and ran over… but all was still.

A single bubble rose to the surface and then popped.

And then a cloud of blood swirled up through the water, dark and ugly.

Ariel

“No...” she sobbed.

Flounder leapt up out of the water, which flew from his body in viscous, sparkling red and black drops.

“Eric is all right! Help him out, he’s all tangled and trapped under her body!”

Ariel stumbled over to the fountain, her father still clutched in her arms. In the blurry depths she could see Ursula’s massive body... and Flotsam’s dagger somehow buried in her chest. The witch’s face was growing pale, and her mouth hung open slackly. Her servant was stunned, entangled around her in ccl form. Underneath the two of them Eric struggled weakly.

"Here!" she commanded, thrusting her father into Vareet's hands. "Guard him with your life!"

Trying not to choke on water polluted with the sea witch's foul ichor, Ariel dove in, reverting to her real body immediately. Tentacles and arms and legs were everywhere. She wrestled with the slick cecaelia body, heaving it aside. Grabbing the front of Eric's shirt, she pulled him away from Ursula, wedging her tail against the dead woman's midriff.

All the years she had thought about what she would do when she finally defeated Ursula, what she would say or experience... and now the sea witch was just an object, a blunt obstacle that was keeping her from saving Eric.

With a mighty heave Ariel managed to fling Eric out onto the side of the fountain, his chest cracking against the marble. He coughed and water came streaming out of his mouth.

"She did it! She defeated the terrible sea monster!" the apple seller cried.

The crowd screamed and cheered and clapped and went berserk.

Eric was a *mess*, all broken and bloody and barely upright, legs still dragging under the water. But he was alive. Flounder kept his distance, not wanting to breathe in any more blood.

Everything around them was bruised and broken but the confusion seemed to be slowly clearing up. There was a pile of mostly unconscious soldier bodies on the dais – ones with tiny black octopus insignia on their sleeves. A triumphant ragtag crew stood above them: Argent with her stained and cracked walking stick, which she now held like a club; Grimsby, who had somehow managed to acquire a musket and was holding it quite steadily; two seagulls; several loyal soldiers and their captain; a soprano and two bass clarinetists.

Vareet stood by the fountain, Triton cradled safely in her small arms.

"So this is what winning feels like," Ariel said. "I think I like it."

Eric groaned and would have slipped back underwater if she hadn't grabbed him.

Eric

If it had been up to the prince, there would have been happily ever afters right then. The bad guy had been defeated, the love of his life was holding him, she had just said something funny, the crowd was cheering, the perfect place for an opera to end.

Alas, real life was a little more complicated than that.

And real blood, not stage blood, was continuing to leak out his nose.

The captain and the remaining loyal guards, who would all be rewarded richly later, scanned the situation and reacted appropriately, placing themselves between the prince and the confused, curious, adoring crowd. "You,

Decard," he said weakly. "Send two men to go find Carlotta in the castle… in the basement…"

"Yes, Your Highness, immediately." The captain saluted and spun off.

With that last order given, Eric succumbed to a wave of weakness and began to slip back into the water.

"Nope, no, you don't," Ariel said, hoisting him back up and all the way out of the fountain. Grimsby was there instantly, offering his shoulder to lean on. Even in his current state Eric couldn't help watching the mermaid with her glorious tail thrown out for balance, sparkling in the sunlight. Behind them he could hear oohs and gasps as the townspeople saw her clearly for the first time.

He couldn't blame them. She was magnificent.

He tried not to put all his weight on the old butler. Things shifted perspective and swam before him, unsurprisingly, there was water in his ears.

"Well done, Prince Eric!" Grimsby said, voice shaking with excitement. "Good show!"

"It was you and Vareet and Max who really got the ball rolling," he said with a grin. Then he put his arm round the other man and gave him a good squeeze. "You mean so much to me, Grims. Have I ever said that before? I was so worried about you."

"O-oh, well, there, there," Grimsby stuttered, smiling but looking around with embarrassment. "You're a bit out of your head. Shh."

Ariel was saying something to the fish in the fountain. Eric felt a strange sense of loss. The fish was truly incredible, unusual by any account. But all he saw was a glaze-eyed animal who apparently was saying something in its silent fishy language, and it made Ariel throw back her head and laugh like a girl. She kissed it on its head and then slipped off the fountain, legs forming as she did.

"I'm getting better at this," she said, turning to face her human friends and twirling the trident.

"I think this is yours," Vareet said, handing her the glass ampoule and curtsying. "What is it?"

"This, brave girl, is my father," Ariel said, kissing her on the forehead. She carefully set the jar down on the ground, then shot a bolt at it.

Smoke, no, water vapor, swirled up and up and up into the sky. On the ground, the polyp grew and lengthened and stretched and hardened into a man.

A man that Eric now remembered: he must have been seven or eight feet tall, broad and somehow lit from within. He seemed more real than the petty humans around him, the cobbled streets, the fountain; as though they were all a child's drawings while he was the original, badly copied. His beard was white and flowed down over him, looking the way Eric had always imagined the patriarchs in the Old Testament. His skin was a coppery shade, more precious metal than flesh. His eyes were almost hidden beneath a bushy brow, but sparks shone there.

When Eric saw him last, that fateful wedding day, Triton had the tail of a fish. Now he had two broad, strong legs.

"Father," Ariel said, and a thousand meanings were in that word: apology, sorrow, joy, love.

"Ariel," her father breathed, choking on the first word he had said in years. Then without a moment's hesitation he wrapped his arms round her and began to cry.

All the humans around them felt similarly to Eric, he could tell: amazed but vaguely uncomfortable, wanting to leave the two alone. Even in his emotions, the king of the merfolk was mightier than mortals.

"I am so sorry," Ariel whispered. She, oddly, was *not* crying, though she hugged her father back firmly. "For everything."

"You are forgiven. For everything," he said, stroking her hair.

"How?" she asked in wonder.

"Some day, you will understand," Triton said with a

smile. "Perhaps when you are a mother."

Then he looked around and seemed to notice the small crowd of mortals.

"Father, this is Prince Eric," Ariel said smoothly, taking Triton's hand and indicating Eric with her other. "He has been a great help in your rescue and defeating Ursula."

"Eric," Triton said neutrally, "I thank you for all the service you have rendered to my royal self and the mer of the sea."

"King Triton," Eric said, bowing his head. "It is an honour to meet you."

"All of these people, all of these *humans,* helped save you," Ariel said. "This is Grimsby, Eric's right-hand man. This is Vareet, who, despite her age and size, risked her life to get us valuable information. This is Argent, who knew about mermaids and can apparently wield a shillelagh with no small skill. Sebastian and Flounder you already know. Jona the seagull and Max the dog were both instrumental in defeating Ursula. Scuttle is the reason we are all here today, and why you are now free!"

"I did what I could," Sebastian said modestly from her pocket.

"I thank you all," Triton said with a bow. "Would that I could stay and reward you as you so honourably deserve right now, but I miss my home, and must return to the sea at once. Ariel, my trident."

She handed it over gracefully and formally, but might have been gritting her teeth a little.

"You will be recipients of my gratitude shortly," the king added, addressing the townspeople in front of him. "The sea does not forget."

He put his arm out and Ariel took it. But not until after she gave Eric a quick kiss on the cheek. It was so familiar, so *Honey, I'm going out for a few minutes, back soon*, that Triton, and not a few other people, gasped. Grimsby looked as delighted as a gossipy old hen. Vareet looked embarrassed, disgusted and vaguely amused. Max barked.

"See you in a few tides," she whispered.

Eric grinned and then kissed her back firmly on her lips, tipping her head back so he wouldn't accidentally bleed onto it.

The townsfolk cheered.

When they were done, Ariel scooped Flounder out of the fountain, holding him under her arm. She and her father walked through the crowds, which parted, almost everyone bowing to the mer couple. They went straight to the docks and leapt off together, tails slapping the water as they dove down.

"HA!" shouted the old woman with the club. "I got to see *two*! *TWO* mermaids!"

Jona

This was the second time in a month that she had been conscripted by a foreign entity to carry a message of grave importance. The gull winged her way out over the sea laden with a sense of historic gravity, the special roll of paper tied to her leg and tucked up into her feathers. She was probably the only bird in the world who carried regular communiqués between two of the major, though somewhat self-important, civilized races of the world. It was something to think about.

Crazy joy overtook her, and she allowed herself exactly one loop-the-loop and a single long *whoop!* before returning to her original heading and task.

She was, after all, her great-grandfather's great-grandgull. Sometimes the crazy was hard to keep in.

Eric

There were terrible, terrible messes to clean up afterwards.

For the first and perhaps only time in history, a seagull was used to deliver a message to the ships sent out to sea, to prevent them from bombing Atlantica. While the prince was fairly certain Ariel and her dad would stop it in time, it didn't hurt to offer an official order to prevent them before another deadly storm was unleashed.

Carlotta was rescued and royally thanked. She was given a holiday (which she didn't take), a snug country house (which she did) and a significant raise.

Eric had his men chain Flotsam and Jetsam together and toss them into the ocean. Either they would be found and treated appropriately by the mer, or… not. Not really his problem.

Then he oversaw a careful scripting of the official record of events of the day, to be read, announced, distributed, shared and generally understood by all the good citizens of Tirulia who had borne witness to the events. There was no mass hypnosis spell to make everyone forget the existence of mermaids this time. Now everyone knew. It was important that they all knew the *same* thing, and didn't concoct potentially dangerous fake news about what happened.

Except that he *did* have to draft a fake formal announcement for the death of Princess Vanessa. Tirulians would understand what really happened; the rest of the continent would only know the faintest details: she died. Possibly drowned.

Troops from everywhere had to be recalled immediately.

Ambassadors and emissaries had to be thoroughly debriefed, and in some cases exiled.

It was endless and exhausting work. Eric stayed up until the wee hours of the night trying to get everything done. Sometimes, given a spare moment, he would glance ironically at the moon and think about how he used to compose music at that time. But that was all right. He had a duty to his kingdom. Being prince wasn't just fun and games.

There *were* a few bright moments, like when he summoned Vareet into his office.

The little maid had passed out from exhaustion the afternoon after everything happened, and slept for over a day. Eric couldn't imagine what was going on in the poor girl's head, in thrall to a witch-princess for years and then saved by a mermaid girl.

She came in wide-eyed and understandably suspicious when the prince smiled at her and shook her hand. "Nice to meet you, formally."

She continued to look confused, but her eyes widened in interest.

"Vareet, you have borne more than any of us, in some ways, and come through it all bravely, helping us out in our darkest hour. Of course you shall have whatever you like, *fresh*, ahem, drawing paper, toy soldiers, a pony, you have but to name it.

"But also: I have hired a tutor from the Academia to come live at the castle. She will teach you how to read and write and do maths. And probably Latin. Sorry about that, but it's part of the package. Then you can make a choice, when you are caught up: either stay here as my personal secretary, or go to university and attain whatever else you wish to do with your life."

Vareet remained silent.

The prince suddenly felt awkward, something he had rarely experienced. He had no idea what the little girl was thinking. Should he repeat what he had said, slower? Would that be insulting?

Then suddenly she flung her arms round his neck and buried her head in his chest.

Eric laughed and hugged her back. *That* was the happily-ever-after moment he had been waiting for, and it wasn't even his.

Ariel

Triton's arrival was epic, although a *truly* epic official parade was planned for the next day. Flounder, once returned to the sea, shot ahead and told every fish he met. By the time Ariel and her father got close to Atlantica, a massive crowd had already formed: most of the mer, and many, many other people of the sea. Whales and sharks and minnows and sardines and tuna and cod and octopodes... even all the little corals, anemone and barnacles came out to wave their fronds.

"FATHER!"

Five slippery, sparkling mergirls shot out of the crowd

and wrapped themselves round him like the fat tentacles of a kraken. Attina hugged Ariel.

"You did it," she whispered, pressing her forehead to her sister's like they used to when sharing secrets. "You actually did it."

"I did," Ariel said with a smile.

"You really are something." The oldest mer princess smiled and shook her head. When the others regretfully disengaged, she too, went to greet her father, with a solid, if slightly more formal, embrace.

"Good people of Atlantica," Triton said, holding his trident aloft, *"I have returned!"*

His voice boomed out through the water, far more commanding even than Ariel's newly regained voice. The crowd went wild: cheering, flapping their tails, slapping, bubbling, gurgling, swimming in circles.

The king himself was only too happy to retire quietly that first night, drink goldenwine with his closest friends, swim lustily through the kingdom and generally stretch his tail, arms and fins the way he hadn't in years. When his daughters finally forced him into his coral bed, he only resisted a little.

The celebrations, feasting and partying the next day were like nothing mortal eyes had ever witnessed. Old rivalries were forgotten; the barracuda even brought gifts of apology. Ariel surprised everyone by singing some of what Sebastian had composed so far for his "Tribute to the Return of the King."

And on the third day, everyone finally got back to work.

Triton sat at the throne, reviewing all the policies and paperwork Ariel had managed while he was gone. He did not use a desk, instead having people hold tablets, decrees and documents *for* him while he read. The king frowned and muttered and said things like "Mmmh. Good point about the right-of-way" and "I would have told the rays to consider an alternate breeding ground" and "Bah, the Rites. I always hated dealing with those. Always made Threll and Sebastian do it."

At this Ariel raised her eyebrows at Sebastian. The little crab shrugged, chagrined. The seahorse coughed nervously.

"Overall, a very impressive job," Triton said, raising his eyebrows as he studied his youngest daughter. "Please don't take this the wrong way, Ariel, but I am pleasantly surprised by how you have matured. Your time ruling has shown wisdom, pragmatism, quick thinking and unique solutions to difficult problems. You might even have surpassed your old man."

"Thank you, Father."

"You know," he added, speculatively, "I *could* use a hand with all of this. A right-fin man, or mer. I know you probably want to be off again with your sisters, or singing—"

"Nope. No," Ariel interrupted immediately.

"Well, then, it's settled," the old mer said with a grin. "Father-daughter day! Every day! What a team!"

Ariel cleared her throat. Her thumbs passed over her fingers and back, as if thinking of something to sign.

"Actually, Father, I had another idea…"

"This isn't about you going to the surface again, is it? Because let me tell you—"

"Hang on," Ariel said, putting her hand up to stop him – something she never would have done before. She did it calmly, without anger or a sudden burst of temper at his attitude; also something new. "We'll get to my career options in a moment. Let me first make it absolutely clear, however, that I love Eric and want to be with him. And I can do that for at least one week a month, with your help."

"WITH MY HELP? IF YOU THINK FOR ONE SECOND I—"

Ariel fixed him with a cool eye. "Remember what happened last time I had to find an alternate solution for walking on land? I'm sure there are other ways out there, and I'm sure I could find them. Do you really want me doing that?"

"Are you threatening me?"

"I am merely stating what will inevitably happen if you resist this. I *will* see Eric. If you want to turn him into a mer for a week every month, I'm fine with that too. However, currently he is a prince with actual duties, and I doubt he has the time for such things."

"And what about *you*? A *princess* with actual duties?"

"Father, I've ruled, and while I might be good at it, I don't like it. I want to do what I've *always* wanted to do." She pointed out at the dark ocean. "*Explore.* Meet new people. Learn new languages. Discover new *things* and the artists who make them. I want to find out what happened to the Hyperboreans. I want to re-engage trade with the Tsangalu. I want to know if there's anyone else out there like Ursula..."

Triton and Sebastian and Flounder shuddered.

"Maybe they're not all *like* her," she said quickly. "Father, the world of the mer has been getting smaller and smaller, consumed with ourselves and our own arts, thoughts and philosophies for far too long. Humans have conquered most of the Dry World, we need to unite the World Under the Sea, for survival if nothing else."

Triton frowned, but not sceptically. He scratched his left eyebrow.

"But this is the job for an ambassador or an emissary, not a princess…"

"Who better? I have royal blood. I have interacted with humans. No one, *no* one of the mer is more qualified."

"But… you're my youngest daughter…"

"Dad, let her go," Attina said softly. "She doesn't want to be here. If you want to keep her at all, this is the only way. Otherwise she will just leave. And not come back."

"It's true," Flounder agreed. "She's got itchy fins."

"As much as I'm probably gonna regret what I'm about to say," the eldest princess continued hesitantly, "what about this? I'm no Ariel, but if you need help now and then, and it needs to be from a royal princess, I'll swim up to the task."

"Really?" Ariel asked in surprise. "You mean it?"

Her father looked doubtful. "But—"

"Let Ariel start by being our official envoy to the idiot humans whom her idiot prince rules. That will give her time with him, and we can see how good her negotiating skills are, like keeping them out of our hair and the Great Tides that feed us."

Triton and Ariel both looked at her in surprise.

"Well, that's…" Triton said, scratching his beard. "That's…"

"A really good idea," Ariel finished, smiling. "An excellent compromise."

"Yeah, well, I'm second in line to rule, you know, so…" Attina said, stretching. "I'm sort of a natural at this." She winked at Flounder.

"I haven't agreed to anything yet," Triton growled.

"It's okay," Attina said, kissing him on the cheek. "*We* have. Say, do I get a necklace or day-crown or something for my new job? I need to look the part."

Triton looked at Sebastian helplessly. "I thought I was getting my kingdom back. I don't even have my *daughters* back listening to me."

"Ah, women. What can you do?" Sebastian said in displeasure.

"Listen to them," Flounder suggested. "Since they both outrank you."

Ariel laughed, and so did Attina.

And eventually even Triton joined in with a chuckle.

Ariel and Eric

A full moon gleamed over the bay. Eric leapt onto the banister of the long stairs that led to the beach and slid down it, balanced on his stocking feet with arms outstretched. Ariel, standing in the shallows, laughed softly.

"Aren't you getting a little old for that sort of thing?"

"I feel like a kid again," he said, scooping her up in his arms. He spun her around and she laughed again, drips of water flying off her toes like diamonds in the moonlight. Then he put her down and they kissed. Properly. For a long time. For the first time Ariel understood the human expression 'making one's toes curl'.

"So what's the story?" Eric asked when they finally parted.

Ariel shrugged and sighed. "I'm to negotiate a path for your ships to take when entering the open sea, past the coastal shelf, to not disturb us. Also to work out a schedule so humans avoid the beaches at turtle and plover nesting times. After this week is up, I then get to make an exploratory trip to the territory held by the Neraide. We never lost complete contact with them, but we haven't exchanged diplomatic pleasantries in a long time, or officially visited."

"Neraide... Greek? Are they like the ancient Greeks?"

"No, they are mer," she said with a smile.

"Of course." Eric bowed. "I should absolutely know better than to say things like that now. Forgive me!"

"Forgiven. And you? What have you been doing?"

"I'm trying to set things in order too, so *I* can eventually make a trip... to the islands of Arawakania in the lands to the west. My father would prefer I go to Ranahatta, but I want to see what tropical waters are like. I hear there are reefs you can just walk out to, as colourful as a rainbow."

"You'll have to tell me all about it," Ariel said with a touch of jealousy.

"I thought you would come along and lead our ship into safe harbours," he said, tweaking her nose.

"Maybe. Mer move slower than human ships, and mer kings slowest of all."

"So is there a chance? That we could ever be together? Forever?" Eric asked, trying not to sound childish. Trying not to sound desperate.

It was adorable.

"There is always a chance," Ariel said, kissing him on the cheek. "And each day, it looks better and better."

"I'd leave Tirulia to my sister in a heartbeat. Say the word and I'm mer forever."

"I'm… exploring that option as well. But what would your people think?"

"What, are you kidding me? They're already positively moony over the story of you and me, and the defeat of Ursula. The only thing better than having an official mermaid ambassador would be having her marry their besotted Mad Prince and the two living happily ever after. Especially if I gave 'em an opera or two about it."

"I can see it now. Sebastian and Eric: *A Tale of Two Worlds*," Ariel said, putting her hand up as if reading a sign.

"I work alone."

"Yes, so does Sebastian. Ah well, another great idea tossed into the Great Tide…"

"*Hey*, check this out," Eric said, pulling up his sleeve and holding out his arm.

The name *Ariel* was written out – in mer runes! It circled his arm like the sort of band a warrior would wear, and glistened with oil he had rubbed into it.

"Eric! What did you *do*?"

"What? Don't you like it?"

"I love it, but…"

"Until we have wedding rings, I thought it was a nice permanent commitment. Argent did it! Sebastian helped me with the letters."

"It… must have hurt."

"You have *no* idea. That's how much I love you," he said, kissing her on the forehead.

They held hands and walked down the beach under the moon, talking about nothing important. Not mermaids, not armies, not sea witches, not fathers, not kingdoms, not distant lands to the west. What they *did* talk about, no one could much hear; there was a breeze, and the lapping of waves, and the cry of a strangely alert gull. And when they kissed in the light of the moon again, no one saw, and no one cared, except for themselves.

And they were very, very happy.

Vareet

The moon was just waning. Ariel had gone.

Vareet looked out her window grumpily. She knew the mermaid would be back soon, but it was still hard. Eric was nice, and awfully cute, but she didn't feel as close to him. Her tutor was endlessly patient. Carlotta was doting and Grimsby spoilt her rotten… but none of them was Ariel.

At least the seagulls were a constant presence. Scuttle had been moved to a comfy nook in a belfry near her, extremely happy with his glittering medal, luxurious retirement and doting great-grandgull. Jona was made official bird emissary and messenger, keeping lines open between the mer and

Eric until Ariel returned. And when Jona wasn't needed, she tended to stick around Vareet. They couldn't talk, but they did communicate in their own way. The gull even rode on her shoulder sometimes like a falcon.

Still, Vareet felt a little lonely.

She sighed and climbed into bed, wondering how she would ever get to sleep with all these thoughts in her head.

Then she noticed something on her pillow.

A beautiful, swirled brown and white shell like the one Ursula used to wear, but larger. A whelk, not a nautilus. Vareet picked it up in wonder, turning it over in her hands, admiring its gleam in the moonlight. On a whim she put it to her ear.

Her eyes widened.

In the depths of the shell, she could hear what must have been the echo of distant waves… and also the song of a mermaid.

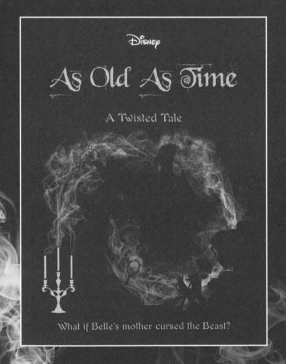

A Whole New World

What if Aladdin had never found the lamp?

Evil Jafar has possession of the magical lamp and the power-mad ruler is determined to take control of life and death.

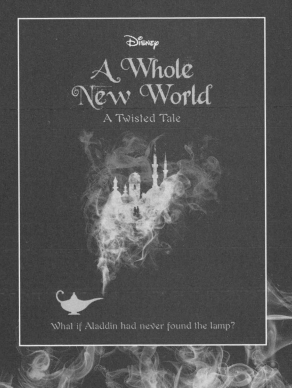

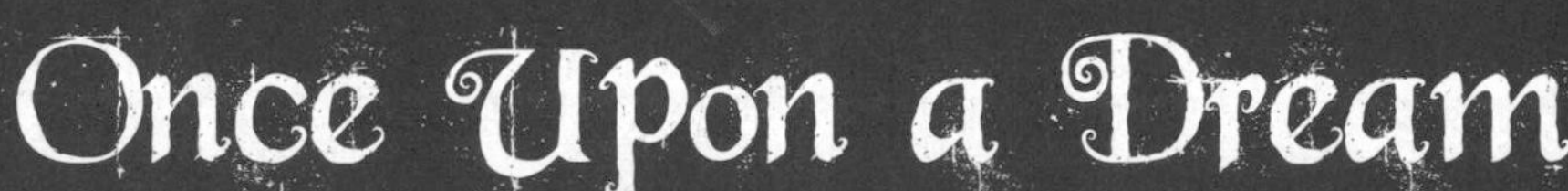

What if the sleeping beauty never woke up?

As the prince prepares to kiss the sleeping princess, he too falls into a deep sleep and the fairytale is far from over.

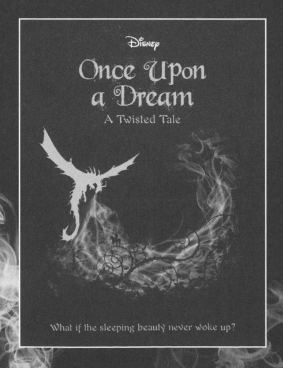

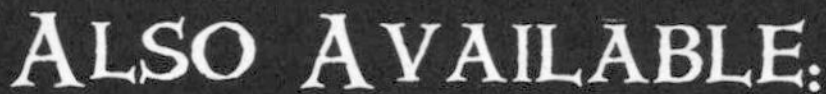

ALSO AVAILABLE:

VILLAIN TALES

CLASSIC STORIES RE-TOLD
BY THE VILLAINS.

Mistress of All Evil

WHY DID MALEFICENT CURSE THE PRINCESS?

Delve into the dark and mysterious world of one of the biggest villains of all time, Maleficent.

Discover why she cursed the princess to fall into an eternal sleep in this tale of love, betrayal, fantasy and magic.

Also Available:

Villain Tales
classic stories re-told
by the villains.

Fairest of All

How did the Wicked
Queen become so evil?

When the King asks the beautiful daughter of a cruel mirror-maker for her hand in marriage, she accepts, hoping her fortunes will change for the better… but will they?

This is the untold tale of love, loss and dark magic behind the classic story of Snow White.

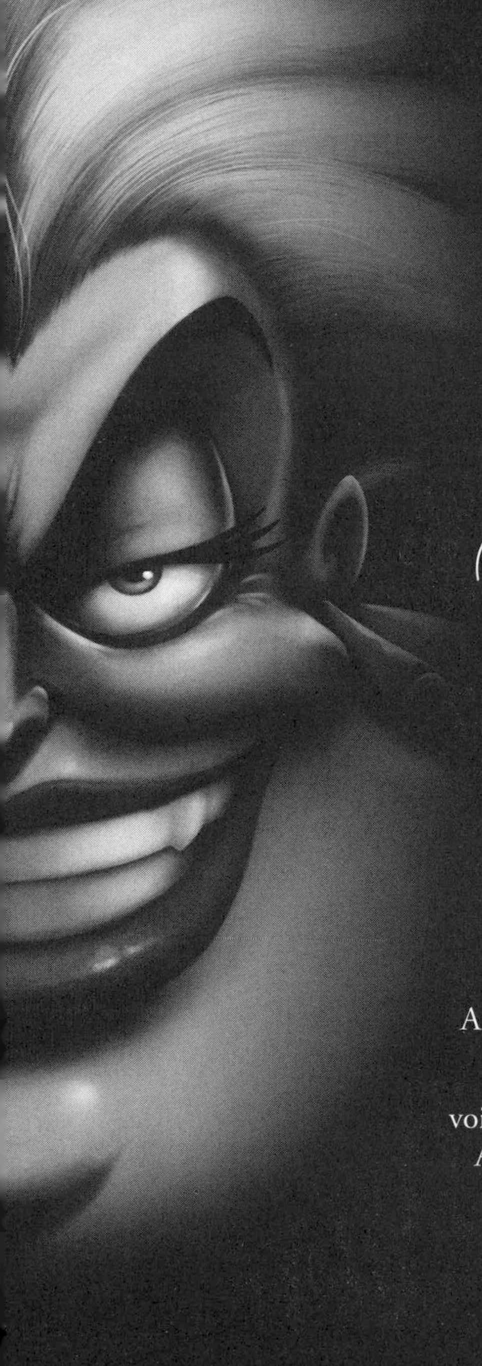

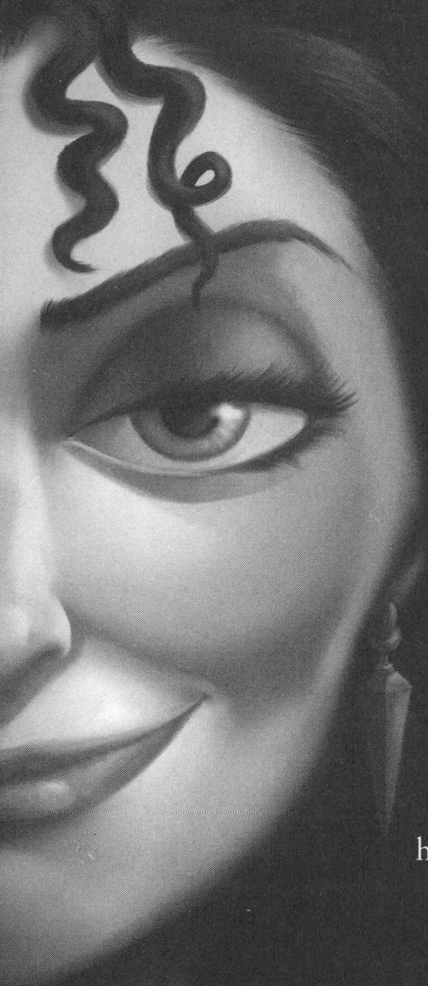